MICROBIAL PATHOGENESIS AND IMMUNE RESPONSE II

ANNALS OF THE NEW YORK ACADEMY OF SCIENCES
Volume 797

MICROBIAL PATHOGENESIS AND IMMUNE RESPONSE II

Edited by Edwin W. Ades, Stephen A. Morse, and Richard F. Rest

The New York Academy of Sciences
New York, New York
1996

Cover: The art for the softcover version of this volume was supplied by H. Kirk Ziegler.

Library of Congress Cataloging-in-Publication Data

Microbial pathogenesis and immune response ii/edited by Edwin W.
    Ades, Stephen A. Morse, and Richard F. Rest.
        p.   cm.—(Annals of the New York Academy of Sciences, ISSN
0077-8923; v. 797)
        Includes bibliographical references and indexes.
        ISBN 1-57331-016-6 (cloth: alk. paper).—ISBN 1-57331-017-4
(pbk.: alk. paper)
        1. Host-bacteria relationships—Congresses.   2. Virulence
(Microbiology)—Congresses.   3. Pathogenic microorganisms—
Congresses.   4. Immune response—Congresses.   I. Ades, Edwin W.
II. Morse, Stephen A.   III. Rest, Richard F.   IV. Series.
        [DNLM: 1. Bacteria—pathogenicity—congresses.   2. Bacterial
Infections—immunology—congresses.   3. Bacterial Infections—
microbiology—congresses.   W1 AN626YL v.797 1996/QZ 65 M6262
        1996]
Q11.N5   vol. 797
[QR175]
500 s—dc20
[616′ .01]
DNLM/DLC   96-43704
for Library of Congress   CIP

SP
Printed in the United States of America
ISBN 1-57331-016-6 (cloth)
ISBN 1-57331-017-4 (paper)
ISSN 0077-8923

ANNALS OF THE NEW YORK ACADEMY OF SCIENCES
Volume 797
October 25, 1996

MICROBIAL PATHOGENESIS AND IMMUNE RESPONSE II[a]

Editors and Conference Chairs
EDWIN W. ADES, STEPHEN A. MORSE, AND RICHARD F. REST

CONTENTS

[a]This volume is the result of a conference entitled **Microbial Pathogenesis and Immune Response II** which was sponsored by the New York Academy of Sciences and held on October 25–28, 1995 in New York, New York.

viii

***

Financial assistance was received from:

Supporters
- AMGEN INC
- CENTERS FOR DISEASE CONTROL AND PREVENTION

Contributors
- BRISTOL-MYERS SQUIBB PHARMACEUTICAL RESEARCH INSTITUTE
- MERCK RESEARCH LABORATORIES
- PFIZER INC
- SMITHKLINE BEECHAM PHARMACEUTICALS

Preface

RICHARD F. REST

Department of Microbiology and Immunology
Allegheny University for the Health Sciences
2900 Queen Lane
Philadelphia, Pennsylvania 19129

These are the proceedings of the second "Microbial Pathogenesis and Immune Response" meeting sponsored by the New York Academy of Sciences, held in New York City on October 25–28, 1995. The purpose of the meeting, following that of the first meeting in the fall of 1993, was to gather a few preeminent researchers in the fields of microbial pathogenesis and microbial immunity and have them interact in a short intense meeting. So often these days, the themes of scientific conferences focus on particular microbes, or aspects of pathogenesis, such as adhesion, invasion, or toxicity, or aspects of host immune response. Infrequently, however, do investigators interested in molecular and cellular microbial pathogenesis get a chance to interact with those interested in the molecular and cellular mechanisms of host immune response. This conference offered such a forum. It was hoped that bringing together such diverse groups, with sufficient time for discussion during meals, free time, and poster presentations, would foster better understanding of host-parasite interactions and would engender collaborative interactions among researchers attending the meeting.

The presentations in this volume represent only brief glimpses of a few areas of intense research in the field. The researchers who presented papers at this meeting represented a global spectrum of infection and immunity research, coming from universities, government agencies, and corporate laboratories from the United States and Europe. It is impossible, at this point, to have an all-inclusive meeting of those interested in microbial pathogenesis and host response; however, just as we hoped that the meeting would spark new ideas and approaches to the problems of microbial pathogenesis and immunity, it is hoped that reading the articles in this volume will spark ideas for your own research. Good luck.

The organizers are sincerely indebted to the companies and agencies, including the New York Academy of Sciences, whose contributions made the meeting possible. Without such contributions, our meetings could not be held.

Structure and Function of the *Toxoplasma gondii* Vacuole

K. A. JOINER,[a] D. BERMUDES, A. SINAI, H. QI,
V. POLOTSKY, AND C. J. M. BECKERS

Section of Infectious Disease
Yale University School of Medicine
New Haven, Connecticut 06520–8022

Toxoplasma gondii is an obligate intracellular protozoan that resides within a specialized vacuole inside host cells. The vacuolar space and surrounding parasitophorous vacuole membrane (PVM) are the interface between the parasite and the host cell. Establishment and maintenance of the vacuole and PVM are dependent on temporally regulated secretion from three different secretory organelles, the rhoptries, micronemes, and dense granules. Understanding the process of secretion and the localization and function of secreted parasite proteins provides important insights into the pathogenesis of infections with *T. gondii.*

For this reason, we have been studying the structure and function of the PVM and of secreted parasite proteins in the vacuolar space and membrane. Our initial results showed that the newly formed PVM is fusion incompetent, being incapable of fusing with any vesicular organelle of the host endocytic apparatus.[1] These experiments extended the pioneering work of Jones and Hirsch[2] as well as the later experiments of Sibley *et al.,*[3] showing the absence of fusion of *T. gondii* vacuoles with lysosomes and the lack of vacuolar acidification. We hypothesized[4] that vacuolar fusion incompetence results from the unique entry mechanism of the parasite into cells[5] and the associated exclusion from the PVM of host cell membrane proteins that could serve as signals for fusion. The PVM, however, is modified during and after invasion by parasite proteins that behave as integral membrane proteins in the PVM and are presumed to play important roles in PVM function. Our focus over the last several years has been the identification and characterization of selected secreted parasite proteins that are associated with the PVM or with the vacuolar space as well as with the basic function that the PVM and vacuolar proteins play in nutrient salvage and protein traffic events.

PVM PERMEABILITY

Although the formation of a PVM lacking host cell plasma membrane proteins including transporters may be responsible for preventing fusion, the absence of transporters poses a dilemma for nutrient access and metabolite exchange. For this reason, we were particularly interested in examining the permeability of the PVM to small molecules. By microinjection of different sized fluorescent tracers into the cytoplasm of infected host cells, we demonstrated a functional pore across the PVM sufficient to allow the rapid bidirectional exchange of molecules of less than 1300

[a] Address for correspondence: LCI 808, Section of Infectious Disease, Yale University School of Medicine, 333 Cedar St., P.O. Box 208022, New Haven, CT 06520-8022.

1

daltons.[6] It is our hypothesis that this is the route by which the parasite acquires small nutrients such as amino acids and purines.

PVM-ASSOCIATED PARASITE PROTEINS AND ORGANELLES

GRA3. The first *T. gondii* protein shown to be associated with the PVM was the dense granule protein, GRA3. After examining the kinetics and the morphology of the association,[7] we used GRA3 as a marker for PVM purification and to study the mechanism of GRA3 association with the PVM. GRA3 shifted from a soluble, hydrophilic molecule in dense granules to an amphiphilic, oligomeric integral membrane protein in the PVM.[8] Many features of the conformational change were reminiscent of pore-forming proteins, but there is as yet no direct evidence to incriminate GRA3 as a pore-forming molecule. The predicted amino acid sequence deduced from molecular cloning experiments[9] suggested the potential involvement of amphiphilic helices in posttranslational insertion into the PVM.

ROP2, 3, 4, and 7. Because any PVM-associated parasite protein that could serve as a pore-forming molecule or interact with host cell organelles would by definition need to be exposed on the host cell side of the PVM, we initiated experiments to identify parasite proteins with this orientation. The plasma membrane of infected cells was permeabilized under conditions that left the PVM intact, and the parasite proteins exposed on the host cell side of the PVM were sought. A complex of rhoptry proteins (ROP2/3, and ROP4/7) were identified. The sequence of ROP2 was completed and the topology of the protein in the PVM was determined.[10] These data provide the first direct evidence for the involvement of rhoptry proteins in PVM formation.

Association of Host Cell Organelles. Immediately after cell entry, host cell mitochondria and host cell endoplasmic reticulum begin to associate with the PVM. This association, at the electron microscopic level, consists of intimate contact between the mitochondrial membrane and the PVM as well as intimate contact between endoplasmic reticulum membrane and the PVM.[11] Ribosomes are present on the contralateral but not the ipsilateral face facing the PVM.

Of interest, host cell mitochondria and endoplasmic reticulum associate with the vacuolar membrane surrounding both *Legionella pneumophila*[12] and Chlamydia, two other pathogens which, like *T. gondii,* reside inside vacuoles that fail to fuse with lysosomes and/or to acidify.[13] With Legionella, the mitochondrial binding is transient, whereas association with endoplasmic reticulum is a consequence of microbial induction of the autophagic pathway in host cells, as described by Swanson *et al.* in this volume.

Despite the long-standing recognition of this event, little investigation has been done on either the mechanism or function of the association for *T. gondii.* Endo *et al.*[14] reported that mitochondrial association occurred when lethally irradiated *T. gondii* entered cells. In this circumstance, the entry process is morphologically identical to that with wild-type parasites. Fusion of the vacuole with host cell lysosomes does not occur, but the parasite gradually involutes and disappears. This is likely to be mechanistically similar to the results we previously reported, indicating that killing parasites after cell entry does not reverse the fusion incompetence of the parasitophorous vacuole.[1]

Recently, we explored basic aspects of the organelle association with the *T. gondii* vacuole membrane.[15] Viable parasites are necessary to establish the association. Parasites must enter cells by active invasion, because no association is observed with phagocytosed organisms. Once live parasites invade cells, they can be killed intracellularly with the dihydrofolate reductase inhibitor pyrimethamine, yet the mitochondria and endoplasmic reticulum (ER) association with the PVM is maintained. There is no contribution from the host cell microtubule network (both mitochondria and ER are associated with microtubules in normal cells) or from the host cell microfilament network.

Taken as a whole, these results strongly suggest that an intermolecular interaction between components in the PVM and organelle membranes is established as a consequence of active parasite entry. Membrane fractions containing the host cell endoplasmic reticulum marker calnexin and the PVM markers GRA3 and ROP2,3,4 have been purified from infected cells. These fractions are currently being used to identify and characterize the components from parasite and host that mediate the association.

NUTRIENT ACCESS BY INTRACELLULAR *T. GONDII*

Because *T. gondii* is an obligate intracellular parasite, components provided by the host cell are obviously essential for parasite survival and growth. It has long been suspected that one function of proteins secreted by parasite dense granules into the vacuolar space is to participate in nutrient salvage. No evidence to support that contention exists.

Several years ago, we began experiments to understand the contribution of *T. gondii* vacuole organization to purine salvage. *T. gondii* is completely incapable of de novo purine synthesis and must salvage purines from the host cell[16,17] (reviewed in ref. 18). Adenosine is the preferred substrate for salvage, with rates of incorporation more than 10-fold higher than those for any other substrate, in part due to an extremely active adenosine kinase.[17]

To gain access to parasite salvage enzymes, purines must cross the PVM, vacuolar space, and parasite plasma membrane. Because purine nucleotides, nucleosides (reviewed in ref. 19), and probably nucleobases will not spontaneously diffuse across lipid bilayers and require the involvement of specific transporters, our initial experiments focused on transport of purines across the PVM and across the parasite plasma membrane. These experiments led in an unexpected way to subsequent experiments on a secreted dense granule protein, the nucleoside triphosphate hydrolase.

Plasma Membrane Adenosine Transporter. The functional PVM pore just described was initially identified during experiments evaluating purine transport across the PVM. This pore should permit ready diffusion of purine bases, nucleosides, and nucleotides from the host cell cytosol into the vacuolar space. By contrast, the parasite plasma membrane is intrinsically impermeant. Working collaboratively with Dr. Robert Handschumacher, an authority on nucleoside transport, we identified a single plasma membrane, high capacity, low affinity ($K_m > 200$ μM) transporter for adenosine, with alternative transport pathways for inosine, hypoxanthine, and adenine.[20] Like other protozoan transport pathways, the inhibition profile for the *T. gondii* adenosine transporter was unusual, suggesting that it may be amenable to specific inhibition.

The Nucleoside Triphosphate Hydrolase. The high K_m for adenosine transport at the parasite plasma membrane was surprising, because cytoplasmic concentrations of adenosine in the host cell should be < 1 μM. By contrast, ATP levels in the host cell cytosol are in the 5–10 mM range, and these levels should be equilibrated with levels in the vacuolar space. Given the knowledge that ATP can also be salvaged by

T. gondii, but that all three phosphates must be removed first,[16] we questioned whether a mechanism existed to generate adenosine from ATP in the vacuolar space.

This called our attention to one of the most prevalent proteins produced by the parasite (1–2% of total parasite protein), the nucleoside triphosphate hydrolase (NTPase). As first described by Asai and O'Sullivan[21] in 1983, the NTPase sequentially cleaves all nucleoside triphosphates to the diphosphate and monophosphate form. Acting in conjunction with a 5'nucleotidase, we hypothesized that the NTPase, if secreted into the vacuolar space, could generate adenosine at high levels for purine salvage (FIG. 1). To pursue this possibility, we undertook experiments to characterize the NTPase at the molecular level and to understand the localization of the enzyme in infected cells.

Based on a published partial cDNA sequence,[22] genomic and cDNA clones for the NTPase were identified from the virulent RH strain of *T. gondii.*[23] Three tandemly repeated genomic copies of the NTPase were identified (NTP1, 2, and 3). NTP2 appears to be a pseudogene, because it contains a deletion at the 5' end relative to NTP1 and NTP3 and lacks a 400 base region upstream of NTP1 and NTP3 which is likely to contain the promoter (Nakaar, Bermudes, Peck, and Joiner, unpublished observations). No cDNAs for NTP2 have been identified. NTP1 and NTP3 are over 97% identical at the nucleotide level and amino acid level, but can easily be distinguished from one another by two-dimensional gel electrophoresis. Of interest, the intergenic regions between the NTP genes are equally conserved. Recently, Asai *et al.*[24] confirmed the cDNA sequences of NTP1 and NTP3 (termed NTPII and NTPI, respectively, in their study) and also provided the sequence of the NTPase from the avirulent Beverly strain, which differs in only 3 of 628 residues when compared to NTP1 (NTPII in the Asai designation).

Analysis of the NTP1 and NTP3 sequence provides only limited clues as to the residues involved in nucleotide binding and hydrolysis. The enzyme lacks a complete glycine-rich loop (P loop or Walker motif) present in many nucleotide binding proteins such as adenylate kinase, Ras, and EF-Tu.[25] NTPase does contain a motif that fits the β-phosphate binding site within the hsp70-actin-hexokinase family.[26] There are a surprisingly small number of apyrases in the nucleotide data base with which to compare the NTPase sequence. Of interest, the NTPase shares the β-phosphate binding loop as well as several other short stretches with a recently cloned apyrase from pea (S. Verjovski-Almeida, personal communication). The significance of these identities remains to be determined.

Antiserum was prepared to a GST-fusion protein containing the amino terminal 70% of NTP3. This antiserum was used in immunofluorescence and immunoelectron microscopy to show that the enzyme resides in dense granules within the parasite and is secreted in large amounts into the vacuolar space, in association with the tubuloreticular network within the vacuolar space. Interestingly, immunofluorescence also shows a rim of punctate perinuclear staining, suggestive of ER localization within the parasites themselves. The significance of this latter finding is under investigation.

An early clue as to the potential importance of the NTPase in parasite virulence came from the observation that parasites from the mouse virulent clonal lineage described by Sibley and Boothroyd[27] contained both NTP1 and NTP3, whereas parasites from avirulent lineages expressed only NTP1. Earlier work had demonstrated the presence of enzymatically active NTPase in both virulent and avirulent strains of *T. gondii.*[28] The observation assumed even more importance with the recognition that recombinant NTP1 and NTP3 expressed in *E. coli* had markedly different enzymatic specificities.[29] Whereas NTP1 is a true apyrase, capable of cleaving ATP sequentially to ADP and AMP, NTP3 has minimal activity in mediating the ADP to AMP cleavage event. Similar observations were recently made by Asai *et al.*[24] with enzyme purified by native parasites. This has set up some testable hypotheses on the role of the NTPase in parasite virulence and adenosine salvage, including the idea (albeit somewhat unlikely) that expression of NTP3 in avirulent

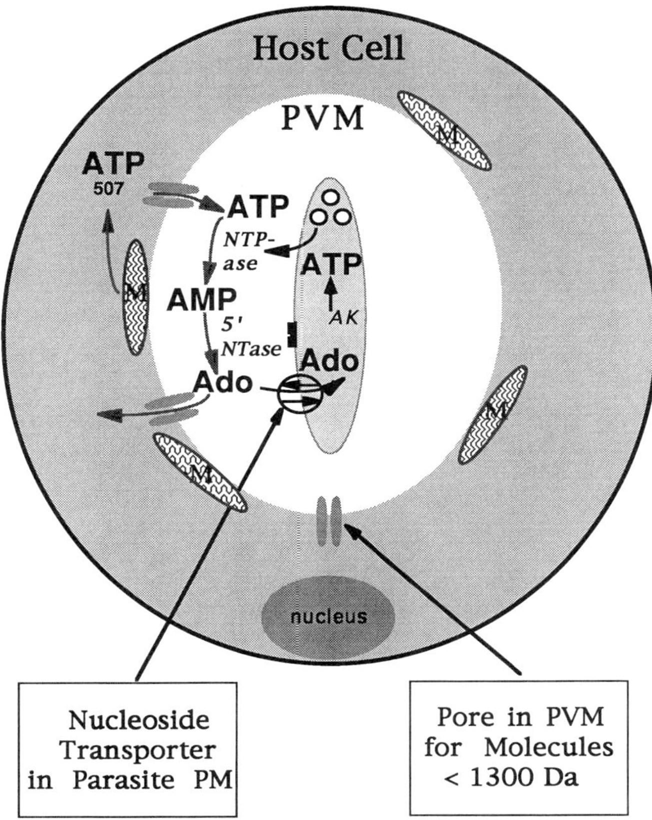

FIGURE 1. Hypothetical scheme for adenosine salvage pathways in *T. gondii*-infected cells. ATP equilibrates between the host cell cytoplasm and the vacuolar space through the functional pore in the parasitophorous vacuole membrane (PVM). The NTPase within the vacuolar space generates AMP from ATP. AMP is then further hydrolyzed to adenosine by the ubiquitous plasma membrane enzyme 5' nucleotidase (reviewed in ref. 31) already identified in other protozoans[32] and also present in the *T. gondii* plasma membrane (D. Dwyer, personal communication). Adenosine is transported into the parasite by the low affinity, high capacity adenosine transporter in the *T. gondii* plasma membrane.

strains expressing only NTP1 will render these parasites mouse virulent and that knockout of NTP3 but not NTP1 in the virulent RH strain will render the parasite incapable of adenosine salvage. These hypotheses are currently under investigation in our laboratory.

Many interesting questions remain to be addressed regarding the activity and function of the NTPase. For example, the NTPase requires dithiols for activation. Glutathione and other monothiols are ineffective. The physiologic dithiol activator is unknown. Asai and Kim[30] demonstrated that mammalian thioredoxin inefficiently activates the NTPase; nonetheless, the vacuolar space should not contain host cell thioredoxin. We showed by liberating NTPase from the vacuolar space of infected cells that a proportion of the secreted enzyme within the vacuolar space is activated. Nonetheless, most of the NTPase liberated under these conditions is inactive but can be activated by the addition of dithiols. Understanding not only the mechanism of dithiol-dependent activation but also the physiologic dithiol required for activation is an important issue to be addressed in the future. Similarly, defining the residues that control the difference in enzymatic specificity between NTP1 and NTP3 should give substantial insight into the residues involved in nucleotide binding and catalysis. Ultimately, we hope to identify either inhibitors or subversive substrates for the NTPase that might have therapeutic use.

REFERENCES

1. JOINER, K. A., S. A. FUHRMAN, H. MIETINNEN, L. L. KASPER & I. MELLMAN. 1990. *Toxoplasma gondii:* Fusion competence of parasitophorous vacuoles in Fc receptor transfected fibroblasts. Science **249:** 641–646.
2. JONES, T. C. & J. G. HIRSCH. 1972. The interaction between *Toxoplasma gondii* and mammalian cells. II. The absence of lysosomal fusion with phagocytic vacuoles containing living parasites. J. Exp. Med. **136:** 1173.
3. SIBLEY, L. D., E. WEIDNER & J. L. KRAHENBUHL. 1985. Phagosome acidification blocked by intracellular *Toxoplasma gondii.* Nature **315:** 416–419.
4. JOINER, K. A. 1992. Toxoplasmosis. J. L. Smith, Ed. :73–81. Springer-Verlag. Berlin.
5. SCHWARTZMAN, J. D. & L. D. SAFFER. 1992. How *Toxoplasma gondii* gets into and out of host cells. Subcell. Biochem. **18:** 333–364.
6. SCHWAB, J. C., C. J. M. BECKERS & K. A. JOINER. 1994. The parasitophorous vacuole membrane surrounding intracellular *Toxoplasma gondii* functions as a molecular sieve. Proc. Natl. Acad. Sci. **91:** 509–513.
7. DUBREMETZ, J. F., A. ACHBAROU, D. BERMUDES & K. A. JOINER. 1993. Kinetics of apical organelle exocytosis during *Toxoplasma gondii* host cell interaction. Parasitol. Res. **79:** 402–408.
8. OSSORIO, P. N., J. F. DUBREMETZ & K. A. JOINER. 1994. A soluble secretory protein of the intracellular parasite *Toxoplasma gondii* associates with the parasitophorous vacuole membrane through hydrophobic interactions. J. Biol. Chem. **269:** 15350–15357.
9. BERMUDES, D., J. F. DUBREMETZ & K. A. JOINER. 1994. Molecular characterization of the dense granule protein GRA3 from *Toxoplasma gondii.* Mol. Biochem. Parasitol. **68:** 247–257.
10. BECKERS, C. J. M., J. F. DUBREMETZ, O. MERCEREAU-PUIJALON & K. A. JOINER. 1994. The *Toxoplasma gondii* rhoptry protein ROP2 is inserted into the parasitophorous vacuole membrane, surrounding the intracellular parasite, and is exposed to the host cell cytoplasm. J. Cell Biol. **127:** 947–961.
11. PORCHET-HENNERE, E. & G. TORPIER. 1983. Relations entre Toxoplasma et sa cellule-hote. Protistologica **19:** 357–370.
12. HORWITZ, M. A. 1983. Formation of a novel phagosome by the Legionnaires disease bacterium (*Legionella pneumophila*) in human monocytes. J. Exp. Med. **158:** 1319–1331.
13. MOULDER, J. W. 1985. Comparative biology of intracellular parasitism. Microbiol. Rev. **49:** 298–337.
14. ENDO, T., B. PELSTER & G. PEIKARSKI. 1981. Infection of murine peritoneal macrophages with *Toxoplasma gondii* exposed to ultraviolet light. Z. Parasitenk. **65:** 121–129.
15. SINAI, A., P. WEBSTER, P. OSSORIO & K. JOINER. 1995. Association of the *T. gondii*

parasitophorous vacuole membrane with host cell organelles. Molecular Parasitology Meeting, 1995. Woods Hole, MA.

16. SCHWARTZMAN, J. D. & E. R. PFEFFERKORN. 1982. *Toxoplasma gondii:* Purine synthesis and salvage in mutant host cells and parasites. Exp. Parasitol. **53:** 77–86.

17. KRUG, E. C., J. J. MARR & R. L. BERENS. 1989. Purine metabolism in *Toxoplasma gondii.* J. Biol. Chem. **264:** 10601–10607.

18. PFEFFERKORN, E. R. 1988. The Biology of Parasitism. P. Englund & A. Sher, Eds. :479–502. A. R. Liss. New York.

19. PLAGEMANN, P. G. W., R. M. WOHLHUETER & C. WOFFENDIN. 1988. Nucleoside and nucleobase transport in animal cells. Biochem. Biophys. Acta. **947:** 405–443.

20. SCHWAB, J. C., M. AFIFI-AFIFI, G. PIZZORNO, R. E. HANDSCHUMACHER & K. A. JOINER. 1995. *Toxoplasma gondii* tachyzoites possess an unusual plasma membrane adenosine transporter. Mol. Biochem. Parasitol. **70:** 59–69.

21. ASAI, T. & W. J. O'SULLIVAN. 1983. A potent nucleoside triphosphate hydrolase from the parasitic protozoan *Toxoplasma gondii.* J. Biol. Chem. **258:** 6816–6822.

22. JOHNSON, A. M., S. ILLANA, P. J. MCDONALD & T. ASAI. 1989. Cloning, expression and nucleotide sequence of the gene fragment encoding an antigenic portion of the nucleoside triphosphate hydrolase of *Toxoplasma gondii.* Gene **85:** 215–220.

23. BERMUDES, D., K. R. PECK, M. AFIFI-AFIFI, C. J. M. BECKERS & K. A. JOINER. 1994. Tandomly repeated genes encode nucleoside triphosphate hydrolase isoforms secreted into the parasitophorous vacuole of *Toxoplasma gondii.* J. Biol. Chem. **269:** 29252–29260.

24. ASAI, T., S. MIURA, D. SIBLEY, H. OKABAYASHI & T. TSUTOMU. 1995. Biochemical and molecular characterization of nucleoside triphosphate hydrolase isozymes from the parasitic protozoan *Toxoplasma gondii.* J. Biol. Chem. **270:** 11391–11397.

25. WALKER, J. E., M. SARASTE & N. J. GAY. 1984. The unc operon. Nucleotide sequence, regulation, and structure of ATP-synthase. Biochim. Biophys. Acta **768:** 164–200.

26. FLAHERTY, K. M., D. B. MCKAY, W. KABSCH & K. HOLMES. 1991. Similarity of the three dimensional structures of actin and the ATPase fragment of a 70kDa heat shock cognate protein. Proc. Natl. Acad. Sci. **88:** 5041–5045.

27. SIBLEY, L. D. & J. C. BOOTHROYD. 1992. Virulent strains of *Toxoplasma gondii* comprise a single clonal lineage. Nature **359:** 82–85.

28. ASAI, T. & Y. SUZUKI. 1990. Remarkable activities of nucleoside triphosphate hydrolase in the tachyzoites of both virulent and avirulent strains of *Toxoplasma gondii.* FEBS Microbiol. Lett. **72:** 89–92.

29. BECKERS, C. J. M., V. POLOTSKY, H. QI, E. ROSENBERG & K. JOINER. 1995. The expression of enzymatically distinct nucleoside triphosphate hydrolases in virulent and avirulent strains of *Toxoplasma gondii:* A possible correlation between virulence and efficiency of purine salvage. Molecular Parasitology Meeting. Woods Hole, MA.

30. ASAI, T. & T. KIM. 1987. Possible regulation mechanism of potent nucleoside triphosphate hydrolase in *Toxoplasma gondii.* Zentralbl. Bakteriol. Mikrobiol. Hyg. A. **264:** 464–467.

31. ZIMMERMAN, H. 1992. 5'Nucleotidase: Molecular structure and functional aspects. Biochem. J. **285:** 345–365.

32. GOTTLIEB, M. & D. M. DWYER. 1988. The Biology of Parasitism. P. Englund & A. Sher, Eds. Alan R. Liss. New York.

Analysis of the Intracellular Fate of
Legionella pneumophila Mutants[a]

MICHELE S. SWANSON AND RALPH R. ISBERG[b]

*Department of Molecular Biology and Microbiology
and
Howard Hughes Medical Institute
Tufts University School of Medicine
136 Harrison Avenue
Boston, Massachusetts 02111*

Legionella pneumophila is a member of a class of pathogens that survive and replicate in human macrophages.[1] Commonly found associated with fresh water amebae, this gram-negative bacterium can cause opportunistic infections of the lung when aerosols of contaminated water are inhaled by individuals with impaired immune defenses. Histologic studies indicate that *L. pneumophila* colonizes alveolar macrophages,[2] and the ability of *L. pneumophila* to cause disease correlates with its ability to replicate in macrophages.[3]

Serologic studies indicate that healthy individuals can clear *L. pneumophila* infections.[4] Cell-mediated immunity is the primary means of defense against this intracellular pathogen.[5] Results of *in vitro* studies indicate that macrophages activated by gamma interferon restrict *L. pneumophila* replication by at least two mechanisms. First, activated macrophages internalize fewer bacteria, thereby restricting access to a niche favorable for replication.[6] Second, activated macrophages downregulate transferrin receptors, reducing the intracellular supply of iron which is required by *L. pneumophila* for growth.[7]

Two obvious challenges faced by intracellular macrophage pathogens are evasion of the macrophage bactericidal activities and acquisition of the metabolites needed for replication. We have little insight as to how *L. pneumophila* meets these demands. Many factors have been classified as important for *L. pneumophila* virulence, as judged by quantitative growth studies of mutants lacking these factors in animal or tissue culture models.[8–12] However, elucidation of the mode of action of each of these factors in *L. pneumophila* pathogenesis requires further study. Instead, our current understanding of how *L. pneumophila* establishes a protected niche for growth in the macrophage is based predominantly on detailed morphologic descriptions of its intracellular pathway.

L. pneumophila is taken up within coils of macrophage plasma membrane, which soon resolve to form a vacuole with a single membrane.[13] The *L. pneumophila* phagosome neither acidifies nor fuses with the lysosomes.[14] Instead, the cytoplasmic face of the vacuole appears decorated first with small vesicles, next with mitochondria, and then with endoplasmic reticulum.[13] In both macrophages and ameba, *L. pneumophila* replicates in a compartment bounded by endoplasmic reticulum.[13,15,16] After approximately 24 hours, the host cell lyses, releasing the bacteria for a new round of infection.[13]

[a]This work was supported by the Howard Hughes Medical Institute. MS is an American Cancer Society Post-doctoral Fellow.
[b]To whom correspondence should be addressed. (Tel: 617/636–7393; fax: 617/636–0337.)

Functional roles for the interactions between the *L. pneumophila* phagosome and host organelles are suggested by morphologic analysis of *L. pneumophila* mutants defective for intracellular growth. First, *icm*[8,17] and *dotA*[10,18] mutants, which do not replicate intracellularly, fail to evade the endocytic pathway. Second, a correlation between intracellular replication and association with the endoplasmic reticulum was observed in both genetic and kinetic studies of *L. pneumophila* growth in macrophages.[8,10,15]

A number of the morphologic hallmarks of the *L. pneumophila* intracellular pathway have been observed for other intracellular pathogens. *Leishmania donovani* is taken up within coils of macrophage plasma membrane,[19] the *Toxoplasma gondii* vacuole associates with mitochondria and endoplasmic reticulum,[20] and phagosomes containing *Mycobacterium tuberculosis*[21] and *Chylamidia psittaci*[22] do not fuse with host lysosomes. Although the benefits of avoiding the degradative lysosomes seem obvious, the functional significance of the interactions between these pathogens and the host mitochondria and endoplasmic reticulum remains obscure.

The results of previous genetic studies of *L. pneumophila* growth in macrophages, as well as the shared morphologic features of its intracellular pathway, suggest that one class of avirulent mutants may be defective for particular phagosome-organelle interactions. This type of bacterial mutant could be used to identify the bacterial factor(s) that mediate specific stages of the *L. pneumophila* intracellular pathway. To facilitate identification and analysis of this class of mutants, we have characterized macrophages derived from the bone marrow of A/J mice as a tissue culture model of *L. pneumophila* infection.[15] Here we describe a series of quantitative fluorescence microscopic assays that can be used to classify avirulent mutants according to their traffic pattern in macrophages.

MATERIALS AND METHODS

Cell Culture. Mouse macrophages were derived from the bone marrow exudate of female A/J mouse femurs (Jackson Laboratories, Bar Harbor, Maine), as described previously.[15] Cells were plated in tissue culture wells or on coverslips (12 mm diameter, #1 thickness, Fisher Scientific) as indicated in RPMI containing 10% fetal bovine serum (RPMI/FBS) without antibiotics.

Bacterial Strains and Medium. The *L. pneumophila* strains used in this study are derived from the Philadelphia-1 strain, serogroup 1. Lp02, a thymine auxotroph, served as the wild-type strain.[10] Lp046 is a mutant that grows slowly in macrophages and is slow to associate with the endoplasmic reticulum.[10,15] Lp120, Lp126, Lp147, and Lp172 were isolated after ethlymethane sulfonate treatment of Lp02 and were identified on the basis of a defective intracellular growth phenotype (Swanson and Isberg, manuscript in preparation). *Legionella micdadei* strain D-2676 is a clinical isolate obtained from Barry S. Fields; it has been passaged on CYE medium fewer than 10 times.

Phenotypic Screens for Intracellular Growth Mutants. The ability of *L. pneumophila* strains to grow in macrophages can be judged by a single plaque assay, as previously described.[10] In this assay, 3×10^5 macrophages in 0.5 ml RPMI/FBS were plated per well of a Falcon 24-well tissue culture plate (Becton Dickinson). After overnight incubation, serial dilutions of a suspension of bacteria in RPMI/FBS were added to each well to achieve a low multiplicity of infection. Thus, the plaque size indicates the degree of intracellular replication of individual bacteria.

Immunofluorescence Microscopy. The distribution of markers for the late endosomal and lysosomal compartments and for the endoplasmic reticulum in macrophages infected with wild-type and mutant *L. pneumophila* was analyzed by immuno-fluorescence microscopy. For these studies, macrophages were cultured, infected, fixed, stained, and photographed as described previously.[15] The interaction of *L. pneumophila* with the late endosomal and lysosomal compartment was assessed 2 hours after infection by immunofluorescence localization of the protein lgp120 (mLAMP-1) using a 1:100 dilution of the rat monoclonal antibody ID4B. This reagent was developed by Thomas August of Johns Hopkins University School of Medicine and was obtained from the Developmental Studies Hybridoma Bank maintained by the Department of Pharmacology and Molecular Sciences at Johns Hopkins University School of Medicine, Baltimore, Maryland, and the Department of Biology at the University of Iowa, Iowa City, Iowa under contract number N01-HD-2-3144 from the NICHD. The association of *L. pneumophila* with the endoplasmic reticulum (ER) was assayed 4–5 hours after infection by immunofluo-rescence localization of the ER lumenal protein BiP using a 1:250 dilution of a rat monoclonal antibody[23] (kind gift of David Bole). Intracellular and extracellular bacteria were stained differentially, as described previously.[15]

Phagosome-Lysosome Fusion Assay. Interaction between *L. pneumophila* and the lysosomal compartment was assessed 1.5 and 5 hours after infection using the soluble fluorescent protein Texas Red-ovalbumin (TRov).[24] The macrophage endocytic pathway was first labeled by incubating the macrophages with 50 μg of TRov per milliliter of RPMI/FBS for 30 minutes at 37°C. To allow the TRov to accumulate specifically in the lysosomes, the labeling medium was removed, the monolayers were washed with three changes of 37°C medium, and the cells were incubated in RPMI/FBS for an additional 30 minutes at 37°C. Suspensions of bacteria in RPMI/FBS were added to the well; then, in an effort to synchronize the infection, the mixed culture was centrifuged for 10 minutes at $100 \times g$ before incubating the cultures for 0.5 hours at 37°C. The monolayers were washed three times with 37°C RPMI to remove most the bacteria not associated with macrophages, fresh 37°C media was added, and the incubation was continued for the times indicated. The cultures were then incubated for 20 minutes at room temperature with either of two fixatives, prewarmed to 37°C. To preserve both the tubular morphology and the fluorescent labeling of the lysosomal compartment in methanol-extracted cells, the preparations were treated with GF fixative[25] (3.7% formaldehyde, 0.05% glutaralde-hyde, 250 mM sucrose, 1 mM EGTA, 0.5 mM EDTA, 20 mM HEPES, pH 7.4). To reduce the TRov staining of lysosomes that did not contain bacteria, cells were fixed with periodate-lysine-paraformaldehyde[26] containing 5% sucrose. This fixative pre-served the compartmentalization of the TRov label in cells that were not methanol-extracted. However, in methanol-extracted preparations, the TRov could be washed out of the permeabilized lysosomal compartment with three changes of phosphate-buffered saline solution (PBS). By contrast, this fixative efficiently cross-linked TRov to bacteria present in the lysosomes, and the label remained bound to lysosomal bacteria after methanol extraction and washes with PBS. Thus, this treatment greatly reduced the labeling of the extensive lysosomal network of the macrophages and facilitated scoring phagosome-lysosome fusion.

In these experiments, bacteria were visualized by immunofluorescent staining with *L. pneumophila*-specific antiserum, rather than the DNA stain DAPI. This was necessary because we observed that macrophages incubated with formalin-killed *L. pneumophila* contained lysosomal, non-rod shaped particles that stained with *L. pneumophila*-specific serum but not with the DNA stain DAPI. As the length of the infection period increased, the ratio of rod to non-rod shaped particles decreased, the size of the particles recognized by the *L. pneumophila*-specific antiserum de-creased, and the distribution of the particles in each infected macrophage increased.

Therefore, once formalin-killed *L. pneumophila* are delivered to the lysosomes, the bacteria are degraded, the rod-like morphology is lost, the particles no longer stain with DAPI, and fragments of bacteria are dispersed as the lysosomal network is redistributed.

We also observed an effect of the bacterial growth state on the efficiency of phagosome-lysosome fusion. In particular, cells taken from early log phase liquid broth cultures or from thin patches grown overnight on CYET plates were less competent to evade the lysosomes, and both intracellular and extracellular bacteria had less uniform morphology. Reproducible results were obtained when the cells were collected from thicker patches after overnight growth on CYET plates.

Extracellular and intracellular bacteria were distinguished by incubating the cells before methanol extraction with rabbit serum specific for *L. pneumophila,* followed by a 1:5000 dilution of Cascade Blue-conjugated goat anti-rabbit IgG. The cells were then methanol-extracted, and the intracellular and extracellular bacteria were stained with *L. pneumophila*-specific antiserum and FITC-conjugated anti-rabbit IgG. By this method, extracellular bacteria fluoresced both blue and green, whereas intracellular bacteria fluoresced only green.

Intracellular bacteria were defined as rod- and non-rod-shaped particles that were stained by the *L. pneumophila*-specific antiserum. In each experiment, viable cells from wild-type strain Lp02 were included as the positive control. The negative control strains for the quantitative experiments were formalin-fixed Lp02 cells. In pilot experiments as well as the micrographs shown in FIGURE 3, viable *L. micdadei* cells were included as a second negative control strain. In mouse bone marrow-derived macrophages, the number of *L. micdadei* colony-forming units decreases approximately 10-fold during each 24 hours in culture, consistent with the observed colocalization with TRov (Swanson and Isberg, unpublished data).

RESULTS

Intracellular Growth Phenotype of the L. pneumophila *Mutants.* To facilitate identification of the factors required by *L. pneumophila* to evade the lysosomes and to form replication vacuoles in macrophages, we recently isolated a new collection of *L. pneumophila* mutants that are defective for growth in macrophages (Swanson and Isberg, manuscript in preparation). The aim of this study was to determine if the mutants were defective for evasion of the lysosomes, formation of the replication vacuole, or both.

The intracellular growth phenotype of four mutants is shown in FIGURE 1. Three days after infection of mouse macrophages, the wild-type strain Lp02 forms visible plaques. Mutant Lp046, which has a weak intracellular growth phenotype,[10,15] served as a negative control strain. Strain Lp172 formed plaques that were somewhat smaller than wild-type, whereas mutants Lp120 and Lp147 did not make discernible plaques (FIG. 1).

The intracellular growth defect of the mutant strains was confirmed by quantitative time course experiments. The yield of the wild-type strain Lp02 increased about 100-fold during a 2- or 3-day incubation. The yield of the weakest mutant, Lp172, was approximately 10-fold lower than the wild type, whereas the number of colony-forming units for mutant Lp147 remained constant during a 2- or 3-day incubation. Mutant strain Lp120 exhibited a more complex intracellular growth phenotype; this strain appeared to replicate normally early in the incubation, but not at later times. The results of the quantitative experiments were consistent with the data obtained from the single plaque assays and indicated that the single plaque assay is sufficiently sensitive to detect relatively subtle defects in intracellular growth.

Intracellular Trafficking Phenotype of the Mutants. Previous studies demonstrated that the *L. pneumophila* phagosome does not acquire lysosomal markers, but does associate intimately with the macrophage ER.[13,15] Therefore, the interactions between each of the mutant strains and both the host endocytic pathway and the endoplasmic reticulum were analyzed using fluorescence microscopy.

The interaction between intracellular bacteria and the endocytic pathway was assessed first by immunolocalization of the protein lgp120, a membrane glycoprotein that resides in the late endosomes and lysosomes of macrophages. For most strains, the ability to replicate intracellularly correlated with residence in an lgp120-negative

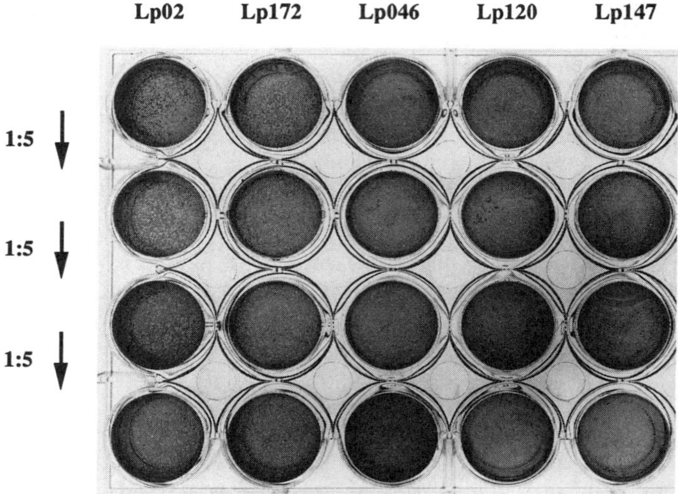

FIGURE 1. Plaque formation on macrophage monolayers by *L. pneumophila* as a visual assay for intracellular growth. Monolayers of mouse macrophages were infected with a series of fivefold dilutions of each of the bacterial strains indicated, then incubated for 3 days before plaques were visualized with the macrophage vital stain, Neutral Red (Materials and Methods). The number of viable counts of bacteria added to the wells was determined for each strain and found to be within a fivefold range.

compartment. Most intracellular wild-type bacteria did not colocalize with the late endosomes or lysosomes (Fig. 2A and B). Lp172, which has a minor intracellular growth defect, also had an intermediate phenotype in this assay. Most of the phagosomes containing the severely defective intracellular growth mutant Lp126 were brightly stained by antibodies specific for lpg120 (FIG. 2C to F), as were most phagosomes containing mutant Lp120. Interestingly, mutant Lp147, which also has a severe intracellular growth defect, frequently occupied an lgp120-negative compartment (FIG. 2G and H).

The ability of each of the intracellular growth mutants to bypass fusion with lysosomes was assessed in microscopy experiments using the soluble endocytic probe, Texas Red-ovalbumin (TRov). As shown in FIGURE 3, bone marrow-derived mouse

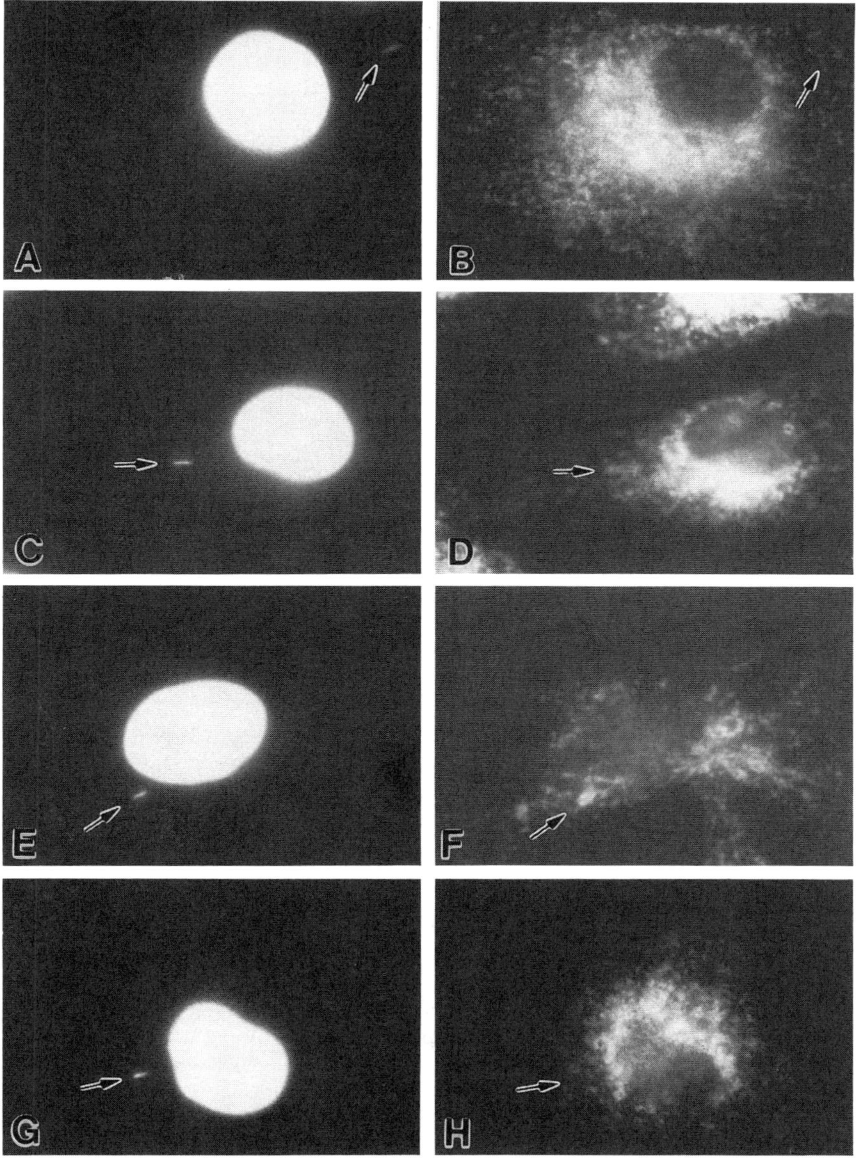

FIGURE 2. Immunofluorescence localization of the late endosomal protein lgp120 in macrophages infected with *L. pneumophila*. Mouse macrophages incubated for 2 hours with the wild-type strain Lp02 (**A** and **B**) or the intracellular growth mutants Lp126 (**C** to **F**) or Lp147 (**G** and **H**) were fixed and stained with DAPI to localize macrophage and bacterial DNA (**A, C, F,** and **G**) and with a monoclonal antibody specific to lgp120 to identify the macrophage late endosomes (**B, D, F,** and **H**). Mutant Lp126 was frequently associated with lgp120 (**C–F**), whereas wild-type (**A** and **B**) and mutant Lp147 cells (**G** and **H**) were not. *Arrows* indicate positions of bacteria.

macrophages contain an extensive network of tubular lysosomes. The abundant fluorescently-labeled lysosomes frequently obscured *L. pneumophila* phagosomes, making quantification of phagosome-lysosome fusion difficult (for example, see FIG. 3B). This problem was circumvented by changing the fixation procedures as described in Materials and Methods. When the preparations were fixed with periodate-lysine-paraformaldehyde,[26] partially degraded bacteria identified by the *L. pneumophila*-specific antiserum colocalized with TRov (FIG. 4C to F). By contrast, bacteria

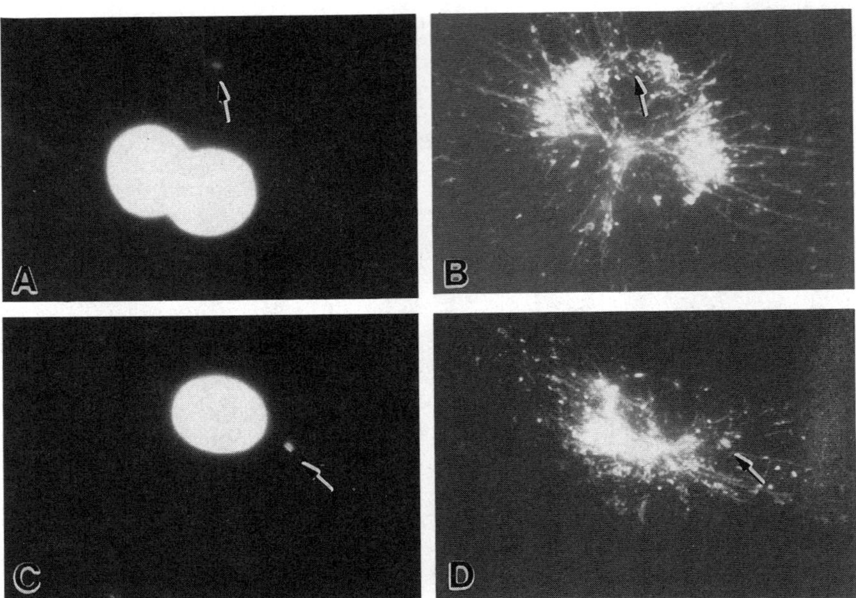

FIGURE 3. Fluorescent labeling of the macrophage lysosomal compartment with Texas Red-ovalbumin (TRov). The macrophage endocytic pathway was labeled with the soluble fluorescent protein TRov (**B** and **D**), the cells were infected for 1.5 hours with either wild-type *L. pneumophila* (**A** and **B**) or *L. micdadei* (**C** and **D**), and then the cells were treated with GF fixative and stained with DAPI to localize macrophage and bacterial DNA (**A** and **C**). The extensive network of lysosomes in macrophages is visualized by this method, but phagosomes are frequently obscured by the abundant staining, and scoring of phagosome-lysosome fusion was difficult. Colocalization of *L. micdadei* with the lysosomal TRov marker is clear (**C** and **D**), while the absence of TRov in the *L. pneumophila* phagosome (**A** and **B**) is more difficult to determine because of the adjacent lysosomes. *Arrows* indicate positions of bacteria.

with a typical rod-like morphology identified by the *L. pneumophila*-specific antiserum did not colocalize with TRov (FIG. 2A to D).

Most phagosomes containing wild-type *L. pneumophila* did not colocalize with the lysosomal marker TRov 1.5 or 5 hours after infection (FIG. 4A and B). By contrast, most formalin-killed *L. pneumophila* colocalized with TRov after a 1.5- or 5-hour incubation (FIG. 4C and D). By this assay, Lp126, a severely defective intracellular growth mutant, appeared to be delivered to the lysosomes (FIG. 4E and F). Mutant Lp147 appeared to evade fusion with the lysosomes as efficiently as did

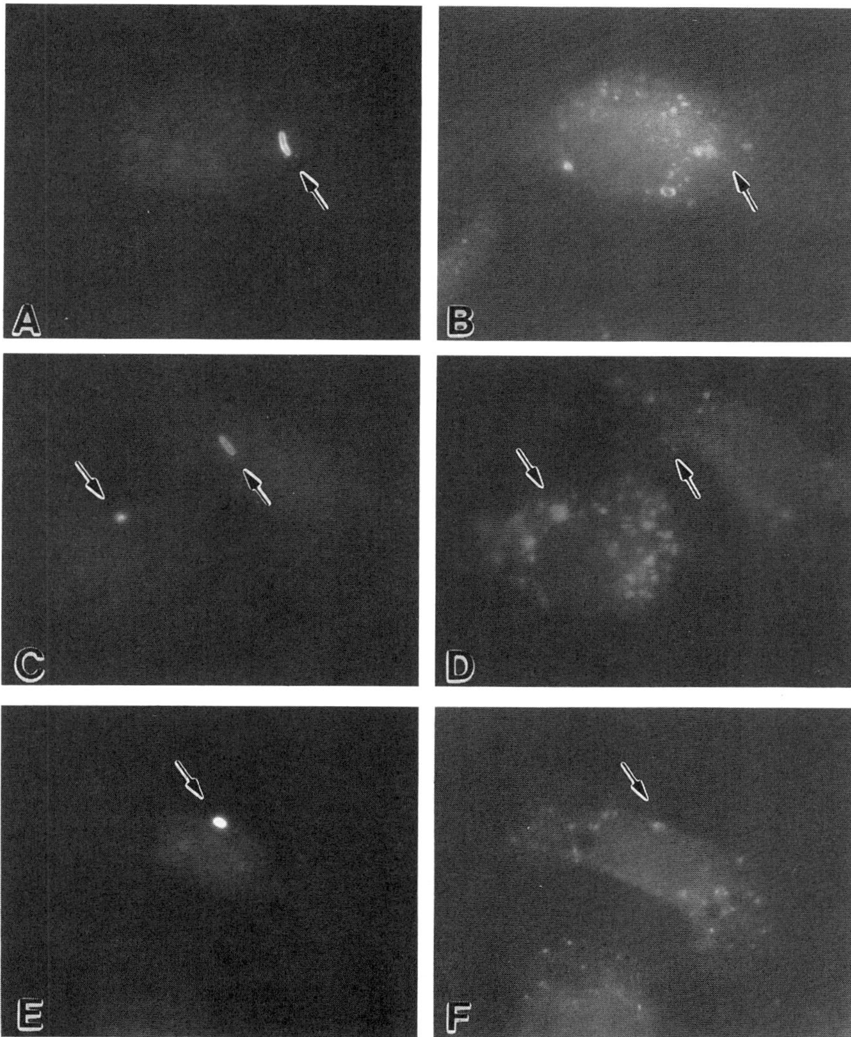

FIGURE 4. Phagosome-lysosome fusion can be visualized clearly in macrophages labeled with Texas Red-ovalbumin (TRov) after treatment with PLP-sucrose fixative. Macrophages labeled with the endocytic probe TRov (**B, D,** and **F**) were infected with bacteria strains Lp02 (**A** and **B**), formalin-killed Lp02 (**C** and **D**), or the mutant Lp126 (**E** and **F**) as described for FIGURE 3, then the preparations were fixed with PLP-sucrose and stained with *L. pneumophila*-specific antiserum to localize intact and degraded bacteria (**A, C,** and **E**). Under these conditions, TRov was cross-linked efficiently to lysosomal bacteria, but not to lysosomal membranes. Unbound TRov was washed away after methanol extraction, and phagosome-lysosome fusion was readily scored. The bacterial rods (panels **A** and **D**) were not stained with lysosomal TRov, whereas the degraded *L. pneumophila* particles (**C** and **F**) colocalized with TRov. *Arrows* indicate positions of bacterial particles.

wild-type, whereas mutant Lp120 had an intermediate phenotype; 5 hours after infection, about half of the intracellular bacteria colocalized with the lysosomal marker.

Association of the *L. pneumophila* phagosomes with the host ER appears to be required for intracellular replication.[2,7,8,10,15] Therefore, we determined whether the mutants were competent to form this specialized vacuole, as judged by immunolocalization by fluorescence microscopy of the ER lumenal protein BiP.[15] The ability to replicate in macrophages correlated with the ability to associate with the ER. Nearly 80% of wild-type bacteria associate with the ER 5 hours after infection of macrophages.[15] The mutant with the least pronounced intracellular growth defect, Lp172, appeared to be partially defective for formation of the replication vacuole, as only approximately 40% of the intracellular bacteria colocalized with BiP after 5 hours. The mutant Lp120, which replicates early in infection but not later, associated with the ER infrequently. Interestingly, mutant Lp147, which is severely defective for intracellular growth, appears to associate with the ER with near wild-type efficiency.

DISCUSSION

Using a series of fluorescence microscopy assays, we have classified a new collection of intracellular growth mutants according to their intracellular fate in macrophages. Further characterization of these mutants and their respective gene products may provide insight to the mechanisms used by *L. pneumophila* to establish a protected niche for intracellular replication.

One intracellular growth mutant fails to evade the endocytic pathway. Vacuoles containing Lp126 frequently colocalized with lgp120 and TRov, markers for the late endosomes and the lysosomes, respectively. This intracellular fate is consistent with results of intracellular growth assays, which indicated that Lp126 cells die in macrophage cultures.[28]

Another mutant bypasses the endocytic pathway nearly as well as does wild-type, but associates with the ER less efficiently. This mutant, Lp172, replicates intracellularly, but produces about 10-fold fewer progeny than does wild-type. This phenotype is shared by mutant Lp046, which was shown previously to be partially defective for both intracellular growth and formation of the replication vacuole.[10,15] Identification of the bacterial factor(s) altered in this class of mutants may facilitate experimental tests of the hypothesis that *L. pneumophila* exploits the autophagy machinery of macrophages to establish an intracellular niche favorable for replication.[15]

Two of the strains had more complex phenotypes. Mutant Lp147 evaded the endocytic pathway and associated with the ER nearly as efficiently as did the wild-type bacteria, but no net increase in bacterial colony-forming units occurred during a 2- or 3-day infection. Perhaps this strain cannot obtain a particular nutrient from its intracellular environment, and its replication is limited by the size of its metabolic stores. The majority of Lp120 bacteria were delivered to the late endosomes or lysosomes, whereas a minority associated with the ER. Presumably it is this minority population that accounts for the increase in colony-forming units seen early in infection. The Lp120 mutation may partially reduce the activity of a factor to near the threshold required for virulence. Thus, most cells contain subthreshold levels and are avirulent, whereas a minority are above the threshold and replicate at normal rates.

The utility of characterizing the intracellular fate of bacterial mutants is illustrated by considering two strains, Lp126 and Lp147. Both mutants were defective for plaque formation, but their intracellular fates were different: most of the mutant

Lp126 cells entered the lysosomes, whereas the majority of mutant Lp147 cells associated with the ER.

This work demonstrates that fluorescence microscopy is a feasible approach to analysis of the intracellular fate of *L. pneumophila* in macrophages. Knowledge of the pathway followed by avirulent mutants can be used to place the mutants into phenotypic groups. In addition, this information allows representative strains to be chosen from each phenotypic group for future molecular and genetic analyses of *L. pneumophila* growth in macrophages.

SUMMARY

L. pneumophila is a model organism for investigating the mechanisms by which intracellular pathogens acquire the metabolites needed for replication while evading the microbicidal mechanisms of the macrophage. We determined that intracellular *L. pneumophila* replicate in close association with the endoplasmic reticulum and suggest that *L. pneumophila* exploits the macrophage autophagy pathway to establish this specialized vacuole. To identify the bacterial factors required at this step as well as the factors important for other stages of the intracellular pathway, we isolated a collection of bacterial mutants that are defective for growth in macrophages. The ability of the mutant strains to evade fusion with the lysosomes and to establish replication vacuoles was examined by fluorescence microscopic localization of markers for the late endosomes (lgp120), lysosomes (Texas Red-ovalbumin), endoplasmic reticulum (BiP), and *L. pneumophila*. By this approach, we identified mutants with distinct intracellular fates; one type does not evade the endocytic pathway, another forms replication vacuoles less efficiently than does wild-type, and a third type forms replication vacuoles but replicates poorly. These mutants are likely to facilitate identification and characterization of the bacterial factors required by *L. pneumophila* to establish a protected niche for intracellular replication.

REFERENCES

1. HORWITZ, M. A. & S. C. SILVERSTEIN. 1980. Legionns' disease bacterium (*Legionella pneumophila*) multiplies intracellularly in human monocytes. J. Clin. Invest. **66:** 441–450.
2. GLAVIN, F. L., W. C. WINN, JR. & J. E. CRAIGHEAD. 1979. Ultrastructure of lung in Legionnaires' disease. Ann. Intern. Med. **90:** 555–559.
3. CIANCIOTTO, N., B. I. EISENSTEIN, N. C. ENGLEBERG & H. SHUMAN. 1989. Genetics and molecular pathogenesis of *Legionella pneumophila*, an intracellular parasite of macrophages. Mol. Biol. Med. **6:** 409–424.
4. MCDADE, J. E., C. C. SHEPARD, D. W. FRASER, T. R. TSAI, M. A. REDUS & W. R. DOWDLE. 1977. Legionnaires' disease: Isolation of a bacterium and demonstration of its role in other respiratory diseases. N. Engl. J. Med. **297:** 1197–1203.
5. HORWITZ, M. A. 1983. Cell-mediated immunity in Legionnaires' disease. J. Clin. Invest. **71:** 1686–1696.
6. HORWITZ, M. A. & S. C. SILVERSTEIN. 1981. Activated human monocytes inhibit the intracellular multiplication of Legionnaires' disease bacteria. J. Exp. Med. **154:** 1618–1635.
7. BYRD, T. F. & M. A. HORWITZ. 1988. Interferon gamma-activated human monocytes downregulate transferrin receptors and inhibit the intracellular multiplication of *Legionella pneumophila* by limiting the availability of iron. J. Clin. Invest. **83:** 1457–1465.
8. HORWITZ, M. A. 1987. Characterization of avirulent mutant *Legionella pneumophila* that survive but do not multiply within human monocytes. J. Exp. Med. **166:** 1310–1328.

9. MARRA, A., M. A. HORWITZ & H. A. SHUMAN. 1990. The HL-60 model for the interaction of human macrophages with the Legionnaires' disease bacterium. J. Immunol. **144:** 2738–2744.

10. BERGER, K. H. & R. R. ISBERG. 1993. Two distinct defects in intracellular growth complemented by a single genetic locus in *Legionella pneumophila.* Mol. Microbiol. **7:** 7–19.

11. CIANCIOTTO, N. P., B. I. EISENSTEIN, C. H. MODY, G. B. TOEWS & N. C. ENGLEBERG. 1989. A *Legionella pneumophila* gene encoding a species-specific surface protein potentiates the initiation of intracellular infection. Infect. Immun. **57:** 1255–1262.

12. ARROYO, J., M. C. HURLEY, M. WOLF, M. S. McCLAIN, B. I. EISENSTEIN & N. C. ENGLEBERG. 1994. Shuttle mutagenesis of *Legionella pneumophila:* Identification of a gene associated with host cell cytopathicity. Infect. Immun. **62:** 4075–4080.

13. HORWITZ, M. A. 1983. Formation of a novel phagosome by the Legionnaires' disease bacterium (*Legionella pneumophila*) in human monocytes. J. Exp. Med. **158:** 1319–1331.

14. HORWITZ, M. A. & F. R. MAXFIELD. 1984. *Legionella pneumophila* inhibits acidification of its phagosome in human monocytes. J. Cell Biol. **99:** 1936–1943.

15. SWANSON, M. S. & R. I. ISBERG. 1995. Association of *Legionella pneumophila* with the macrophage endoplasmic reticulum. Infect. Immun. **63:** 3609–3620.

16. FIELDS, F. S. 1993. *Legionella* and Protozoa: Interaction of a pathogen and its natural host. *In* Legionella: Current Status and Emerging Perspectives, J. M. Barbaree, R. F. Breiman & A. P. Dufour, Eds. :129–136. American Society for Microbiology, Washington, DC.

17. MARRA, A., S. J. BLANDER, M. A. HORWITZ & H. A. SHUMAN. 1992. Identification of a *Legionella pneumophila* locus required for intracellular multiplication in human macrophages. Proc. Natl. Acad. Sci. USA **89:** 9607–9611.

18. BERGER, K. H., J. J. MERRIAM & R. I. ISBERG. 1994. Altered intracellular targeting properties associated with mutations in the *Legionella pneumophila dotA* gene. Mol. Microbiol. **14:** 809–822.

19. CHANG, K. P. 1979. *Leishmania donovani* promastigote-macrophage surface interactions *in vitro.* Exp. Parasitol. **48:** 175–189.

20. JONES, T. C. & J. G. HIRSCH. 1972. The interaction between *Toxoplasma gondii* and mammalian cells. J. Exp. Med. **136:** 1173–1194.

21. ARMSTRONG, J. A. & P. D. HART. 1971. Response of cultured macrophages to *M. tuberculosis* with observations on fusion of lysosomes with phagosomes. J. Exp. Med. **134:** 713–740.

22. FRIIS, R. R. 1972. Interaction of L cells and *Chlamydia psittaci:* Entry of the parasite and host responses to its development. J. Bacteriol. **110:** 706–721.

23. MACHAMER, C. E. R., W. DOMS, D. G. BOLE, A. HELENIUS & J. K. ROSE. 1990. Heavy chain binding protein recognizes incompletely disulfide-bonded forms of vesicular stomatitis virus G protein. J. Biol. Chem. **265:** 6879–6883.

24. SWANSON, J. A. 1989. Fluorescent labeling of endocytic compartments. Meth. Cell. Biol. **29:** 137–151.

25. RACOOSIN, E. L. & J. L. SWANSON. 1994. Labeling of endocytic vesicles using fluorescent probes for fluid-phase endocytosis. Cell Biology: A Laboratory Handbook. :375–380. Academic Press, Inc.

26. McLEAN, I. W. & P. K. NAKANE. 1974. Periodate-lysine-paraformaldehyde fixative. A new fixative for immunoelectron microscopy. J. Histochem. Cytochem. **22:** 1077–1083.

27. HORWITZ, M. A. 1987. Characterization of avirulent mutant Legionella pneumophila that survive but do not multiply within human monocytes. J. Exp. Med. **166:** 1310–1328.

28. SWANSON, M. & R. R. ISBERG. 1996. Infect. Immun. In press.

Genetic and Tissue Culture Systems for the Study of Bacterial Pathogenesis

FREDERICK D. QUINN, KRISTIN A. BIRKNESS,
LYNNE C. KIKUTA-OSHIMA, GALE W. NEWMAN,
EFRAIN M. RIBOT, AND C. HAROLD KING

*Division of AIDS, STD, and TB Laboratory Research
Centers for Disease Control and Prevention
Atlanta, Georgia 30333*

The universal goal of a pathogenic microorganism is its establishment within the host by multiplication through transient or long-term colonization with eventual transmission to a new susceptible host. Infection and disease are inadvertent and unfavorable outcomes of such microbial colonization. Nevertheless, identifying the factors responsible for infection and disease is central to understanding how to control or prevent microbial infections.

Bacterial pathogenesis is a process by which the infectious agent is constantly sensing its surroundings and responding in an appropriate manner. The response often involves coordinate alterations in the expression of sets of bacterial genes encoding virulence factors and components for other standard biochemical pathways. Therefore, understanding the precise genetic regulation of the bacterium, as well as the physiologic alterations that can occur in the host, permitting the bacterium to change its status from colonizer to pathogen, needs to be understood. To this end, a variety of tools have been developed. Factors expressed by bacteria grown under artificial conditions or in association with physiologically inappropriate host cells are not necessarily identical to those expressed during association with the tissues of the actual host. Identifying these differentially expressed bacterial genes and gene products may be the key to developing new forms of diagnosis, treatment, and disease prevention. Therefore, in addition to the development of genetic tools, the concomitant development of model systems that more accurately reflect human physiology needs to be a key component in the study of human bacterial pathogenesis.

PHYSIOLOGICALLY APPROPRIATE *IN VITRO* VIRULENCE MODELS

Most bacterial pathogens are highly adapted microorganisms with survival strategies that require multiplication on or within a particular living organism, tissue, or cell type. To identify all but the most basic constitutively expressed biochemical pathways, appropriate virulence model systems may be required. Although animal models remain the "gold standard" in the study of many bacterial pathogens, physiologically appropriate alternative systems are gaining acceptance.

Primary and Transformed Tissue Culture Monolayers. Since the 1950s, tissue culture monolayers have played a crucial role in the understanding of the bacterial-host cell interaction. Human tissue culture monolayers are easy to work with, can be maintained under controlled conditions, and are relevant to human disease. Although many primary and transformed cell lines have been examined over the years to study bacterial virulence, the most common cell types used in monolayer studies have been epithelial cells and cells of the macrophage/monocyte lineage. This was primarily due to the fact that epithelial cells are most likely the cells that first come in contact with pathogenic bacteria, while macrophages and other professional phagocytes function to limit the spread of many bacterial infections.[1,2] Using these cells of both human and animal origin, researchers have examined bacterial adhesion, mechanisms of phagocytosis, invasion and host cell membrane trafficking, mechanisms for bacterial intracellular survival, and the production of factors necessary for extracellular survival and extracellular colonization in the host.[1,2]

Recently, as the complexity of the cellular immune response to infections from bacteria such as *Shigella* spp.[3] and *Listeria monocytogenes*[4] has begun to be understood, it has become evident that not only macrophages and neutrophils contribute to the inflammatory process, but also cell types, such as lung and intestinal epithelial cells and vascular endothelial cells, may be infected and/or at least involved in the production of cytokines and chemokines.[5,6]

Multiple Layer Tissue Culture Systems. Monolayer systems, although immensely useful, have limitations for the study of host-bacterial interactions. When infecting a human host, the bacteria must interact with multiple layers of cells, including epithelial cells, fibroblasts, vascular endothelial cells, basement membranes, and fibrous connective material. Several tissue culture systems available through Collaborative Biomedical Products (Becton Dickinson, Bedford, Massachusetts) are composed of immortalized or primary cells overlaid onto a porous membrane coated with adhesion molecules or Matrigel. This permits the study of bacterial association with an epithelial or endothelial cell layer that has differentiated in response to the presence of the associated cellular matrix material.

A more relevant model incorporates the added complexity of cell-to-cell interactions associated with multiple layers. Alexander *et al.*[7] reported the addition of a second tissue culture layer, in this case smooth muscle cells, to the surface of the plastic tissue culture dish. The endothelial cell layer remained attached to the filter surface but separate from the second cell type.

Birkness *et al.*[8] recently developed an artificial tissue system incorporating epithelial and endothelial monolayers separated by the microporous membrane (FIG. 1A). This construction may be more appropriate for examining the process of attachment and passage occurring as the bacterium makes its way from the mucosal surface through the epithelial cells and into the vascular system. The layering of one cell type over another allows the cells to communicate and interact, essential components for the polarization, growth, and differentiation of cell types *in vivo*. In an initial report,[8] the interaction of *Neisseria meningitidis, Yersinia enterocolitica, Shigella flexneri, Salmonella typhimurium,* and *Haemophilus influenzae* type b with the bilayer system was examined.

Subsequently, a bilayer composed of A549 human lung pneumocytes and human lung microvascular endothelial cells (HULEC) was constructed. *Mycobacterium tuberculosis* was added to the upper chamber and peripheral blood mononuclear cells were added to the lower chamber. Although only a small portion of the initial bacterial inoculum ($<0.01\%$) passed from the apical to the basal cell surfaces within the initial 3 days, a significant number of mononuclear cells successfully migrated from the basal endothelial surface, through the filter membrane, and ultimately through the epithelial cells to interact with the bacterial inoculum on the pneumocyte cell surface by 4 hours postinfection (FIG. 1B) (Birkness *et al.,* manuscript in preparation). Levels of inflammatory mediators produced by the various cell types can also be measured during different stages of the infectious process. Fibroblasts and other components are being added to this system, and the importance of each of

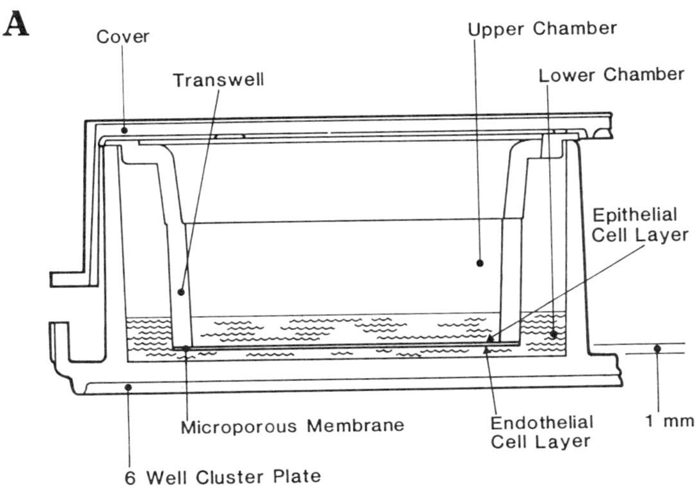

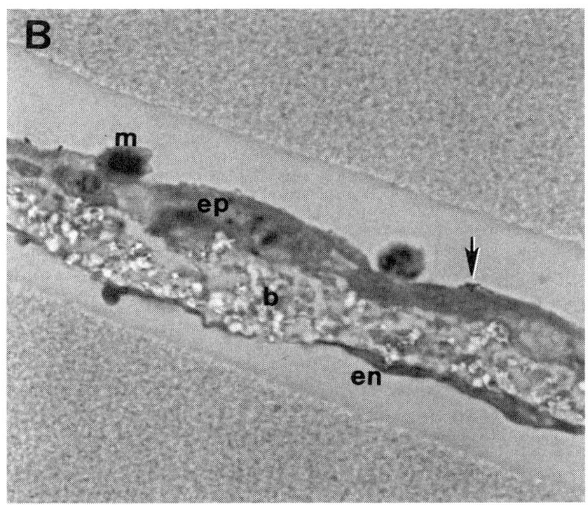

FIGURE 1. (A) Schematic diagram of a Transwell-COL chamber (Costar, Cambridge, Massachusetts) with layers of epithelial and endothelial cells in one well of a six-well tissue culture dish. **(B)** A549 and HULEC bilayer. *M. tuberculosis* has been added to the upper chamber, and peripheral blood mononuclear cells have been added to the lower chamber. Bacteria (*arrows*) are seen on the pneumocyte epithelial (ep) cell surface. Mononuclear cell (m) has migrated from beneath the endothelial (en) cell layer, through a 3.0-μm microporous membrane (b), and through the epithelial cell surface within 4 hours of bacterial addition (magnification ×1,000).

the individual components is being assessed during the early stages of the infectious process.

DIFFERENTIAL GENE EXPRESSION

In fulfilling molecular Koch's postulates[9] for demonstrating that a phenotype, such as virulence, is caused by the presence and expression of a specific gene, three conditions need to be met: (1) virulence mutants must be identified, (2) the responsible virulence gene must be cloned, and (3) the mutant phenotype must be complemented through introduction of the wild-type gene. Although modern research has brought us closer to defining some of these pathogenic factors, molecular Koch's postulates only have been fulfilled for a small number of virulence genes mostly from less fastidious bacterial pathogens.

The host-microbe interaction that occurs during pathogenesis is a dynamic process in which the infecting organism encounters many diverse environmental conditions. Competitive growth and survival in different anatomic locations within the host, as well as the transition to and from an external reservoir, require adaptive responses on the part of the bacterium. These and other selective pressures apparently direct the evolution of specialized bacterial regulatory systems controlling virulence factor expression during critical points in the course of an infection. Early on, researchers manipulated laboratory conditions to try to induce the bacteria into expressing or overexpressing these host-associated, temporally expressed virulence factors without understanding the underlying genetic regulation. Under these conditions, several bacterial toxins were identified,[10] as were the environmental conditions required to optimally produce them.[11] However, the identification of many of these products has required that the pathogen be cultured on artificial media, have a detectable *in vitro* phenotype, possess virulence factors stable enough to assay *in vitro,* and produce its virulence factors constitutively so as to permit the identification of the relevant gene and gene product. Factors identified in this manner include bacterial cytolysins from *Escherichia coli*[12] and *L. monocytogenes,*[13–15] that have been shown to produce profound pleiotropic effects on eukaryotic cells. Therefore, these toxins, under defined conditions, can act as single determinants to produce disease.

Even in these cases, however, the actual contribution of the toxin to the overall pathogenic processes of infection remains poorly defined. Microbial pathogenesis is usually complex and multifactorial. Bacterial pathogens have several biochemical mechanisms that may act individually or in concert to produce infection and disease. Removal of any one of these components may or may not render the organism avirulent. Furthermore, microbiologists have often neglected the complex role of the host, and only recently have cellular and immunologic components been added to studies of microbial pathogenesis.

In Vivo Gene Expression Assays Using Auxotrophs. An alternative approach to the traditional molecular and genetic tools are methodologies based on the direct identification of *in vivo* differentially expressed genes. These technologies focus on previously unknown genes induced in the bacterium during infection in an appropriate virulence model system. The underlying assumption of this technology is that genes expressed when the organism is growing *in vivo* may encode products required for survival and multiplication in the host, that is, virulence factors. Regardless of whether the identified genes code for so-called housekeeping factors or actual known virulence factors, the identified genes may be necessary to cause disease in the particular virulence model being examined.

Mahan *et al.*[16] published the first of these new methodologies. In the *in vivo* expression technology (IVET) genetic system, a promoter fusion library is constructed in an auxotroph of the host strain. The desired fusion will only express the auxotrophic marker under proper *in vivo* conditions. Several genes from *S. typhimurium* that are expressed exclusively during murine infection have been identified and sequenced. However, for use with many fastidious pathogens such as *M. tuberculosis,* several components are required before this system can be successfully utilized, including the identification of selectable and auxotrophic markers, plasmid systems that can be transformed and stably maintained, and the identification of an appropriate virulence model for inducing the bacterial genes under consideration.

Subtractive Hybridization. A technique known as RNA-based subtractive hybridization has been developed specifically to identify eukaryotic and prokaryotic genes expressed differentially under defined conditions[17–20] (FIG. 2). RNA from the positive strain (strain with the phenotype of interest, such as virulence) and the negative strain (possessing a negative phenotype, such as avirulence) is extracted. The RNA species are subsequently reverse transcribed and hybridized. The remaining cDNA molecules from the positive population contain the differentially expressed target genes of interest. For example, a RNA-cDNA based subtractive hybridization procedure was described that identified a single genetic difference between two isogenic strains of *L. monocytogenes* engineered to differ in only one virulence gene.[21] Recently, two studies with *M. tuberculosis,* one by Kinger and Tyagi[22] and the second by our laboratory, Kikuta-Oshima *et al.,*[23] used similar cDNA-cDNA hybridization methods to identify chromosomal fragments containing genes differentially expressed between *M. tuberculosis* H37Rv and H37Ra strains. Another study by Plum and Clark-Curtiss[24] identified a putative heat shock gene that was expressed by *M. avium* during tissue culture infection. Kikuta-Oshima *et al.* (manuscript in preparation) are identifying genes differentially expressed by *M. tuberculosis* during association with human peripheral blood-derived macrophages.

Arbitrary Primed and Differential Display Polymerase Chain Reaction. Arbitrary primed polymerase chain reaction (AP-PCR) is a modified PCR amplification method that was initially developed to obtain a DNA fingerprint for the analysis of polymorphisms in plant and animal cells.[25] Unlike the typical PCR reaction in which conditions are optimized to amplify a single target sequence, in AP-PCR a single primer containing an arbitrary sequence is used at low stringency so that multiple sequences are simultaneously amplified. This fingerprint of multiple amplified bands on a gel is specific (for the primer and template) and reproducible. Thus in one run, up to 90 bands can be seen, each representing a DNA sequence at a specific region of the genome. Another key feature of this technique is that it is sequence dependent, that is, if either a primer of a different sequence is used or the sequence of the template is altered, the fingerprint will change. Wong and McClelland[26] modified and successfully used this technique to isolate differentially expressed genes from *S. typhimurium.*

Differential display PCR (dd-PCR), developed by Liang and Pardee,[27] is also based on the use of random primers and has been used to identify differences in gene expression between two target cell populations. The bacterial mRNA is first reverse transcribed into cDNA, and the cDNA is subjected to PCR using two 10–12 nucleotide long random degenerate oligonucleotide primers in the presence of ^{35}S-dATP. The multiple PCR fragments are resolved by polyacrylamide gel electrophoresis. The bands on an autoradiogram represent a random but limited sample of the genome. Different primer sets can be used until significant pattern differences are observed and until a significant portion of the genome has been analyzed. Both the AP-PCR and dd-PCR procedures are rapid and sensitive and can be performed with small amounts of sample materials.

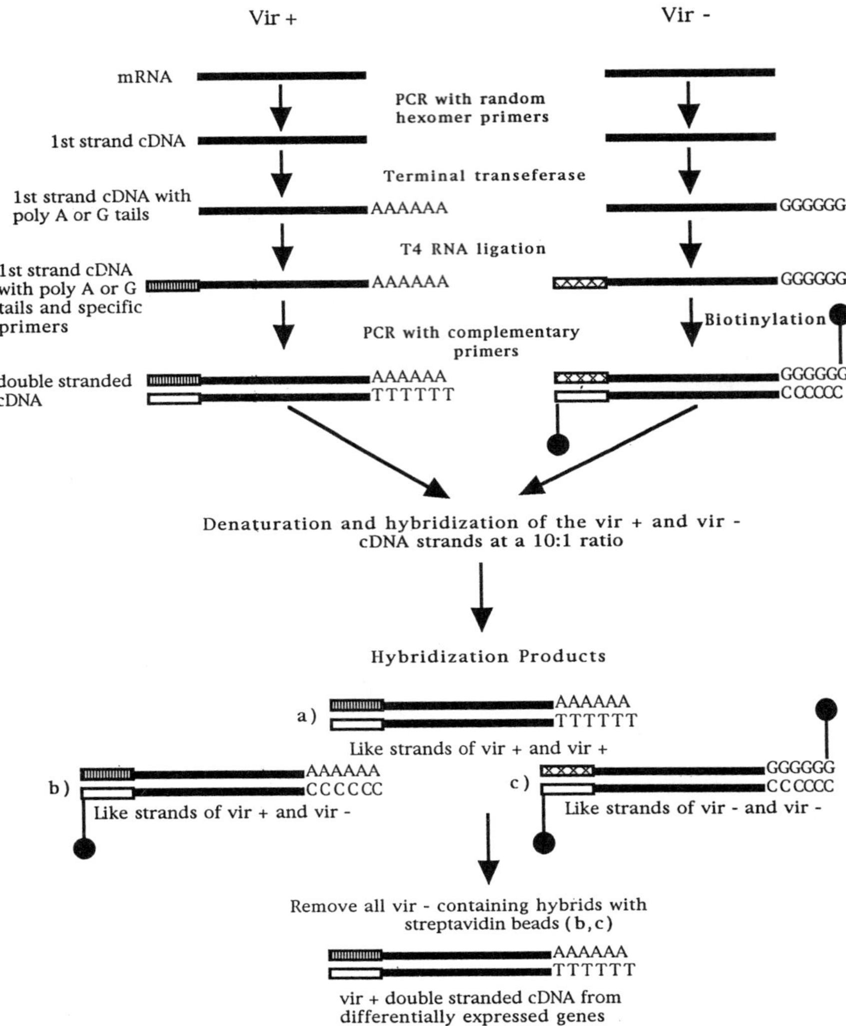

FIGURE 2. Schematic representation of bacterial cDNA-based subtractive hybridization.

CONCLUSION

We stand at the crossroads in our search for bacterial disease-causing mechanisms. Although the development of molecular tools for the identification and study of bacterial genes and gene products has progressed steadily for nearly 30 years, most of these systems have severe limitations for their routine use in the study of specific yet unknown virulence factors from nonenteric pathogens. Virulence models, until recently, consisted of animal and monolayer systems and were limited in their ability to accurately represent human physiology. However, a recent philosophical change in how researchers study virulence mechanisms has occurred. With this new holistic approach have come technological innovations that permit the identification of bacterial genes differentially expressed during various stages of human disease. With still more innovations in recombinant DNA technology, cell biology, and immunology, our abilities to quickly identify virulence-associated genes, modify them, and study their efficacy as in novel diagnostic tests and therapies stand optimistically on the horizon.

REFERENCES

1. ROTH, J. A., C. A. BOLIN, K. A. BROGDEN, F. C. MINION & M. J. WANNEMUEHLER. 1995. Virulence Mechanisms of Bacterial Pathogens. ASM Press. Washington, DC.
2. MOULDER, J. W. 1985. Microbiol. Rev. **49:** 298–337.
3. ZYCHLINSKY, A., J. J. PERDOMO & P. J. SANSONETTI. 1994. Ann. N.Y. Acad. Sci. **730:** 197–208.
4. PORTNOY, D. A., T. CHAKRABORTY, W. GOEBEL & P. COSSART. 1992. Infect. Immun. **60:** 1263–1267.
5. STADNYK, A. W. 1994. FASEB J. **8:** 1041–1047.
6. LUKACS, N. W., S. L. KUNKEL, R. ALLEN, H. L. EVANOFF, C. L. SHAKLEE, J. S. SHERMAN, M. D. BURDICK & R. M. STRIETER. 1995. Am. J. Physiol. **268:** L856–L861.
7. ALEXANDER, J. J., R. MIGUEL & D. GRAHAM. 1991. J. Vasc. Surg. **13:** 444–451.
8. BIRKNESS, K. A., B. L. SWISHER, E. H. WHITE, E. G. LONG, E. P. EWING, JR. & F. D. QUINN. 1995. Infect. Immun. **63:** 402–409.
9. FALKOW, S. 1988. Rev. Infect. Dis. **10:** 5274–5276.
10. ALOUF, J. E. & J. FREER. 1991. Source Book of Bacterial Toxins. Academic Press. New York.
11. FREER, J., R. AITKEN & J. E. ALOUF. 1994. Bacterial Protein Toxins. Gustav Fischer Verlag. New York.
12. WELCH, R. A., T. FELMLEE, F. PELLETT & D. E. CHENOWETH. 1986. The *Escherichia coli* haemolysin: Its gene organization and interaction with neutrophil receptors. *In* Protein-Carbohydrate Interactions in Biological Systems: The Molecular Biology of Microbial Pathogenicity. D. L. Lark *et al.,* eds.: 431–438. Academic Press. New York.
13. CLUFF, C. W., G. GARCIA & H. K. ZIEGLER. 1990. Infect. Immun. **58:** 3601–3612.
14. CLUFF, C. W. & H. K. ZIEGLER. 1987. J. Immunol. **139:** 3808–3812.
15. BERCHE, P., J. L. GAILLARD & P. L. SANSONETTI. 1987. J. Immunol. **138:** 2266–2271.
16. MAHAN, M. J., J. M. SLAUCH & J. J. MEKALANOS. 1993. Science **259:** 686–688.
17. DUGUID, J. R. & J. C. DINAUER. 1989. Nucl. Acid Res. **18:** 2789–2792.
18. LISITSYN, N., N. LISITYN & M. WIGLER. 1993. Science **259:** 946–951.
19. STRAUS, D. & F. M. AUSUBEL. 1990. Proc. Natl. Acad. Sci. **87:** 1889–1893.
20. TIMBLIN, C., J. BATTEY & W. M. KUEHL. 1990. Nucl. Acids Res. **18:** 1587–1593.
21. UTT, E. A., J. P. BROUSAL, L. C. KIKUTA-OSHIMA & F. D. QUINN. 1995. Can. J. Microbiol. **41:** 152–156.
22. KINGER, A. K. & J. S. TYAGI. 1993. Gene **131:** 113–117.
23. KIKUTA-OSHIMA, L. C., C. H. KING, T. M. SHINNICK & F. D. QUINN. 1994. Ann. N.Y. Acad. Sci. **730:** 263–265.
24. PLUM, G. & J. E. CLARK-CURTISS. 1994. Infect. Immun. **62:** 476–483.
25. ZHANG, L. & D. MEDINA. 1993. Mol. Carcinog. **8:** 123–136.
26. WONG, K. K. & M. MCCLELLAND. 1994. Proc. Natl. Acad. Sci. USA **88:** 639–643.
27. LIANG, P. & A. B. PARDEE. 1992. Science **257:** 967–971.

Enteropathogenic *E. coli* Exploitation of Host Epithelial Cells[a]

B. BRETT FINLAY,[b,c] SHARON RUSCHKOWSKI,
BRENDAN KENNY, MARKUS STEIN,
DIETER J. REINSCHEID, MURRY A. STEIN,
AND ILAN ROSENSHINE[d]

*Biotechnology Laboratory and
Departments of Biochemistry & Molecular Biology and
Microbiology & Immunology
University of British Columbia
Vancouver, BC, Canada, V6T-1Z3*

ENTEROPATHIC E. COLI-MEDIATED DISEASE

Escherichia coli is an extremely versatile pathogen. In addition to being a member of the normal intestinal flora, *E. coli* also causes bladder infections, meningitis, and diarrhea. Diarrheogenic *E. coli* contain at least five types of *E. coli,* which cause various symptoms ranging from cholera-like ones to extreme colitis.[1] Each type of diarrheogenic *E. coli* possesses a particular set of virulence factors, including specific adhesins, invasins, and/or toxins, which are responsible for causing a specific type of diarrhea. One of these groups, enteropathogenic *E. coli* (EPEC), is a predominant cause of infant diarrhea worldwide. In addition to isolated outbreaks in day-care centers and nurseries in developed countries, EPEC poses a major endemic health threat to young children (<6 months) in developing countries, where it has a high mortality rate.[2] Worldwide, EPEC is the leading cause of bacteria-mediated diarrhea in children, and it is estimated to kill up to one million children each year. EPEC disease is characterized by watery diarrhea of varying severity, while vomiting and fever often accompany fluid loss.

Despite the significance of EPEC-mediated disease, little is known about how this pathogen actually causes disease. Unlike other *E. coli* diarrheas such as enterotoxigenic *E. coli,* EPEC diarrhea is not mediated by a toxin. Instead, EPEC binds to intestinal surfaces of the small bowel. A characteristic histologic lesion, called the attaching and effacing (A/E) lesion, occurs.[3] A/E lesions are marked by dissolution of the intestinal brush border surface and loss of epithelial microvilli (effacement) at the sites of bacterial attachment. Once bound, EPEC reside upon a

[a]B.K. was supported by a fellowship from the Human Frontiers Science Program, M.S. by a studentship from Gottlieb Daimler- und Karl Benz-Stiftung, D.J.R. by a fellowship from the Chemical Industry Grant (Germany), M.A.S. by a fellowship from the Medical Research Council of Canada, and I.R. by a Canadian Gastroenterology Fellowship. This work was supported by a Howard Hughes International Research Scholar Award and an operating grant from the Canadian Bacterial Diseases Network Center of Excellence to B.B.F.

[b]To whom correspondence should be addressed.

[c]Tel: 604/822-2210; fax: 604/822-9830; e-mail: bfinlay@unixg.ubc.ca.

[d]Current Address: Department of Biotechnology and Molecular Genetics, The Hebrew University, Faculty of Medicine, POB 12272, Jerusalem 91120, Israel (tel: 972 2 758754; fax: 972 2 784010; e-mail: ilanro@md2.huji.ac.il).

cup-like projection or pedestal upon which adherent bacteria reside. Underlying this pedestal in the epithelial cell are several cytoskeletal components, including actin, alpha-actinin, ezrin, talin, and myosin light chain.[4,5] Formation of the A/E lesion appears to be responsible for fluid secretion and diarrhea; however, mechanistically this remains to be proven. It has been suggested that disruption of the brush border and microvilli may be responsible for diarrhea. Although EPEC can enter (invade) tissue culture cells,[6] it does not normally cause invasive disease and rarely penetrates the intestinal barrier.

EPEC belongs to a group of pathogenic organisms that form A/E lesions, including enterohemorrhagic *E. coli* (EHEC), several EPEC-like animal pathogens that cause disease in rabbits (RDEC), dogs, pigs (PEPEC), and the like, and some isolates of *Citrobacter freundii, Hafnia alvei,* and probably *Helicobacter pylori.* These organisms all cause cytoskeletal rearrangement and pedestal formation on relevant host epithelial cells. EHEC, which causes enteric colitis (hamburger disease), can also cause hemolytic uremic syndrome in approximately 10% of cases. EHEC

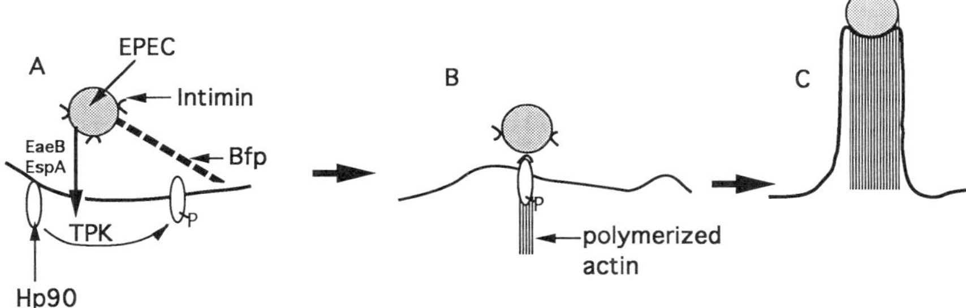

FIGURE 1. Model of the various stages of enteropathogenic *E. coli* (EPEC) interaction with epithelial cells. (**A**) EPEC initially binds to epithelial cells via its bundle-forming pilus. At least two EPEC-secreted proteins (EaeB and EspA) cause activation of host signal transduction pathways, including a tyrosine protein kinase (TPK) which phosphorylates a host membrane protein (Hp90). (**B**) Once Hp90 is phosphorylated, EPEC intimin then binds to it, and polymerized actin and related cytoskeletal proteins accumulate beneath the adherent bacteria. (**C**) Actin polymerization continues beneath adherent bacteria, developing into a fully developed attaching/effacing lesion.

appears to possess all of the EPEC virulence factors needed for A/E lesion formation, but it has an additional shiga-like toxin that contributes to its increased pathogenesis.

MECHANISMS OF PATHOGENICITY

Initial Adherence. Recently, significant progress has been made in defining the bacterial and host factors involved in formation of attaching and effacing lesions. (See FIG. 1 for an outline.) Initial bacterial adherence is dependent on the presence of a 55–70 MD plasmid that is common to EPEC strains. This process is mediated by a plasmid-encoded bundle-forming pilus (BFP) and possibly other factors.[7] Mutants in EPEC that are defective in initial adherence produce fewer A/E lesions on epithelial cells, but these lesions are indistinguishable from those caused by parental EPEC.

Signal Transduction. When EPEC interact with cultured epithelial cells, several signal transduction pathways are activated in the epithelial cells, including the release of the eukaryotic secondary messengers, IP$_3$, and intracellular calcium.[8,9] EPEC binding to cultured epithelial cells also causes tyrosine phosphorylation of a host 90-kD membrane protein, Hp90, which is not normally phosphorylated in uninfected cultured cells.[10] The addition of tyrosine kinase inhibitors inhibits the phosphorylation of Hp90 and EPEC uptake into epithelial cells. Hp90 phosphorylation appears to precede IP$_3$ fluxes and cytoskeletal rearrangements.[8]

All of the EPEC genes known to be involved in A/E formation (except the plasmid-encoded regulator *per*) are found within a unique contiguous region in the EPEC chromosome.[3] Several bacterial loci have been identified that are involved in activating epithelial signal transduction. Strains containing mutations in *eaeB,* a gene found downstream of the intimin gene *eaeA* (see below), do not stimulate signal transduction or cytoskeletal rearrangement.[11] Strains cured of the EPEC virulence plasmid are still capable of activating epithelial signal transduction pathways and organizing the underlying cytoskeletal structure; however, their efficiency at these events is significantly decreased, presumably because of the loss of the plasmid-encoded bundle-forming pilus and a plasmid-encoded positive regulator. In addition to *eaeB,* Tn*phoA* mutants belonging to Class 4 (*cfm* mutants) are also unable to stimulate signal transduction.[10] We recently found that another locus upstream of *eaeB,* called *espA* (*E. coli*-secreted protein A), is also needed to stimulate epithelial signals.[12]

We recently showed that when EPEC is grown in tissue culture media, five bacterial proteins (110, 40, 39, 37, and 25 kD) are secreted into the supernatant medium.[13] Amino terminal sequencing identified the 37 kD as EaeB (a protein needed to trigger signal transduction[11]), and the 25 kD protein matched the predicted product of *espA,* EspA.[12] The 39-kD protein is homologous to glyceraldehyde-3-phosphate dehydrogenase (GAPDH), with 14 of 16 amino acids at its amino terminus being identical to GAPDH. *cfm* mutants were unable to secrete any of these proteins except the 110-kD protein.[13] We recently cloned and sequenced the gene encoding the 110-kD protein (Stein and Finlay, manuscript in preparation). This protein is homologous to a hemagglutinin found in an avian pathogen *E. coli* and uses an IgA protease secretion mechanism. However, by constructing internal gene deletions, we found that the 110-kD protein is not needed for signal transduction and is not secreted by several A/E-causing organisms such as RDEC, *C. freundii,* and *H. alvei* (Stein and Finlay, manuscript in preparation). It also appears that the 39- and 40-kD proteins are not encoded within the 35-kb locus of the enterocyte effacement region, based on DNA hybridization studies and DNA sequence analysis. This region encodes all the factors necessary for A/E formation when placed in HB101 (J. Kaper, personal communication), and thus these two proteins are probably not needed for A/E lesion formation. Characterization of the *cfm* insertions led to the identification of a "Type III" secretion system in EPEC, encoded by the *sep* genes.[13,14] Such secretion systems are used by several bacterial pathogens to export virulence factors out of the bacteria and into contact with mammalian cells. Examples include the invasion systems of *Shigella* and *Salmonella* species, the *Yersinia*-secreted proteins including a tyrosine phosphatase that enters phagocytic cells, and harpins from plant pathogens.[15] Collectively, this information indicates that EPEC secretes at least two molecules (EaeB and EspA) that are critical for activating signal transduction and cytoskeletal rearrangement in epithelial cells, and EPEC has a specialized secretion system for exporting these molecules.

Intimate Adherence. Intimin is the product of a bacterial chromosomal locus, *eaeA,* and is a 94-kD EPEC outer membrane protein that is needed for intimate adherence.[16] We found that *eaeA* mutants form immature A/E lesions and do not organize phosphotyrosine proteins and cytoskeletal components beneath adherent bacteria, although epithelial signal transduction is still activated.[10] Intimin appears to participate in reorganization of the underlying host cytoskeleton after other bacterial factors stimulate epithelial signal transduction.[10] Although cloned intimin in non-pathogenic *E. coli* does not mediate adherence,[16] we recently showed that if an *eaeA* defective strain of EPEC is added to epithelial cells (to stimulate signal transduction) before the addition of the cloned intimin expressed in *E. coli* HB101, bacteria expressing the cloned intimin now adhere to epithelial cells.[17] If EPEC mutants that are defective for stimulating signal transduction (such as *eaeB* or *cfm*) are used to preinfect monolayers, organisms containing the cloned intimin do not adhere. This indicates that EPEC-induced signal transduction pathways are needed before successful intimin-mediated adherence to epithelial cells.

Further support for this hypothesis comes from studies using a purified fusion peptide consisting of 280 amino acids of the carboxyl terminus of intimin fused to the maltose-binding protein (MBP).[17,18] We found that this fusion peptide (MBP/Int) adheres to epithelial cells *only* when the monolayer is previously infected with EPEC (or the *eaeA* mutant) to preinduce signals.[17] If these signals are blocked with a tyrosine kinase inhibitor (which blocks signaling), binding of the fusion peptide to epithelial cells is also blocked. Not surprisingly, peptide binding is not affected by treatment of the monolayer with cytochalasin D, indicating that actin rearrangement is not needed for intimin-mediated binding.

Hp90 is an epithelial membrane-localized protein that localizes beneath adherent organisms at the tip of extended pseudopods.[17] This protein interacts with intimin and is a candidate for the intimin receptor. If EPEC is added to epithelial cells and then removed by detergent extraction, Hp90 remains associated with the bacteria; however, if an *eaeA* mutant is used, Hp90 is not isolated with the bacteria.[17] Hp90 is also coimmunoprecipitated with the intimin-maltose binding protein fusion peptide, but only if prior signals are induced in the epithelial cells by EPEC strains.

Cytoskeletal Rearrangement and Pedestal Formation. As just described, the A/E lesion (or pedestal) formed by EPEC on association with epithelial cells is associated with the assembly of highly organized cytoskeletal structures in the epithelial cells immediately beneath adherent bacteria. Although this pedestal usually raises the bacterium slightly above the epithelial cell surface, we recently showed that EPEC can trigger extended pseudopod formation, with projections extending up to 10 μ above the epithelial cell surface with the bacteria located extracellularly at the tip of these extensions.[17] The stalk of these extended pseudopods contains polymerized actin, whereas Hp90 is localized only at the tip of these structures beneath EPEC. Extended pedestals are not seen when strains containing mutations in *eaeA, eaeB,* or *cfm* are used, reinforcing the linkage between signal transduction events and cytoskeletal rearrangement.

The product of the *eaeA* gene, intimin, appears to be critical for organizing cytoskeletal rearrangements. *eaeA* mutants trigger signals in epithelial cells and cause generalized actin accumulation near adherent organisms, but they are unable to organize the cytoskeleton into defined structures that lead to pedestal and extended pseudopod formation. Additionally, they do not invade epithelial cells, even if complemented with signal transduction-defective EPEC mutants. Further support for the role of intimin comes from experiments performed with the cloned EPEC intimin expressed in nonpathogenic *E. coli* HB101. If EPEC containing a defective *eaeA* gene are first added to epithelial cells followed by strains containing cloned intimin, only HB101 harboring intimin, but not the *eaeA* mutant, organize the cytoskeleton into pedestals and extended pseudopods.[17] This indicates that intimin molecules direct the final condensation and organization of the host cytoskeleton from their outer membrane location on the adherent *E. coli*. In addition to mediating intimin binding, Hp90 also probably plays a significant role in organizing the host cytoskeleton. It may even serve as a bridge, linking intimin in the bacterial outer membrane to the host cytoskeleton on the other side of the epithelial cell membrane.

Production of Diarrhea? Despite our increasing knowledge of the bacterial factors and host molecules that mediate EPEC interactions with epithelial cells, the actual molecular mechanisms that cause diarrhea remain undefined. EPEC strains lacking intimin are significantly decreased in their ability to cause diarrhea in human volunteers.[19] One or more of the events associated with the formation of A/E lesions also cause diarrhea. However, signal transduction mutants such as *eaeB* or *espA* have not been tested for virulence in humans or relevant animal models. In addition to the morphologic rearrangements that occur on the apical surface of epithelial cells, EPEC also causes a large decrease in transepithelial resistance in polarized Caco-2 epithelial cell monolayers.[20] This disruption does not appear to be due to alterations in tight junctions, but instead it affects a transcellular pathway. Mutants defective for signal transduction and *eaeA* mutants do not cause this loss in transepithelial resistance, indicating that this process is linked to these events. It is possible that such transepithelial disruptions occur *in vivo,* which would lead to ionic imbalances and possibly diarrhea.

By using whole cell patch clamping technology, we recently found that EPEC causes significant depolarization of individual HeLa cells (Stein, Mathers, and Finlay, in preparation). Although *eaeA* mutants still caused depolarization, both *eaeB* and *cfm* mutants did not depolarize cells, indicating that EPEC-secreted proteins that affect epithelial signaling are needed for these events. The occurrence of such a process in the gut would reduce the electrochemical gradient available for sodium ion absorption from the gut lumen, thereby contributing to ionic imbalance, fluid loss, and diarrhea.

SUMMARY

Enteropathogenic *E. coli* (EPEC) is a leading cause of neonatal diarrhea worldwide. These organisms adhere to the intestinal cell surface, causing rearrangement in the epithelial cell surface and underlying cytoskeleton, resulting in a structure termed an attaching/effacing (A/E) lesion. A/E lesion formation is thought necessary for EPEC-mediated disease. EPEC secretes several proteins that trigger signal transduction, intimate adherence, and cytoskeletal rearrangements in epithelial cells. Additionally, it produces intimin, an outer membrane product that mediates intimate adherence. Together these various bacterial molecules contribute to the intimate relationship that is formed by EPEC with host epithelial cells which results in A/E lesion formation and diarrhea.

REFERENCES

1. HART, C. A., R. M. BATT & J. R. SAUNDERS. 1993. Diarrhoea caused by *Escherichia coli*. Ann. Trop. Paediatr. **13:** 121–131.

2. LEVINE, M. M. & R. EDELMAN. 1984. Enteropathogenic *Escherichia coli* of classic serotypes associated with infant diarrhea: Epidemiology and pathogenesis. Epidemiol. Rev. **6:** 31–51.
3. MCDANIEL, T. K., K. G. JARVIS, M. S. DONNENBERG & J. B. KAPER. 1995. A genetic locus of enterocyte effacement conserved among diverse enterobacterial pathogens. Proc. Natl. Acad. Sci. USA **92:** 1664–1668.
4. FINLAY, B. B., I. ROSENSHINE, M. S. DONNENBERG & J. B. KAPER. 1992. Cytoskeletal composition of attaching and effacing lesions associated with enteropathogenic *Escherichia coli* adherence to HeLa cells. Infect. Immun. **60:** 2541–2543.
5. KNUTTON, S., T. BALDWIN, P. H. WILLIAMS & A. S. MCNEISH. 1989. Actin accumulation at sites of bacterial adhesion to tissue culture cells: Basis of a new diagnostic test for enteropathogenic and enterohemorrhagic *Escherichia coli.* Infect. Immun. **57:** 1290–1298.
6. DONNENBERG, M. S., A. DONOHUE-ROLFE & G. T. KEUSCH. 1990. A comparison of HEp-2 cell invasion by enteropathogenic and enteroinvasive *Escherichia coli.* FEMS Microbiol. Lett. **57:** 83–86.
7. GIRON, J. A., A. S. HO & G. K. SCHOOLNIK. 1993. Characterization of fimbriae produced by enteropathogenic *Escherichia coli.* J. Bacteriol. **175:** 7391–7403.
8. FOUBISTER, V., I. ROSENSHINE & B. B. FINLAY. 1994. A diarrheal pathogen, enteropathogenic *Escherichia coli* (EPEC), triggers a flux of inositol phosphates in infected epithelial cells. J. Exp. Med. **179:** 993–998.
9. DYTOC, M., L. FEDORKO & P. M. SHERMAN. 1994. Signal transduction in human epithelial cells infected with attaching and effacing *Escherichia coli* in vitro. Gastroenterology **106:** 1150–1161.
10. ROSENSHINE, I., M. S. DONNENBERG, J. B. KAPER & B. B. FINLAY. 1992. Signal transduction between enteropathogenic *Escherichia coli* (EPEC) and epithelial cells: EPEC induces tyrosine phosphorylation of host cell proteins to initiate cytoskeletal rearrangement and bacterial uptake. EMBO J. **11:** 3551–3560.
11. FOUBISTER, V., I. ROSENSHINE, M. S. DONNENBERG & B. B. FINLAY. 1994. The *eaeB* gene of enteropathogenic *Escherichia coli* is necessary for signal transduction in epithelial cells. Infect. Immun. **62:** 3038–3040.
12. KENNY, B., L.-C. LAI, B. B. FINLAY & M. S. DONNENBERG. 1996. EspA, an enteropathogenic *Escherichia coli* (EPEC) secreted protein, is required for activating signal transduction in epithelial cells. Mol. Microbiol. **20:** 313–323.
13. KENNY, B. & B. B. FINLAY. 1995. Protein secretion by enteropathogenic *Escherichia coli* is essential for transducing signals to epithelial cells. Proc. Natl. Acad. Sci. USA **92:** 7991–7995.
14. JARVIS, K. G., J. A. GIRON, A. E. JERSE, T. K. MCDANIEL, M. S. DONNENBERG & J. B. KAPER. 1995. Enteropathogenic *Escherichia coli* contains a putative Type III secretion system necessary for the export of proteins involved in attaching and effacing lesion formation. Proc. Natl. Acad. Sci. USA. **92:** 7996–8000.
15. VAN GIJSEGEM, F., S. GENIN & C. BOUCHER. 1993. Conservation of secretion pathways for pathogenicity determinants of plant and animal bacteria. Trends Microbiol. **1:** 175–180.
16. JERSE, A. E., J. YU, B. D. TALL & J. B. KAPER. 1990. A genetic locus of enteropathogenic *Escherichia coli* necessary for the production of attaching and effacing lesions on tissue culture cells. Proc. Natl. Acad. Sci. USA **87:** 7839–7843.
17. ROSENSHINE, I., S. RUSCHKOWSKI, M. STEIN, D. J. REINSHEID & B. B. FINLAY. 1996. A pathogenic bacterium triggers epithelial signals to form a functional bacterial receptor that mediates actin pseudopod formation. EMBO J. **15:** 2613–2624.
18. FRANKEL, G., D. C. CANDY, P. EVEREST & G. DOUGAN. 1994. Characterization of the C-terminal domains of intimin-like proteins of enteropathogenic and enterohemorrhagic *Escherichia coli, Citrobacter freundii,* and *Hafnia alvei.* Infect. Immun. **62:** 1835–1842.
19. DONNENBERG, M. S., C. O. TACKET, S. P. JAMES, G. LOSONSKY, J. P. NATARO, S. S. WASSERMAN, J. B. KAPER & M. M. LEVINE. 1993. Role of the *eaeA* gene in experimental enteropathogenic *Escherichia coli* infection. J. Clin. Invest. **92:** 1412–1417.
20. CANIL, C., I. ROSENSHINE, S. RUSCHKOWSKI, M. S. DONNENBERG, J. B. KAPER & B. B. FINLAY. 1993. Enteropathogenic *Escherichia coli* decreases the transepithelial electrical resistance of polarized epithelial monolayers. Infect. Immun. **61:** 2755–2762.

Differentially Expressed Genes
of *Mycobacterium tuberculosis*

BARBARA J. MARSTON[a,b] AND THOMAS M. SHINNICK[b,c]

aDivision of Infectious Diseases
Emory University and
bDivision of AIDS, STD, and TB Laboratory Research
National Center for Infectious Diseases
Centers for Disease Control and Prevention
Atlanta, Georgia 30333

TUBERCULOSIS

The global impact of tuberculosis is enormous. The World Health Organization estimates that as many as a third of the world's population or ~ 1.7 billion persons are or have been infected with *Mycobacterium tuberculosis,* the causative agent of tuberculosis.[1–3] Each year, there are 8 to 10 million new cases of tuberculosis and nearly 3 million deaths due to tuberculosis.[1–3] The social and economic impact of tuberculosis is magnified beyond these impressive numbers, because of the groups affected. About 95% of new cases occur in developing countries, and about 80% of tuberculosis cases affect persons of child-bearing age and during their most productive years, ages 15–59 years.[1–3] Tuberculosis is also an important source of morbidity and mortality among children under the age of 15 years. Infection with *M. tuberculosis* occurred in 1.3 million children and was responsible for 450,000 deaths in 1989.[4] Not surprisingly, the World Health Organization declared tuberculosis to be a global public health emergency in 1993.

Tuberculosis is also reemerging as an important public health problem in many industrialized countries.[5,6] That is, after decades of consistently declining numbers of annually reported cases of tuberculosis, many industrialized countries experienced significant increases in the number of reported tuberculosis cases during the last 5–10 years.[5] For example, the United Kingdom had a 5% increase in annual reported tuberculosis cases from 1987 to 1991, Ireland had a 9% increase from 1988 to 1991, the Netherlands had a 19% increase from 1987 to 1992, and Italy had a 27% increase from 1988 to 1992.[5] In the United States, the number of tuberculosis cases reported to the Centers for Disease Control declined consistently from 84,000 cases in 1953 to a low of 22,201 cases in 1985, before increasing by more than 20% to 26,673 cases in 1992.[7,8] During the last 2 years, the number of reported cases declined to 25,287 in 1993 and 24,361 in 1994, but was still well above the low point.[7,8]

The consistent decline in reported tuberculosis cases led to relaxation of efforts directed at tuberculosis control, less funding for control programs, and the discontinuation of surveillance for drug-resistant isolates of *M. tuberculosis,* all of which contributed to the resurgence of tuberculosis.[6,9] The key factors contributing to the resurgence were the epidemic of infection with human immunodeficiency virus

cAddress for correspondence: T. M. Shinnick, PhD, Mailstop G35, Centers for Disease Control and Prevention, 1600 Clifton Road, N.E., Atlanta, GA 30333 (tel: 404/639–3601; fax: 404/639–1287).

(HIV), deterioration of the public health infrastructure, transmission in congregate settings, and increased immigration from countries with a high incidence of tuberculosis.[6,10–13]

In addition to increases in the number of cases, *M. tuberculosis* organisms resistant to antituberculosis drugs have become relatively common in some places; perhaps as many as a third of all *M. tuberculosis* isolates in New York City are resistant to at least one antituberculosis drug.[14] Of additional concern are recent outbreaks of multidrug-resistant tuberculosis in hospitals and prisons in New York and Florida, which have been characterized by high rates of transmission, rapid development of illness, and poor clinical outcomes.[15,16] These nosocomial outbreaks also involved transmission of tuberculosis to health care personnel. In one nosocomial outbreak, tuberculin skin test conversion was demonstrated for between 22 and 50% of health care workers, and several health care workers developed active tuberculosis.[17]

Because of these concerns, new preventive and therapeutic strategies are needed for tuberculosis. An understanding of the molecular biology of mycobacteria generally and of virulence genes specifically is essential to the development of both new vaccines and new antituberculosis therapies.

TABLE 1. Potential Virulence Factors of *M. tuberculosis*

Virulence Feature	Phenotypic Basis
Failure to fully stimulate host macrophages[19,20]	Mannose capping of cell-wall glycolipids may mimic host tissues
Inactivation of, or resistance to, products of the respiratory burst[21,22]	Respiratory burst products may be scavenged, possibly by glycolipids[23,24] or inactivated by catalase[25] or superoxide dismutase[26]
Resistance to lysosomal enzymes[27]	Diffusion of lysosomal enzymes near mycobacteria may be inhibited by a secreted, protective capsule[27]
Inhibition of phagosome acidification[28]	Proton ATPase may be excluded from phagosomal membrane[29] and pH may be buffered by weak bases such as ammonium chloride[30]
Inhibition of phagosome-lysosome fusion, sequestration in nonfused vacuoles[31–34]	Fusion inhibition may be related to inhibition of phagosome acidification

PATHOGENICITY OF *MYCOBACTERIUM TUBERCULOSIS*

The virulence of an infecting organism is defined by its ability to cause injury or death to the host. It has become clear that for many organisms, virulence is not conferred by a single characteristic (for example, the elaboration of a toxin), but instead depends on an array of bacterial attributes. Virulence factors may include both elements that directly damage host structures and elements that allow the organism to overcome the usual host defense mechanisms. The capacity of *M. tuberculosis* to survive and grow within macrophages is generally considered a defining feature of the virulence of this pathogen.[18] The interactions between tubercle bacilli and host macrophages have been the focus of much attention during the last several decades, and a variety of steps have been proposed as components of the ability of pathogenic mycobacteria to survive within macrophages and avoid host defenses[19–35] (TABLE 1).

Such host defenses may include limitation of the availability of key nutrients such as iron or exposure to a variety of lethal cellular products such as oxygen metabolites, lysozymes, proteases, lipases, cationic proteins, or reactive nitrogen intermediates.

IDENTIFYING VIRULENCE FACTORS AND DIFFERENTIALLY EXPRESSED GENES

A key step in sorting out the survival strategies of the tubercle bacillus will be the identification and characterization of the mycobacterial genes and gene products required for intracellular survival and replication. Approaches taken recently to identify mycobacterial genes associated with virulence include (1) using cosmid vectors to transfer genomic DNA from virulent strains to related attenuated strains to identify genes that complement the defect in the attenuated strains,[36,37] (2) passing clones from recombinant libraries of mycobacterial DNA in *Escherichia coli* through macrophages or HeLa cells to isolate clones with enhanced resistance to killing by macrophages or enhanced ability to enter HeLa cells,[38,39] and (3) using RNA subtractive hybridization techniques to identify genes that are expressed to a greater degree by virulent strains than by related attenuated strains.[39–41]

Another molecular approach to identifying virulence factors is to identify genes that are specifically expressed during intracellular replication.[41–43] Such genes likely encode products required for intracellular survival and thus for virulence. Because expression of these virulence genes is presumably regulated at least in part at the level of transcription, identification of differentially expressed transcription promoters should lead to recognition of differentially expressed gene products. A novel genetic approach to the identification of such differentially expressed genes was developed by Mekalanos and coworkers.[43] The method is termed *in vivo* expression technology (IVET) and is based on the identification of genes that are expressed during growth in the host, but not during growth in axenic media. This approach involves (a) cloning promoters in front of a gene whose product is required for growth *in vivo*, (b) introducing the recombinants into a pathogenic bacterium that does not express the required gene product, and (c) passing the recombinants through an animal host. Recombinants recovered from the animal host should contain promoters that directed expression of the required gene during growth *in vivo*. Unfortunately, the IVET approach cannot yet be applied directly to *M. tuberculosis* because the prerequisite mutant strains of *M. tuberculosis* and complementing genes are not yet available.

To circumvent this problem, we modified the IVET approach to use an easily measured enzymatic activity rather than a selectable marker to investigate differential gene expression. Firefly luciferase was chosen as the reporter activity because (1) its activity (light production) can easily be assayed from relatively large numbers of individual clones using an automated luminometer and 96-well culture plates and (2) lysis of the mycobacteria is not necessary for this enzymatic assay, because luciferin enters intact cells and light production is readily detectable in the absence of cell lysis. Our basic strategy is to (1) clone pieces of the genome of a virulent *M. tuberculosis* strain in front of a promoterless firefly luciferase reporter gene, (2) electroporate the recombinants into *M. tuberculosis* H37Rv, and (3) assay individual transformants for luciferase activity when they are growing in liquid media or inside macrophages. The overall aim is to identify transformants containing promoters whose expression is markedly increased during growth in macrophages (FIG. 1).

CONSTRUCTION OF RECOMBINANT DNA LIBRARY

The first step in this approach was to construct a plasmid vector with the following features (pCL5, FIG. 2): an origin for extrachromosomal replication in *E. coli,* a polylinker cloning site containing a unique *Bam*HI restriction site, the aminoglycoside 3'-phosphotransferase gene from Tn5 (encodes kanamycin resistance), the integrase and attachment site from mycobacteriophage L5 to allow site-specific integration of the plasmid vector into mycobacterial chromosomal DNA and stable replication of a single copy of the insert DNA,[44] the T1T2 ribosomal RNA transcription terminator from *E. coli*[45] to limit transcription from upstream vector sequences, and a promoterless copy of the firefly luciferase gene.[46] A similar plasmid containing a copy of the firefly luciferase gene fused to the *M. tuberculosis cpn60-2* promoter[47] was constructed for use as a positive control (pCL7).

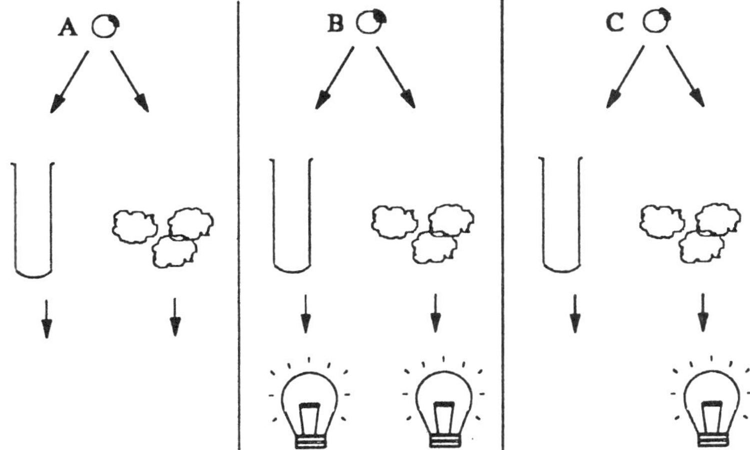

FIGURE 1. Potential patterns of luciferase expression. **A, B,** and **C** show individual *M. tuberculosis* clones in which a test fragment of DNA is cloned upstream of a promoterless firefly luciferase gene. Luciferase expression is depicted as light bulbs for expression during growth in liquid media (*left side of each panel*) and in macrophage cell culture (*right side of each panel*). Clones producing light in neither liquid media nor macrophages (**A**) contain no promoter activity. Clones producing light under both conditions (**B**) probably contain promoters for "housekeeping" genes. Clones producing light during growth in macrophages, but not during growth in liquid media, may contain promoters for potential virulence genes (**C**).

Next, genomic DNA from the virulent H37Rv strain of *M. tuberculosis* was partially digested with the restriction enzyme *Sau*3a to generate fragments of 500 to 2,000 base pairs, the fragments ligated into *Bam*HI-cleaved and phosphatase-treated pCL5, and portions of the ligation mixtures electroporated into *E. coli.* Kanamycin-resistant transformants were harvested after overnight growth, and plasmid DNA was extracted from the pooled bacterial suspension. The purified plasmid DNA was electroporated into *M. smegmatis* strain LR222 and *M. tuberculosis* strain H37Rv to generate libraries of mycobacterial transformants carrying integrated pCL5-based recombinants. Analysis of the *M. tuberculosis* transformants revealed that (1) each

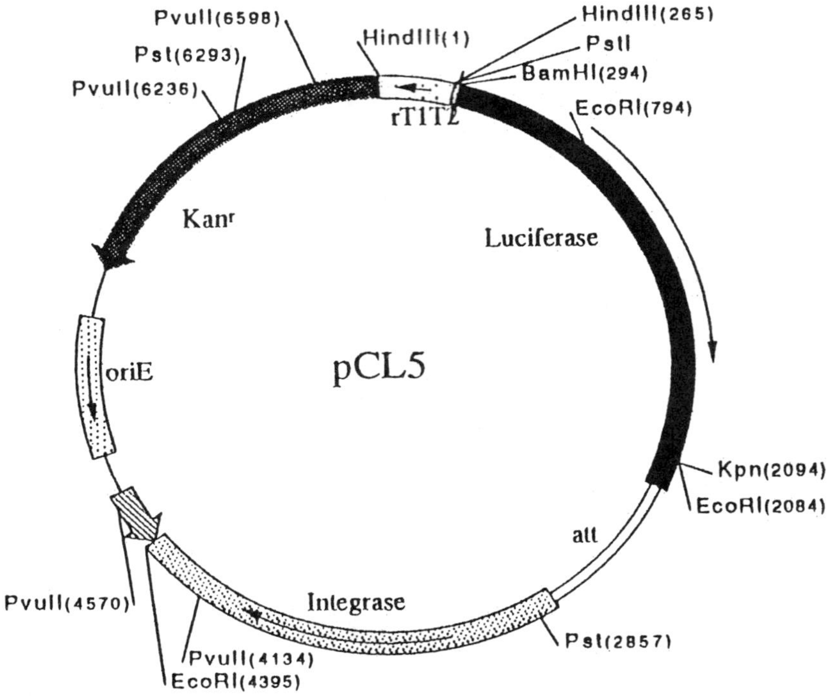

FIGURE 2. Integrating promoter-trap plasmid vector pCL5.

transformant had vector DNA integrated at the L5 attachment site, (2) ~90% of the transformants contained integrated plasmids carrying inserted DNA which ranged in size from 300 to 2,500 base pairs, and (3) the library contained more than 10^5 independent transformants.

LUCIFERASE EXPRESSION DURING GROWTH IN LIQUID MEDIA

To investigate luciferase expression during growth in liquid media, individual mycobacterial transformants were grown in complete Middlebrook 7H10 medium (GIBCO Laboratories, Madison, Wisconsin) to late log phase and assayed for luciferase activity by mixing 100 μl of the bacterial culture with 50 μl of Luciferase Assay Substrate (470 μM luciferin, 270 μM coenzyme A, 530 μM ATP; Promega Corp., Madison, Wisconsin) in a well of a 96-well microdilution plate and measuring light production using a ML 1000 luminometer (Dynatech Laboratories Inc., Chantilly, Virginia). To account for day-to-day variability in the assay, the activities of the transformants were compared to the activity of the negative control, *M. tuberculosis* (pCL5), and the results expressed as a ratio of relative light units (RLU) of luciferase activity produced by the transformant to RLU produced by *M. tuberculosis* (pCL5).

Luciferase expression during growth in liquid media was determined for 84 *M. smegmatis* transformants and 366 *M. tuberculosis* transformants (TABLE 2). Six (7%)

M. smegmatis transformants and 75 (20%) *M. tuberculosis* transformants expressed at least fivefold more luciferase activity than control strains carrying pCL5. *M. tuberculosis* bacilli carrying the pCL7-positive control plasmid, in which luciferase expression is under the control of the strong *cpn60-2* promoter, exhibited more than 1000-fold greater luciferase expression than did *M. tuberculosis* (pCL5).

To identify the mycobacterial promoters/genes directing the expression of luciferase in the light-producing clones, the insert DNAs were recovered by PCR-amplification using primers complementary to the sequences of the kanamycin-resistance gene and the luciferase gene (FIG. 2), and their nucleotide sequences determined using a PRISM™ Ready Reaction DyeDeoxy™ Terminator Cycle Sequencing Kit and Model 373 automated sequencing system (Applied Biosystems, Foster City, California). Initial sequencing was performed using primers complementary to flanking regions of the RNA transcription terminator or the luciferase gene. Subsequently, primers to sites internal to the inserts were synthesized, and sequence analysis and primer synthesis were performed alternately until the entire insert sequence was determined.

Sequence analysis has been completed for inserts from four transformants exhibiting luciferase expression during growth in liquid media (clones 4, 11, 12, and 115). Three of these sequences exhibited no homology to available nucleotide or amino acid sequences. However, the 233 nucleotides of clone 11 immediately adjacent to the luciferase gene displayed 78% identity with the 5'-end of the DNA sequence of an open reading frame encoding a cholesterol dehydrogenase from *Nocardia* sp.[48] The *Nocardia* and *Mycobacterium* genera are taxonomically closely related.[49] The significance of this homology is unclear, but it is likely that we have simply cloned the promoter for a housekeeping gene of *M. tuberculosis.*

LUCIFERASE EXPRESSION DURING GROWTH IN MACROPHAGES

Our initial model for *in vivo* growth is growth in cultured macrophages derived from the human monocytic cell line THP-1.[50] Exposure of THP-1 cells to phorbol myristate 13-acetate (PMA) results in differentiation to macrophage-like cells that adhere to culture plates and display many relevant properties of macrophages such as phagocytosis, antigen presentation, activation, and free radical production.[51]

To investigate luciferase expression during growth within macrophages, bacilli were harvested from a late log-phase culture of an individual *M. tuberculosis* transformant grown in Middlebrook 7H10 medium, washed, resuspended in RPMI1640 (GIBCO) at ~10^7 cells/ml, and used to infect PMA-differentiated THP-1 cells at a ratio of ~10 bacteria per macrophage. After 3 days of incubation at 37°C, the macrophages were lysed with 0.1% Triton X-100, and luciferase activity in the lysate was measured as just described.

To date, we have screened about 300 *M. tuberculosis* transformants for luciferase

TABLE 2. Luciferase Expression during Growth in Liquid Media

Recipient Species	Number (%) Displaying Increase in Activity Relative to *M. tuberculosis* (pCL5)					
	<5-fold	5–10-fold	10–100-fold	100–1,000-fold	>1,000-fold	Total
M. smegmatis	78 (93.0)	2 (2.0)	4 (5.0)	0	0	84
M. tuberculosis	291 (79.5)	25 (6.8)	36 (9.8)	13 (3.6)	1 (0.3)	366

expression during growth in macrophages, and in these initial screens, we identified nine transformants that produce at least fivefold more luciferase activity while growing in macrophages than while growing in liquid medium. Sequence analysis of the insert from one of these clones, which reproducibly produced about 16-fold more light while growing in macrophages than while growing in liquid media, did not reveal any significant matches with previously sequenced genes in the protein and nucleic acid databases. The analysis of the other inserts and the identification of full-length genes are underway.

DISCUSSION AND FUTURE DIRECTIONS

Our library contains clones that express a wide range of luciferase activities during growth in liquid media. The simplest explanation for this variation is differences in promoter strength. However, because of the way the library was constructed, varying luciferase expression may also reflect differences in the efficiency of transcription or translation that relate to the distance between a promoter sequence and the luciferase gene or other factors such as secondary structure associated with intervening DNA or RNA. Studies (e.g., mapping of the transcription start sites by primer extension and fine structure analysis of the promoter regions) of the promoters whose expression is not differentially regulated should allow us to develop consensus sequences for mycobacterial promoters, better understand general transcription mechanisms in mycobacteria, and characterize the variation in luciferase expression in the transformants.

Similar detailed analyses of the upstream regions in the differentially expressed clones should identify the fine structure of differentially expressed promoters and may provide clues as to their regulation (e.g., identification of potential regulatory motifs or sequences). With respect to understanding pathogenesis, a key step will be to isolate and characterize the native gene whose expression is directed by the cloned, differentially expressed promoter.

Finally, the identification of differentially expressed genes should help identify important virulence factors of *M. tuberculosis*. In addition, because these genes are expressed only when the bacterium is growing in the host, these proteins would be good candidates for diagnostic reagents, reagents that may be able to distinguish active disease from inactive infection or prior exposure. Detailed analysis of differentially expressed promoters, their associated genes and gene products, and biologic functions should generate insights into the molecular mechanisms of the intracellular survival and virulence of *M. tuberculosis,* which in turn may facilitate both targeting of antituberculosis drugs and selection of antigens for vaccine development.

REFERENCES

1. SUDRE, P., G. TEN DAM & A. KOCHI. 1992. Tuberculosis: A global overview of the situation today. Bull. W.H.O. **70:** 149–159.
2. MURRAY, C. J. L., K. STYBLO & A. ROUILLON. 1990. Tuberculosis in developing countries: Burden, intervention and cost. Bull. Int. Union Tuberc. Lung Dis. **65:** 2–20.
3. SNIDER, D. E., M. C. RAVIGLIONE & A. KOCHI. 1994. Global burden of tuberculosis. *In* Tuberculosis: Pathogenesis, Protection, and Control. B. R. Bloom, Ed.: 3–11. American Society for Microbiology Press. Washington, DC.
4. WORLD HEALTH ORGANIZATION. 1989. Childhood tuberculosis and BCG vaccine. *In* EPI Update Supplement. World Health Organization. Geneva.

5. RAVIGLIONE, M. C., P. SUDRE, H. L. RIEDER, S. SPINACI & A. KOCHI. 1993. Secular trends of tuberculosis in Western Europe. Bull. W.H.O. **71:** 297–306.

6. CANTWELL, M. F., D. E. SNIDER, G. M. CAUTHEN & I. ONORATO. 1994. Epidemiology of tuberculosis in the United States, 1985 through 1992. JAMA **272:** 535–539.

7. CENTERS FOR DISEASE CONTROL AND PREVENTION. 1994. Expanded tuberculosis surveillance and tuberculosis morbidity—United States, 1993. Morbid. Mortal. Weekly Rep. **43**(RR-20): 361–366.

8. CENTERS FOR DISEASE CONTROL AND PREVENTION. 1995. Tuberculosis Morbidity—United States, 1994. Morbid. Mortal. Weekly Rep. **44**(RR-20): 387–395.

9. WEISS, R. 1992. On the track of "killer" TB, News & Comment. Science **255:** 148–150.

10. HOPEWELL, P. C. 1992. Impact of human immunodeficiency virus infection on the epidemiology, clinical features, management, and control of tuberculosis. Clin. Infect. Dis. **18:** 540–546.

11. BRUDNEY, K. & J. DOBKIN. 1991. Resurgent tuberculosis in New York City: Human immunodeficiency virus, homelessness and the decline of tuberculosis control programs. Am. Rev. Respir. Dis. **144:** 745–749.

12. SMITH, P. G. & A. R. MOSS. 1994. Epidemiology of tuberculosis. *In* Tuberculosis: Pathogenesis, protection, and control. B. R. Bloom, Ed.: 47–59. American Society for Microbiology Press. Washington DC.

13. ELLNER, J. J., A. R. HINMAN, S. W. DOOLEY, M. A. FISCHL, K. A. SEPKOWITZ, M. J. GOLDBERGER, T. M. SHINNICK, M. D. ISEMAN & W. R. JACOBS. 1993. Tuberculosis symposium: Emerging problems and promise. J. Infect. Dis. **168:** 537–551.

14. FREIDEN, T. R., T. STERLING, A. PABLOS-MENDEZ, J. O. KILBURN, G. M. CAUTHEN & S. W. DOOLEY. 1993. The emergence of drug-resistant tuberculosis in New York City. N. Engl. J. Med. **328:** 521–526.

15. EDLIN, B. R., J. I. TOKARS, M. H. GRIECO, J. T. CRAWFORD, J. WILLIAMS, E. M. SORDILLO, K. R. ONG, J. O. KILBURN, S. W. DOOLEY, K. G. CASTRO *et al.* 1992. An outbreak of multidrug-resistant tuberculosis among hospitalized patients with acquired immunodeficiency syndrome. N. Engl. J. Med. **326:** 1514–1521.

16. FISCHL, M. A., G. L. DAIKOS, R. B. UTTAMCHANDANI, R. B. POBLETE, J. N. MORENO, R. R. REYES, A. M. BOOTA, L. M. THOMPSON, T. J. CLEARY, S. A. OLDHAM, M. J. SALDANA & S. LAI. 1992. Clinical presentation and outcome of patients with HIV infection and tuberculosis caused by multiple-drug-resistant bacilli. Ann. Intern. Med. **117:** 184–190.

17. PEARSON, M. L., J. A. JEREB, T. R. FREIDEN *et al.* 1992. Nosocomial transmission of multidrug-resistant tuberculosis. Ann. Intern. Med. **117:** 191–196.

18. JACOBS, W. R. & B. R. BLOOM. 1994. Molecular genetic strategies for identifying virulence determinants of *Mycobacterium tuberculosis. In* Tuberculosis: Pathogenesis, protection, and control. B. R. Bloom, Ed.: 253–268. American Society for Microbiology Press. Washington DC.

19. CHATTERJEE, D., K. LOWELL, B. RIVOIRE, M. R. MCNEIL & P. J. BRENNAN. 1992. Lipoarabinomannan of *Mycobacterium tuberculosis:* Capping with mannosyl residues in some strains. J. Biol. Chem. **267:** 6234–6239.

20. ROACH, T. I. A., C. H. BARTON, D. CHATTERJEE & J. M. BLACKWELL. 1993. Macrophage activation: Lipoarabinomannan from avirulent and virulent strains of *Mycobacterium tuberculosis* differentially induces that early genes c-fos, KC, JE, and TNF-α. J. Immunol. **150:** 1886–1896.

21. MITCHISON, D. A., J. B. SELKON & J. LLOYD. 1964. Virulence in the guinea-pig, susceptibility to hydrogen peroxide and catalase activity of isoniazid-sensitive tubercle bacilli from South Indian and British patients. Pathol. Bacteriol. **86:** 377–386.

22. JACKETT, P. S., V. R. ABER & D. B. LOWRIE. 1978. Virulence and resistance to superoxide, low pH and hydrogen peroxide among strains of *Mycobacterium tuberculosis.* J. Gen. Microbiol. **104:** 37–45.

23. GOREN, M. B., J. M. GRANGE, V. R. ABNER, B. W. ALLEN & D. A. MITCHISON. 1982. Role of lipid content and hydrogen peroxide susceptibility in determining guinea pig virulence of *M. tuberculosis.* Br. J. Exp. Pathol. **63:** 693–700.

24. CHAN, J., X. FAN, S. W. HUNTER, P. J. BRENNAN & B. R. BLOOM. 1991. Lipoarabinoman-

nan, a possible virulence factor involved in persistence of *Mycobacterium tuberculosis* within macrophages. Infect. Immun. **59:** 1755–1761.

25. ZHANG, Y., R. LATHIGRA, T. GARBE, D. CATTY & D. YOUNG. 1991. Genetic analysis of superoxide dismutase, the 23 kilodalton antigen of *Mycobacterium tuberculosis*. Mol. Microbiol. **5:** 381–391.

26. ZHANG, J., B. HEYM, B. ALLEN, D. YOUNG & S. COLE. 1992. The catalase-peroxidase gene of *Mycobacterium tuberculosis*. Nature **358:** 591–593.

27. DRAPER, P. & R. J. REES. 1970. Electron-transparent zone of mycobacteria may be a defense mechanism. Nature **228:** 860–861.

28. CROWLE, A. J., R. DAHL, E. ROSS & M. H. MAY. 1991. Evidence that vesicles containing living, virulent *Mycobacterium tuberculosis* or *Mycobacterium avium* in cultured human macrophages are not acidic. Infect. Immun. **59:** 1823–1831.

29. STURGILL-KOSZYCKI, S., P. H. SCHLESINGER, P. CHAKRABORTY, P. L. HADDIX, H. L. COLLINES, A. K. FOK, R. D. ALLEN, S. L. GLUCK, J. HEUSER & D. G. RUSSELL. 1994. Lack of acidification in mycobacterium phagosomes produced by exclusion of the vesicular proton-ATPase. Science **263:** 678–681.

30. D'ARCY HART, P., M. R. YOUNG, M. M. JORDAN, W. J. PERKINS & M. J. GEISOW. 1983. Chemical inhibitors of phagosome-lysosome fusion in cultured macrophages also inhibit saltatory lysosomal movements. A combined microscopic and computer study. J. Exp. Med. **158:** 477–492.

31. ARMSTRONG, J. A. & P. D'ARCY-HART. 1971. Response of cultured macrophages to *Mycobacterium tuberculosis,* with observations on fusion of lysosomes with phagosomes. J. Exp. Med. **134:** 713–740.

32. RASTOGI, N., ED. 1990. Killing intracellular mycobacteria: Dogmas and realities. Fifth Forum in Microbiology. Res. Microbiol. **141:** 191–270.

33. FREHEL, C. & N. RASTOGI. 1987. *Mycobacterium leprae* surface components intervene in the early phagosome lysosome fusion inhibition event. Infect. Immun. **55:** 2916–2921.

34. CLEMENS, D. L. & M. A. HORWITZ. 1995. Characterization of the *Mycobacterium tuberculosis* phagosome and evidence that phagosomal maturation is inhibited. J. Exp. Med. **181:** 257–270.

35. PASCOPELLA, L., F. M. COLLINS, J. M. MARTIN, M. H. LEE, G. F. HATFULL, C. K. STOVER, B. R. BLOOM & W. R. JACOBS. 1994. Use of in vivo complementation in *Mycobacterium tuberculosis* to identify a genomic fragment associated with virulence. Infect. Immun. **62:** 1313–1319.

36. COLLINS, D. M., R. P. KAWAKAMI, G. W. DELISLE, L. PASCOPELLA, B. R. BLOOM & W. R. JACOBS. 1995. Mutation of the principal sigma factor causes loss of virulence in a strain of the *Mycobacterium tuberculosis* complex. Proc. Natl. Acad. Sci. USA **92:** 8036–8040.

37. SATHISH, M. & T. M. SHINNICK. 1994. Identification of genes involved in the resistance of mycobacteria to killing by macrophages. Ann. N.Y. Acad. Sci. **730:** 26–36.

38. ARRUDA, S., G. BOMFIN, R. KNIGHTS, T. HIUMA-BYRON & L. W. RILEY. 1993. Cloning of an *M. tuberculosis* DNA fragment associated with entry and survival inside cells. Science **261:** 1454–1457.

39. UTT, E. A., J. P. BROUSAL, L. C. KIKUTA-OSHIMA & F. D. QUINN. 1994. The identification of bacterial gene expression differences using mRNA-based isothermal subtractive hybridization. Can. J. Microbiol. **41:** 152–156.

40. KINGER, A. K. & J. S. TYAGI. 1993. Identification and cloning of genes differentially expressed in the virulent strain of *Mycobacterium tuberculosis*. Gene **131:** 113–117.

41. KIKUTA-OSHIMA, L. C., C. H. KING, T. M. SHINNICK & F. D. QUINN. 1994. Methods for the identification of virulence genes expressed in *Mycobacterium tuberculosis* strain H37Rv. Ann. N.Y. Acad. Sci. **730:** 263–265.

42. PLUM, G. & J. E. CLARK-CURTISS. 1994. Induction of *Mycobacterium avium* gene expression following phagocytosis by human macrophages. Infect. Immun. **62:** 476–483.

43. MAHAN, M. J., J. M. SLAUCH & J. J. MEKALANOS. 1993. Selection of bacterial virulence genes that are specifically induced in host tissues. Science **159:** 686–688.

44. LEE, M. H., L. PASCOPELLA, W. R. JACOBS & G. F. HATFULL. 1991. Site-specific integration of mycobacteriophage L5: Integration-proficient vectors for *Mycobacterium*

smegmatis, Mycobacterium tuberculosis, and bacille Calmette-Guérin. Proc. Natl. Acad. Sci. USA **88:** 3111–3115.

45. BROSIUS, J., T. J. DULL, D. D. SLEETER & H. F. NOLLER. 1981. Gene organization and primary structure of a ribosomal RNA operon from *Escherichia coli.* J. Mol. Biol. **148:** 107–127.

46. DEWET, J. R., K. V. WOOD, M. DELUCA, D. R. HELINSKI & S. SUBRAMANI. 1987. Firefly luciferase gene: Structure and expression in mammalian cells. Mol. Cell Biol. **7:** 725–737.

47. SHINNICK, T. M. 1987. The 65 kDa antigen of *Mycobacterium tuberculosis.* J. Bacteriol. **169:** 1080–1088.

48. HORINOUCHI, S., H. ISHIZUKA & T. BEPPU. 1991. Cloning, nucleotide sequence and transcriptional analysis of the NAD(P)-dependent cholesterol dehydrogenase gene from a *Nocardia* sp. and its hyperexpression in *Streptomyces* sp. Appl. Environ. Microbiol. **57:** 1386–1393.

49. SHINNICK, T. M. & R. C. GOOD. 1994. Mycobacterial taxonomy. Eur. J. Clin. Microbiol. Infect. Dis. **13:** 884–901.

50. TSUCHIYA, S., M. YAMABE, Y. YAMAGUCHI, Y. KOBAYASHI, T. KONNO & K. TADA. 1980. Establishment and characterization of a human acute monocytic leukemia cell line (THP-1). Int. J. Cancer **26:** 171–176.

51. AUWERX, G. 1991. The human leukemia cell line, THP-1, a multifaceted model for the study of monocyte macrophage differentiation. Experientia **47:** 22–31.

Molecular and Cellular Mechanisms
of Pneumococcal Meningitis

ELAINE I. TUOMANEN

Laboratory of Molecular Infectious Diseases
Rockefeller University
1230 York Ave
New York, New York 10021

MECHANICS OF TARGETING BLOOD-BORNE PNEUMOCOCCI
TO THE SUBARACHNOID SPACE

Site of the Blood Blood Brain Barrier

Initiation of meningitis requires specific transmigration of bacteria from blood across the blood brain barrier (BBB) into the cerebrospinal fluid (CSF)-filled subarachnoid space. The BBB is formed at two sites. A barrier between blood and CSF arises at the choroid plexus epithelium found in localized areas of each of the four cerebral ventricles. A barrier between blood and brain parenchyma arises at the extensive network of cerebral capillary endothelium. Characteristics of both sites that are important to barrier function are very sparse pinocytotic vesicles and intercellular tight junctions that severely limit the passage of even small molecules from blood into brain or CSF. These functional similarities are also reflected at the molecular level in that the tight junctions at both sites include similar elements such as ZO-1, ZO-2, occludin, and neurothelin.[1–5] Taken together, these morphologic and molecular features indicate that both the endothelial and the epithelial sites of the BBB are substantially similar to peripheral polarized, transporting epithelia.[6,7] Bacteria can cross at both sites (for review see ref. 8). Prolonged, low grade bacteremias (e.g., endocarditis, syphilis) are associated with multiple lesions in the brain parenchyma compatible with exit of the pathogen at many sites along the endothelial BBB. By contrast, bacterial meningitis is preceded by high grade bacteremia, proceeds with highest bacterial densities in the ventricles, and initially spares the brain parenchyma, suggesting entry via the choroid plexus BBB.[9] Regardless of the site of entry into the central nervous system, however, meningeal pathogens require the ability to localize to and cross a BBB which is functionally a polarized epithelium. The mechanisms involved in initiating these events and in subsequently triggering the acute phase meningeal response are discussed in this review.

Glycoconjugates on Resting Cells Initiate Tethering of Pneumococci

Interactions of pneumococci with BBB have not been studied *in vitro*. However, interactions with the polarized epithelium of the lung and endovascular cells have received extensive attention and are likely to have relevance to interactions with central vessels and choroid plexus. The pneumococcus adheres readily to pulmonary epithelial cells and vascular endothelial cells. In both cases, simple attachment on resting cells occurs via two classes of glycoconjugates whose minimal units consist of mannose linked to the disaccharides GalNAcβ1-4Gal or GalNAcβ1-3Gal.[10] The former confirms findings of Krivan *et al.*,[11] whereas the latter receptor is novel. Soluble carbohydrates block pneumococcal adherence to human cells, and immobilized carbohydrates support pneumococcal binding directly. Importantly, bacteria adherent to cultured epithelial and endothelial cells can be dislodged by exposure to glycoconjugates containing these two basic motifs, that is, asialo-GM2 and globoside. A combination of asialo-GM2 and globoside virtually completely elutes adherent bacteria. This additive effect suggests that these glycoconjugates define independent receptors and that application of carbohydrates to elimination of bacteria might be feasible in asymptomatic individuals at risk of progression to disease.

PNEUMOCOCCAL TRANSMIGRATION AND THE PLATELET-ACTIVATING FACTOR RECEPTOR

Activation of Eukaryotic Cells to Display the Platelet-Activating Factor Receptor

The mere presence of pneumococci on a mucosal surface does not assure progression to invasive disease.[12] Similarly, the incidence of invasion of the CSF space, even in the presence of high grade bacteremia, is rare. A molecular mechanism for a transition from a state of simple pneumococcal binding to a state promoting translocation has been proposed to involve activation of the target human cell.[13] By analogy with other cell migration systems, the local generation of inflammatory factors can dramatically alter the presentation of receptors on activated cells. For example, activation of vascular endothelial cells by thrombin, tumor necrosis factor (TNF), or interleukin-1 (IL-1) increases expression of cell adhesion molecules important for leukocyte trafficking.[14,15] Pneumococci appear to take advantage of this scenario and engage one of these new receptors, the platelet-activating factor (PAF) receptor.[13] Coincident with the timing of the appearance of the PAF receptor following a given stimulus, pneumococci undergo waves of enhanced adherence. In the case of thrombin, this occurs in minutes, whereas for IL-1 and TNF, it occurs over hours. Specificity of this interaction is indicated by the observations that binding is inhibitable by PAF receptor antagonists, and COS cells acquire the ability to bind pneumococci upon transfection with PAF receptor cDNA.

Pneumococcal cell wall and, more specifically, the unique phosphoryl choline component of the teichoic acid were critical for pneumococcal adherence to the PAF receptor as evidenced by hapten and antibody inhibition studies.[13] Phosphorylcholine is also essential to the bioactivity of mammalian PAF,[16] a proinflammatory signaling molecule, suggesting that pneumococci may subvert this chemokine pathway by using mimicry to target the PAF receptor.

Numerous tissues, including brain, display specific receptors for PAF.[17] PAF receptors are active in endothelial cell biology, particularly in permeability, and in leukocyte extravasation by modulating integrin activation.[18] The PAF receptor has seven membrane-spanning domains characteristic of G-protein coupled receptors, a family that includes rhodopsin and receptors for chemokines and β-adrenergic agents.[19,20] Although pneumococci bind to the PAF receptor, they do not induce signal transduction[13] nor do they interfere with PAF-induced signaling. Rather, the physiologic importance of pneumococcal binding to the PAF receptor may involve the apparent ability of the PAF receptor to facilitate internalization of pneumococci into endothelial cells, a process that may promote invasion. Pneumococci fail to invade resting cells (0.1%), whereas 2–3% of the inoculum moves to an intracellular compartment in activated cells. This phenomenon is inhibited by PAF receptor antagonists. The PAF receptor is known to be rapidly internalized after interaction with ligand.[21] The significance of this process is now suggested by the ability of a ligand to enter the cell together with the receptor, even in the absence of signaling. These results suggest that pneumococci, at least when bound to the PAF receptor, take a transcellular route across barriers, rather than passing between cells. This is compatible with histologic evidence of pneumococci within vacuoles in human cells[22] and of increased pinocytotic vesicle traffic across the BBB endothelium induced by pneumococcal cell wall components[23] (see below). The prediction of this model of pneumococcal translocation is that PAF receptor antagonists may interfere with the type of pneumococcal attachment that is coupled to invasion of activated eukaryotic cells.

Modulation of Adherence

Aside from involvement of cell wall phosphorylcholine as an adhesive ligand, the proteins involved in pneumococcal attachment remain unknown. Pneumococci harbor a protein Psa A[24] which has sequence similarity to other streptococcal peptide permeases involved in bacterial coaggregation and adherence to teeth, but their direct role as adhesins for eukaryotic cells is undetermined. Genetic strategies are currently being used to identify the important adhesive ligands and regulons of pneumococcus.[25] This analysis has yielded several genetic loci that strongly modulate adherence.

Like other pathogens, pneumococci undergo reversible, high frequency phase variation: opaque colony variants fail to cause disease in a rat model, whereas transparent colonies are virulent.[26] A genetic locus conferring opacity has been identified, but its function has not been clarified.[27] This transition modulates the ability of pneumococci to match its surface adhesins to changes in host cell surface determinants as cells become activated. Opaque and transparent pneumococcal variants adhere to a similar degree to resting epithelial and endothelial cells[28] and appear to cause equal incidence of bacteremia if introduced into the host beyond a mucosal barrier (e.g., intraperitoneally).[26] However, adherence of transparent, but not opaque variants, more than doubles following cytokine stimulation of endothelial cells. This adherence is inhibited by PAF receptor antagonists, and transparent variants adhere to human PAF receptors transfected into COS cells. These results suggest that the transparent phenotype differs strongly from the opaque by the ability to recognize PAF receptors expressed on activated cells. Translated to the *in vivo* situation, this is consistent with the advantage shown by the transparent pneumococci in producing invasive disease.

Genetic studies indicate that two "modulons" affect adherence independent of phase variation. The absence of the production of the second messenger, acetyl phosphate, by pyruvate oxidase (Spx B) completely eliminates all adherence to resting and activated cells, indicating that all three adherence specificities can be coregulated.[29] Two distinct, protein-dependent, peptide permeases, PlpA and AmiA, modulate pneumococcal adherence to resting human cells.[30] Loss of function of PlpA eliminates adherence to GalNac β1-3 Gal, while mutations in AmiA result in loss of binding to GalNac β1-4 Gal. Both mutants adhere normally to the PAF receptor. In contrast to global regulation by Spx B, these permeases are believed to each modulate a single adherence interaction by binding and transporting small peptides.

Transcellular Migration

A step-by-step analysis of the proposed route of transmigration of a pneumococcus from blood across the BBB using the information obtained from lung epithelial and vascular endothelial cells is presented in TABLE 1. The participants and the sequence of steps can be confirmed *in vitro* using the bilayer model of Quinn and colleagues.[31] Pneumococci can be demonstrated to cross pulmonary epithelia overlaid onto vascular endothelia (Rosenow and Tuomanen, unpublished data). Consistent with the model of PAF receptor-dependent internalization, transmigration appears to require the transparent phenotype and is attenuated by PAF receptor antagonists. Preliminary evidence also supports a transcellular route of migration. Adaptation of this model to the reverse direction, that is, passage across a fenestrated endothelium and then a polarized epithelium, will provide a model of the path from blood across the BBB of the choroid plexus.

This model system also presents the bacterium with an intervening extracellular matrix as would be encountered *in vivo*. Pneumococci adhere avidly to immobilized

TABLE 1. Proposed Steps in Transmigration of Pneumococci from Blood across the Blood Brain Barrier[a]

Targeting to cerebral microvascular endothelial cells
- Adherence to resting cells bearing GalNAc β1–4 Gal or GalNac β1–3 Gal glycoconjugates by opaque or transparent pneumococci

Initiation of transmigration
- Activation of eukaryotic cells by thrombin or cytokines with resultant expression of PAF receptor
- Shift in binding of only transparent pneumococci to the PAF receptor involving the cell wall phosphorylcholine
- Internalization of pneumococci by PAF receptor recycling without G-protein signaling
- Transcytosis of pneumococci in vesicles and extrusion on ablumenal surface
- Strong binding to fibronectin of extracellular matrix

---

[a]If these steps occur at the vascular endothelial BBB, pneumococci will gain access to brain parenchymal cells (neurons, glia). If these steps occur at the fenestrated endothelium of the choroid plexus, then pneumococci must complete further steps to traverse the choroid plexus BBB epithelium to enter the CSF. The molecular details of this latter path from cellular base to apex are unknown, but they seem to involve a transcellular rather than an intercellular passage of the bacteria.

fibronectin.[32] Adherence is independent of phase variation. The carboxyterminal heparin binding domain of fibronectin appears to contain the pneumococcal binding site, a region distinct from that supporting attachment of most other bacteria.

THE CELL WALL AS A LIBRARY OF INFLAMMATORY FRAGMENTS

Acute Phase Response in the Brain and the Predominance of the Activity of the Teichoic Acid

When introduced into the subarachnoid space, cell wall has the highest specific inflammatory activity of any intra- or extracellular component of the pneumococcus (TABLE 2).[33,34] The capsule does not shield the underlying cell wall from interacting with host defense systems. When cell wall pieces are present in a density equivalent to $\geq 10^5$ cfu/ml CSF, the host acute phase response is initiated in the CSF space. This implies that significant bacterial growth occurs in CSF before the onset of symptoms associated with inflammation. The signs and symptoms of infection induced by cell wall mimic those of living bacteria in animal models of meningitis, pneumonia, and otitis media.[34–36] Clinical strains and their isogenic laboratory derivatives which have defects in release of cell wall fragments induce an attenuated pattern of disease.[37]

The complete structures of the two major pneumococcal cell wall components, the glycopeptide network and the teichoic acid, have been determined.[38,39] An unusual feature of the pneumococcal cell wall structure is the presence of phosphoryl-choline in the teichoic acid and lipoteichoic acid.[40] The teichoic acid and lipteichoic acid, as opposed to the peptidoglycan, drive the vast majority of the host defense responses associated with acute inflammation. Both strongly activate the alternative pathway of the complement cascade and bind the acute phase reactant C-reactive protein.[41] Phosphorylcholine is also critical for the ability of cell wall to activate procoagulant activity on the surface of endothelial cells and for the induction of cytokines and PAF upon binding to epithelia, endothelia, and macrophages.[22,42–46] Some of these effects arise through the interaction of cell walls with CD14, a cell

TABLE 2. Bioactivities of Pneumococcal Cell Wall Components

Teichoicated cell wall
- Fix complement
- Induce procoagulant activity on endothelial cells
- Activate endothelia, epithelia, and leukocytes to produce IL-1 and TNF
- Chemotactic for leukocytes

Peptidoglycan
- Induce NF-κB
- Induce blood brain barrier permeability by increased vesicle transport
- Cytotoxic to ciliated cells of the choroid plexus
- Cytotoxic to neurons
- Induce sleep

surface receptor known to initiate the inflammatory cascade for endotoxin.[45,47] The IL-1 response is particularly strong, exceeding that for endotoxin on a per bacterial cell basis. Induction of TNF requires > 100 times more cell wall than does the induction of IL-1, even in the presence of putative serum binding components.[44,45]

The influx of leukocytes occurs again in large part due to the proinflammatory activity of the teichoic acid.[48] Leukocyte migration occurs in a manner analogous to that in the periphery in that selectins initiate rolling[49] and CD18 integrins and intercellular adhesion molecules (ICAMs) mediate translocation.[50,51] The unique CD18-independent migration seen in pneumococcal pneumonia is not prominent in brain.[46]

Studies with transgenic mice deficient in various components of the inflammatory cascade have yielded significant insight into the pathogenesis of gram-positive inflammation. Mice deficient in the TNF receptor or p50 of NF-κB are resistant to endotoxin challenge but still die of pneumococcal infection.[52,53] Mice deficient in ICAM-1 have a poorer prognosis for gram-negative meningitis.[51] These findings suggest that the acute phase responses to cell walls and endotoxin might develop differently. When examined for the ability to induce NF-κB, a transcription factor critical to the response to endotoxin, the cell wall of pneumococcus was as potent as endotoxin but the phosphorylcholine moiety was not necessary for the bioactivity. Thus, the cell-signaling mechanism that follows binding of teichoicated, phosphoryl-choline-containing cell wall pieces to PAF receptor or other as yet unknown receptors and engenders the intense acute phase response characteristic of pneumococcal infection remains unclear.

Blood Brain Barrier Permeability and the Bioactivity of Glycopeptides

The teichoic acid of the cell wall drives much of the acute phase response as described above. However, the peptidoglycan portion of the cell wall is also bioactive, particularly as regards induction of BBB permeability. All gram-positive bacteria contain a peptidoglycan composed of a disaccharide tetrapeptide (N-acetylglucosaminyl-N-acetylmuramyl-L-alanyl- D-glutaminyl-L-Lysyl-D-alanine, $\sim 30\%$ of the total wall) and its dimer (another $\sim 30\%$ of the total wall). Other components are structurally variable, creating a unique composition for each pathogen. Differences in the inflammatory capabilities of various bacterial cell walls have been attributed to these structural differences.[54] The bioactivities of bacterial glycopeptides are numerous and depend critically on the structure of the glycopeptide and the nature of the target eukaryotic cell. For instance, modification of the disaccharide moiety to a 1,6 anhydro linkage defines the sleep peptide known to induce slow wave sleep in rabbits upon intravenous administration,[55] whereas a lactyl-tetrapeptide derivative is toxic to respiratory ciliated cells.[56] The most active structure for the BBB is a disaccharide linked to three or four peptides. Modification of the amino acid composition of the peptide side chain was permissible for bioactivity, but multimerization or modification of the disaccharide reduced activity consistent with a restricted structure-activity relationship. The effects of the wall are apparent whether they are introduced intracisternally or intravenously, and bioactivities appear to be topographically restricted to the cerebral microvasculature. The activation of cerebral endothelia results in increased vesicle translocation, leading to enhanced BBB permeability. Tight junctions do not appear to be affected. Permeability is enhanced between 3 and 7 hours after intravenous cell wall challenge and then returns to baseline. Enhanced permeability of the BBB is recognized by the influx of serum proteins into CSF. For some disaccharide tetra- or tripeptides, transient enhancement of BBB permeability, particularly to intravascular markers ≤ 20 kD, occurs without engendering other pathologic elements of meningitis, such as cerebral edema, increased intracranial pressure, or recruitment of leukocytes.[23] The accumulation of penicillin in brain increased up to 250% with a maximum brain uptake of 8% of serum levels. Simultaneous measurement of CSF penicillin penetration indicated an enhancement from 6% in control animals to almost 40% of serum levels in cell wall-treated animals. Relatively few strategies enhance penetration of therapeutic agents into brain. The intravenous application of a glycopeptide provides a simple and readily reversible approach to central nervous system therapeutics.

APPLICATION TO IMPROVEMENT IN OUTCOME OF DISEASE

Interrupting Adherence to Prevent Progression to Invasive Disease

Pneumococcus is a leading cause of hearing loss, resulting from both otitis media as well as the sensorineural hearing loss that follows pneumococcal meningitis. One in 2.5 children carry the pneumococcus in the nasopharynx at any given time. Virtually every child will experience at least one episode of pneumococcal otitis media before the age of 5 years. Based on the current understanding of the pathogenesis of pneumococcal infection, it may be possible to use glycoconjugates or PAF receptor antagonists to prevent the progression from carrier state to overt disease in children at risk for otitis media or bacteremia. For example, coinstillation of pneumococci with α_1 acid glycoprotein or other carbohydrate receptor analogs or the PAF receptor antagonist decreases colonization as much as 100–1000-fold in rat and rabbit models of nasopharyngeal and pulmonary challenge. Furthermore the PAF receptor antagonists strongly attenuate the progression from pneumonia to bacteremia in rabbits.[13]

Attenuation of Neuronal Injury

Multiple mechanisms are recognized whereby sufficient neuronal damage might occur so as to engender permanent sequelae following bacterial meningitis. It is believed that the formation of the acute phase response, and in particular the transmigration of leukocytes, so disrupts the barrier function of the BBB that the neuronal milieu is compromised. Exactly what dysfunction occurs is not known. Penetration into CSF of excitatory amino acids at concentrations present in serum would readily disrupt neuronal function.[57] In addition, pneumococcal cell wall components are directly toxic to neurons.[58] Interestingly, pneumolysin, a pore-forming toxin released as pneumococci lyse,[59,60] is profoundly cytotoxic in the lung,[61] but it does not appear to play a major role in injury during meningitis.[62]

For an individual patient, it is not possible to determine how much damage is irreversible at the time of admission. However, it is also clear that a significant portion of the damage centered around an excessive host response is reversible. For example, profound bilateral meningogenic hearing loss can be completely reversed by intervention over 8–10 hours from the onset of symptoms.[63,64] A major change in the therapy of meningitis arose with the insight that pneumococcal cell wall pieces are bioactive both from intact bacteria and, even more so, from bacteria undergoing antibiotic-induced lysis. This provided an opportunity to mitigate cell wall-associated damage by down-modulating the host response during antibiotic therapy. Over the first few hours of antibiotic therapy, the leukocyte density in CSF can increase one to two orders of magnitude.[65] This burst is sufficiently disruptive as to injure host tissues as evidenced by the significant attenuation of injury upon inhibition of leukocyte recruitment.[50,66] The use of steroids during the early phase of antibiotic therapy to inhibit this response reduces the incidence of sequelae in animals and in patients and has recently become an accepted component of therapy in the clinical setting of childhood meningitis.[65]

REFERENCES

1. STEVENSON, B., J. SILICIANO, M. MOOSEKER & D. GOODENOUGH. 1986. Identification of ZO-1: A high molecular weight polypeptide associated with the tight junction in a variety of epithelia. J. Cell Biol. **103:** 755–766.
2. JESAITIS, L. & G. DA. 1994. Molecular characterization and tissue distribution of ZO-2, a tight junction protein homologous to ZO-1 and the Drosophila discs-large tumor suppressor protein. J. Cell Biol. **124:** 949–961.
3. FURUSE, M., T. HIRASE, M. ITOH, A. NAGAFUCHI, S. YONEMURA, S. TSUKITA & S. TSUKITA.

1993. Occludin: A novel integral membrane prein localizing at tight junctions. J. Cell Biol. **123:** 1777–1788.

4. SCHLOSSBAUER, B. 1993. The blood brain barrier: Morphology molecules, and neurothelin. BioEssays **15:** 341–346.

5. SCHLOSSBAUER, B. & K.-H. HERZOG. 1990. Neurothelin: An inducible cell surface glycoprotein of blood brain barrier specific endothelial cells and distinct neurons. J. Cell Biol. **110:** 1261–1274.

6. LEVINE, S. 1987. Choroid plexus: Target for systemic disease and pathway to the brain. Lab. Invest. **56:** 231–233.

7. DERMIETZEL, R. & D. KRAUSE. 1991. Molecular anatomy of the blood brain barrier as defined by immunocytochemistry. Int. Rev. Cytol. **127:** 57–109.

8. TUOMANEN, E. 1996. Entry of pathogens into the central nervous system. FEMS Micro. Revs. **18:** 289–299.

9. DAUM, R., D. SCHEIFELE, V. SYRIOPOULOU, D. AVERILL & A. SMITH. 1978. Ventricular involvement in experimental Haemophilus influenzae meningitis. J. Pediatr. **93:** 927–930.

10. CUNDELL, D. & E. TUOMANEN. 1994. Receptor specificity of adherence of Streptococcus pneumoniae to human type II pneumocytes and vascular endothelial cells in vitro. Microbiol. Pathog. **17:** 361–374.

11. KRIVAN, H. C., D. D. ROBERTS & V. GINSBURG. 1988. Many pulmonary pathogenic bacteria bind specifically to the carbohydrate sequence GalNacB1-4Gal found in some glycolipids. Proc. Natl. Acad. Sci. USA **85:** 6157–6161.

12. HAMBURGER, M. & O. ROBERTSON. 1940. Studies of the pathogenesis of experimental pneumococcus pneumonia in the dog. J. Exp. Med. **72:** 261–274.

13. CUNDELL, D., N. GERARD, C. GERARD, I. IDANPAAN-HEIKKILA & E. TUOMANEN. 1995. *Streptococcus pneumoniae* anchors to activated eukaryotic cells by the receptor for platelet activating factor. Nature. **377:** 435–438.

14. LASKY, L. A. 1992. Selectins: Interpreters of cell-specific carbohydrate information. Science **258:** 964–969.

15. ZIMMERMAN, G., S. PRESCOTT & T. MCINTYRE. 1992. Endothelial cell interactions with granulocytes: Tethering and signaling molecules. Immunol. Today **13:** 93–100.

16. WISSNER, A., R. SCHAUB, P. SUM, C. KOHLER & B. GOLDSTEIN. 1986. Analogues of platelet activating factor: Some modifications of the phosphorylcholine moiety. J. Med. Chem. **29:** 328–333.

17. CHAO, W. & M. OLSON. 1993. Platelet-activating factor: Receptors and signal transduction. Biochem. J. **292:** 617–622.

18. GENG, J., K. MOORE, A. JOHNSON & R. MCEVER. 1991. Neutrophil recognition requires a Ca-induced conformational change in the lectin domain of GMP-140. J. Biol. Chem. **266:** 22313–22318.

19. HONDA, Z.-I., M. NAKAMURA, I. MIKI, M. MINAMI, T. WATANABE, Y. SEYAMA, H. OKADO, H. TOH, K. IOT, T. MIYAMOTO & T. SHIMIZU. 1991. Cloning by functional expression of platelet activating factor receptor from guinea pig lung. Nature **349:** 342–346.

20. KUNZ, D., N. GERARD & C. GERARD. 1992. The human leukocyte platelet activating factor receptor. J. Biol. Chem. **267:** 9101–9106.

21. GERARD, N. & C. GERARD. 1994. Receptor-dependent internalization of plateletactivating factor. J. Immunol. **152:** 793–800.

22. GEELEN, S., C. BATTACHARYYA & E. TUOMANEN. 1993. Cell wall mediates pneumococcal attachment and cytopathology to human endothelial cells. Infect. Immun. **61:** 1538–1543.

23. SPELLERBERG, B., S. PRASAD, C. CABELLOS, M. BURROUGHS, P. CAHILL & E. TUOMANEN. 1995. Penetration of the blood brain barrier: Enhancement of drug delivery and imaging by bacterial glycopeptides. J. Exp. Med. **182:** 1–8.

24. SAMPSON, J., R. O'CONNOR, A. STINSON, J. THARPE & H. RUSSELL. 1994. Cloning and nucleotide sequence analysis of *psaA*, the *Streptococcus pneumoniae* gene encoding a 37-kilodalton protein homologous to previously reported *Streptococcus* sp. adhesins. Infect. Immun. **62:** 319–324.

25. PEARCE, B., Y. YIN & H. MASURE. 1993. Genetic identification of exported proteins in Streptococcus pneumoniae. Mol. Microbiol. **9:** 1037–1050.

26. WEISER, J., R. AUSTRIAN, P. SREENIVASAN & H. MASURE. 1994. Phase variation in pneumococcal opacity: Relationship between colonial morphology and nasopharyngeal colonization. Infect. Immun. **62:** 2582–2589.

27. SALUGA, S. & J. WEISER. 1995. The genetic basis of colonial opacity in Streptococcus pneumoniae: Evidence for the effect of box elements on phenotypic variation. Mol. Microbiol **16:** 215–227.

28. CUNDELL, D., J. WEISER, J. SHEN, A. YOUNG & E. TUOMANEN. 1995. Relationship between colonial morphology and adherence of Streptococcus pneumoniae. Infect. Immun. **63:** 757–761.

29. SPELLERBERG, B., J. SANDROS, D. CUNDELL, B. PEARCE & H. MASURE. 1996. Pyruvate oxidase as a determinant for virulence of *Streptococcus pneumoniae.* Mol. Microb. **19:** 803–813.

30. CUNDELL, D., B. PEARCE, J. SANDROS, A. NAUGHTON & H. MASURE. 1995. Peptide permeases from Streptococcus pneumoniae affect adherence to eucaryotic cells. Infect. Immun. **63:** 2493–2498.

31. BIRKNESS, K., B. SWISHER, E. WHITE, E. LONG, E. EWING & F. QUINN. 1995. A tissue culture bilayer model to study the passage of Neisseria meningitidis. Infect. Immun. **63:** 402–409.

32. VAN DER FLIER, M., N. CHHUN, T. WIZEMANN, J. MIN, J. MCCARTHY & E. TUOMANEN. 1995. Adherence of Streptococcus pneumoniae to immobilized fibronectin. Infect. Immun. **63:** 4317–4322.

33. TUOMANEN, E. I., A. TOMASZ, B. HENGSTLER & O. ZAK. 1985. The relative role of bacterial cell wall and capsule in the induction of inflammation in pneumococcal meningitis. J. Infect. Dis. **151:** 535–540.

34. TUOMANEN, E., H. LIU, B. HENGSTLER, O. ZAK & A. TOMASZ. 1985. The induction of meningeal inflammation by components of the pneumococcal cell wall. J. Infect. Dis. **151:** 859–868.

35. TUOMANEN, E., R. RICH & O. ZAK. 1987. Induction of pulmonary inflammation by components of the pneumococcal cell surface. Am. Rev. Respir. Dis. **135:** 869–874.

36. RIPLEY-PETZOLDT, M. L., G. S. GIEBINK, S. K. JUHN, D. AEPPLI, A. TOMASZ & E. TUOMANEN. 1988. The contribution of pneumococcal cell wall to the pathogenesis of experimental otitis media. J. Infect. Dis. **157:** 245–255.

37. TUOMANEN, E., H. POLLACK, A. PARKINSON, M. DAVIDSON, R. FACKLAM, R. RICH & O. ZAK. 1988. Microbiological and clinical significance of a new property of defective lysis in clinical strains of pneumococci. J. Infect. Dis. **158:** 36–43.

38. GARCIA-BUSTOS, J. & A. TOMASZ. 1990. A biological price of antibiotic resistance: Major changes in the peptidoglycan structure of penicillin-resistant pneumococci. Proc. Natl. Acad. Sci. USA **87:** 5415–5419.

39. JENNINGS, H., C. LUGOWSKI & N. YOUNG. 1980. Structure of the complex polysaccharide C-substance from *Streptococcus pneumoniae.* Biochemistry **19:** 4712–4719.

40. TOMASZ, A. 1967. Choline in the cell wall of a bacterium: Novel type of polymer-linked choline in pneumococcus. Science **157:** 694–697.

41. WINKELSTEIN, J. & A. TOMASZ. 1978. Activation of the alternative complement pathway by pneumococcal cell wall teichoic acid. J. Immunol. **120:** 174–178.

42. GEELEN, S., C. BHATTACHARYYA & E. TUOMANEN. 1992. Induction of procoagulant activity on human endothelial cells by Streptococcus pneumoniae. Infect. Immun. **60:** 4179–4183.

43. TUOMANEN, E. & S. SANDE. 1989. Inhibition of the binding of penicillin to the pneumococcal penicillin binding proteins (PBPs) by exogenous cell wall peptides. J. Gen. Microbiol. **135:** 639–642.

44. RIESENFELD-ORN, I., S. WOLPE, J. F. GARCIA-BUSTOS, M. K. HOFFMAN & E. TUOMANEN. 1989. Production of interleukin-1 but not tumor necrosis factor by human monocytes stimulated with pneumococcal cell surface components. Infect. Immun. **57:** 1890–1893.

45. HEUMANN, D., C. BARRAS, A. SEVERIN, M. GLAUSER & A. TOMASZ. 1994. Gram positive

cell walls stimulate synthesis of tumor necrosis factor alpha and interleukin-6 by human monocytes. Infect. Immun. **62:** 2715–2721.

46. CABELLOS, C., D. E. MACINTYRE, M. FORREST, M. BURROUGHS, S. PRASAD & E. TUOMANEN. 1992. Differing roles of platelet-activating factor during inflammation of the lung and subarachnoid space. J. Clin. Invest. **90:** 612–618.

47. PUGIN, J., D. HEUMANN, A. TOMASZ, V. KRAVCHENKI, Y. AKAMATSU, M. NISHIJIMA, M. LAUSER, P. TOBIAS & R. ULEVITCH. 1994. CD14 is a pattern recognition receptor. Immunity **1:** 509–516.

48. TOMASZ, A. & K. SAUKKONEN. 1989. The nature of cell wall-derived inflammatory components of pneumococci. Pediatr. Infect. Dis. J. **8:** 902–903.

49. SPELLERBERG, B. & E. TUOMANEN. 1994. The pathophysiology of pneumococcal meningitis. Ann. Med. **26:** 411–418.

50. TUOMANEN, E., K. SAUKKONEN, S. SANDE, C. CIOFFE & S. D. WRIGHT. 1989. Reduction of inflammation, tissue damage, and mortality in bacterial meningitis in rabbits treated with monoclonal antibodies against adhesion-promoting receptors of leukocytes. J. Exp. Med. **170:** 959–969.

51. TAN, T., C. SMITH, E. HAWKINS, E. MASON & S. KAPLAN. 1995. Hematogenous bacterial meningitis in an ICAM-1 deficient infant mouse model. J. Infect. Dis. **171:** 342–349.

52. PFEFFER, K., T. MATSUYAMA, T. KUNDIG & T. MAK. 1993. Mice deficient for the 55kD tumor necrosis factor receptor are resistant to endotoxic shock, yet succumb to L. monocytogenese infection. Cell **73:** 457–467.

53. SHA, W., H. LIOU, E. TUOMANEN & D. BALTIMORE. 1995. Targeted disruption of the p50 subunit of NF-kB leads to multifocal defects in immune responses. Cell **80:** 321–330.

54. BURROUGHS, M., E. ROZDZINSKI, S. GEELEN & E. TUOMANEN. 1993. A structure-activity relationship for induction of meningeal inflammation by muramyl peptides. J. Clin. Invest. **92:** 297–302.

55. KRUEGER, J., D. DAVENNE, J. WALTER, S. SHOHAM, S. KUBILLUS, R. ROSENTHAL, S. MARTIN & K. BIEMANN. 1987. Bacterial peptidoglycans as modulators of sleep. Brain Res. **403:** 258–266.

56. HEISS, L., J. LANCASTER, J. CORBETT & W. GOLDMAN. 1994. Epithelial autotoxicity of nitric oxide: Role in the respiratory cytopathology of pertussis. Proc. Natl. Acad. Sci. USA **91:** 267–270.

57. GUERRA-ROMERO, L., J. TUREEN, M. FOURNIER, V. TAKRIDES & M. TAUBER. 1993. Amino acids in cerebrospinal and brain interstitial fluid in experimental pneumococcal meningitis. Pediatr. Res. **33:** 510–513.

58. TAUBER, M., M. SACHDEVA, S. KENNEDY, H. LOETSCHER & W. LESSLAUER. 1992. Toxicity in neuronal cells caused by cerebrospinal fluid from pneumococcal and gram negative meningitis. J. Infect. Dis. **166:** 1045–1050.

59. PATON, J. C., R. A. LOCK, C. J. LEE, J. P. LI, A. M. BERRY, T. J. MITCHELL, P. W. ANDREW, D. HANSMAN & G. J. BOULNOIS. 1991. Purification and immunogenicity of genetically obtained pneumolysin toxoids and their conjugation to Streptococcus pneumoniae type 19F polysaccharide. Infect. Immun. **59:** 2297–2304.

60. BOULNOIS, G. J., J. C. PATON, T. J. MITCHELL & P. W. ANDREW. 1991. Structure and function of pneumolysin, the multifunctional, thiol-activated toxin of Streptococcus pneumoniae. Mol. Microbiol. **5:** 2611–2616.

61. RUBINS, J. B., P. G. DUANE, D. CLAWSON, D. CHARBONEAU, J. YOUNG & D. E. NIEWOEHNER. 1993. Toxicity of pneumolysin to pulmonary alveolar epithelial cells. Infect. Immun. **61:** 1352–1358.

62. FRIEDLAND, I., M. PARIS, S. HICKEY, S. SHELTON, K. OLSEN, J. PATON & G. MCCRACKEN. 1995. Limited role of pneumolysin in the pathogenesis of pneumococcal meningitis. J. Infect. Dis. **172:** 805–809.

63. BHATT, S., A. LAURETANO, C. H. CABELLOS, R. LEVINE, W. HSU, J. NADOL & E. TUOMANEN. 1993. The progression of hearing loss in experimental pneumococcal meningitis: Correlation with cerebrospinal fluid cytochemistry. J. Infect. Dis. **167:** 675–683.

64. BHATT, S., C. CABELLOS, I. J. NADO, C. HALPIN, A. LAURENTANO, W. XU & E. TUOMANEN.

1994. The impact of dexamethasone on hearing loss in experimental pneumococcal meningitis. Pediatr. Infect. Dis. J. **14:** 93–96.

65. LEBEL, M. H., B. J. FREIJ, G. A. SYROGIANNOPOULOS *ET AL.* 1988. Dexamethasone therapy for bacterial meningitis. N. Engl. J. Med. **15:** 964–971.

66. TUOMANEN, E., B. HENGSTLER, R. RICH, M. BRAY, O. ZAK & A. TOMASZ. 1987. Nonsteroidal anti-inflammatory agents in the therapy of experimental pneumococcal meningitis. J. Infect. Dis. **155:** 985–990.

Posttranslational Modifications
of Meningococcal Pili

Identification of a Common Trisaccharide Substitution
on Variant Pilins of Strain C311[a]

MUMTAZ VIRJI,[b,c] ELAINE STIMSON,[d]
KATHERINE MAKEPEACE,[b] ANNE DELL,[d]
HOWARD R. MORRIS,[d] GAIL PAYNE,[e]
JON R. SAUNDERS,[e] AND E. RICHARD MOXON[b]

[b]Department of Paediatrics
University of Oxford
John Radcliffe Hospital
Oxford, OX3 9DU, UK

[d]Department of Biochemistry
Imperial College
London, SW7 2AY, UK

[e]Department of Genetics and Microbiology
University of Liverpool
Liverpool, L69 3BX, UK

Neisseria meningitidis, the causative organism of one of the most rapidly progressive bacterial diseases, may result in death unless promptly treated with antibiotics. Meningococcal isolates from disseminated infections invariably produce two surface structures, a polysaccharide capsule and polymeric hair-like proteinaceous appendages called pili. Using cultured human cells, it was shown in bacteria with capsulate phenotypes that pili are essential for adherence to both endothelial and epithelial cells.[1-3] In addition, piliated bacteria cause greater damage to human umbilical vein endothelial cells (Huvecs) than do nonpiliated bacteria, and the damage is proportional to the level of bacterial adherence mediated by structurally variant pili.[4] Therefore, structural features that modulate pilus-mediated adhesion may also alter the severity of endothelial necrosis observed *in vivo.* The identification of these features is of importance in understanding meningococcal pathogenesis and ultimately for molecular targeting for intervention during the course of meningococcal infection. To date, the precise nature of the pilus-associated ligand/s or ligand complex/es that may be involved in interactions with host cells is not clearly understood.

Sequence studies of pilins from adherence variants of *N. meningitidis* strains C311 and MC58 suggested that pili might be subject to posttranslational modifications, because the predicted molecular weights of variant pilins were identical, while their

[a]This work was supported by grants from the Wellcome Trust, the MRC, the BBSRC, and the National Meningitis Trust. E.S. and G.P. were supported by BBSRC studentships.

[c]Address for correspondence: Mumtaz Virji, Department of Paediatrics, University of Oxford, John Radcliffe Hospital, Oxford, OX3 9DU, UK (tel: 1865/221072; fax: 1865/220479; e-mail: mumtaz.virji@paediatrics.oxford.ac.uk).

migration on SDS-PAGE was distinct. Chemical techniques (deglycosylation and biotin-hydrazide labeling) provided evidence for glycosylation of these pilins.[3] Our recent study employed both biochemical and molecular biological methods to investigate the glycosylation status of meningococcal pili.

RESULTS

*Mutation in the UDP Galactose-4-Epimerase (*galE*) Gene of Strain C311 Results in Simultaneous Truncation of LPS and Alteration in Pilin* M_r

Galactose epimerase is required in *N. meningitidis* for the production of UDP galactose. Therefore, the absence of GalE could result in the lack of incorporation of galactose into lyopolysaccharide (LPS) (strain C311 LPS is of L3 immunotype and contains several galactose residues) as well as into pili, if these were decorated with galactose moieties. To test this hypothesis, a mutation in the meningococcal *galE* gene was introduced into variants 3 and 16[3] as described in experimental procedures. The resultant mutants were analyzed for their possible concurrent alteration in pilin and LPS M_r. All GalE mutants produced apparently truncated LPS and pili (FIG. 1), indicating that pili contained galactose moiety.

To establish that the observed decrease in M_r of pilins was not a result of deletion or any critical sequence changes in *galE* pilins (see below), polymerase chain reaction (PCR) sequencing of their *pilE* genes was carried out as described previously.[3] Pilin from clone 3 and one of its *galE* mutants had identical predicted amino acid sequences (FIG. 2) but different M_r on SDS-PAGE. The data suggested that galactose must be covalently linked to 3 (GalE$^+$) pili. Limited structural analysis of a GalE mutant of 16 also employed in these studies confirmed that the peptide ^{45}S-K^{75} had identical sequence compared with that of clone 16.

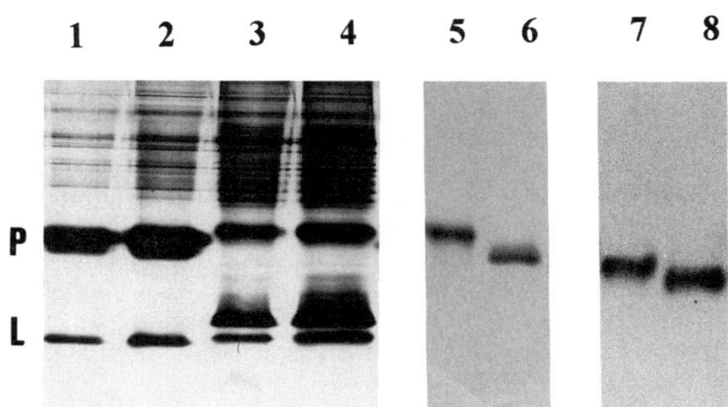

FIGURE 1. (**Left**) Mini-gel analysis of pilins and LPSs of variant 3 (*lanes 3 and 4*) and its *galE* mutants (*lanes 1 and 2*). Electrophoretic separation of crude pilus extracts (1× [*lanes 1 and 3*] and 2.5× [*lanes 2 and 4*] loading) was carried out on 15% SDS-polyacrylamide gels. Silver-stained gel shows pilins (P) as the major protein constituents of the preparations applied in addition to contaminating LPSs (L) and demonstrates the simultaneous reduction of apparent M_r of both pilins and LPSs of the *galE* mutants derived from variant 3. (**Right**) Western blotting of whole cell lysates of variants 3 (*lane 5*) and 16 (*lane 7*) and their *galE* mutants (*lanes 6 and 8*, respectively) after SDS-PAGE. Pilins were located by immunoblotting with mAb SM1 against pilin.

```
     1                                                            50
#3   FTLIELMIVI AIVGILAAVA LPAYQDYTAR AQVSEAILLA EGQKSAVTEY
 1   .......... .......... .......... .......... ..........
 2   .......... .......... .......... .......... ..........
#16  .......... .......... .......... .......... ..........

     51                                                           100
#3   YLNHGEWPGN NTSAGVASSS TIKGKYVKEV TVANGVITAT MLSSGVNKEI
 1   .......... .......... .......... .......... ..........
 2   .......... .......... .......... .......... ..........
#16  .......... .......T.. E.......S. E.K...V... ..........

     101                                                          150
#3   QGKKLSLWAK RQNGSVKWFC GQPVTRNDTD DTVAAVAADN TGNINTKHLP
 1   .......... ..D....... ......AG.. .......... ..........
 2   .......... .......... .......... .......... ..........
#16  .......... ..D....... ......T.AK ADTV.A..KT AD........

     151       160
#3   STCRDASDAS
 1   ..........
 2   ..........
#16  ..........
```

FIGURE 2. Deduced amino acid sequences from the DNA sequence determined by PCR-amplification of *pilE* loci of the relevant variants and mutants. The amino acid sequences of variants 3 and 16 were published previously,[3] and the DNA sequences have Genbank accession numbers L22636 and L22677, respectively. The *underlined sequence in bold* spans the *O*-glycosylation site of C311 pilins. Numbers 1 and 2 represent two GalE mutants of variant 3.

Structural Studies on C311 Pilins

Pilin proteins from variants 3 and 16 and their corresponding *galE* mutants were digested with trypsin, purified by reverse phase HPLC, and fractions were screened by fast atom bombardment mass spectrometry (FAB-MS), electrospray mass spectrometry (ES-MS), and gas phase Edman sequencing. Most tryptic peptides analyzed by FAB-MS produced signals that corresponded to their predicted masses. However, no molecular ions were observed at the calculated masses of ^{45}S-K^{73} (m/z 3041 and 3083 for variants 3 and 16, respectively) or ^{45}S-K^{75} (m/z 3226 and 3268 for variants 3 and 16, respectively) in the fast atom bombardment (FAB) and electrospray (ES) mass spectrometry of HPLC fractions containing these peptides. Instead, many unassigned signals were observed at higher masses (m/z 4300 and 4485 from variant 3; m/z 3913 from variant 16; m/z 3662 and 3816 from the *galE* mutant of variant 3; m/z 3774 from the *galE* mutant of variant 16), indicating that this region of the protein might be posttranslationally modified. Further V8 protease digestion suggested that modification is within amino acid residues 50–73. Experiments addressing the susceptibility of the putative modified peptides to mild base[5] suggested that *O*-linked glycan might be present. This was confirmed by reductive elimination and subsequent FAB-MS analysis of deuteroacetylated, acetylated, or permethylated products. These experiments revealed that a reduced moiety of mass 572 was released from variants 3 and 16, while the corresponding moiety from the *galE* mutant was a Hex_2 interval lower in mass. These data suggested that the parental clones contain Hex_2X, and the *galE* mutant contains X where X is defined as a reducible residue of mass 228 Daltons. Sugar and linkage analyses suggested that the Hex_2 moiety was Gal1–4Gal, and the covalent structure of X was defined as

2,4-diacetamido-2,4,6-trideoxyhexose from the electron impact mass spectrum of its reduced trimethylsilyl derivative.[5]

Determination of Anomeric Stereochemistry

The reductively eliminated trisaccharide from variant 16 was unaffected by treatment with bovine testes β-galactosidase, indicating a possible α-linked terminal galactose which would be consistent with earlier antibody binding experiments in which a Gal α1–3 Gal moiety had been implicated.[6] Surprisingly, however, the trisaccharide was also refractory to digestion with coffee bean α-galactosidase, an enzyme that is known to remove terminal galactose from Gal α1-4 Gal moieties. We considered it probable, therefore, that despite the results from the bovine testes β-galactosidase digestion, the linkage could be beta. Accordingly, we investigated β-galactosidases with different substrate specificities, and convincing data were afforded by *Choronia lampas* β-galactosidase which digested a major portion of the trisaccharide over a period of 48 hours. Digestions were monitored by removal of aliquots at various time points, deuteroacetylating the dried products and subjecting the derivative to FAB-MS analysis. Data are shown in FIGURE 3. At the start of the digestion the sodiated quasimolecular ion for the trisaccharide was observed at m/z 1001 (FIG. 3a). After 48 hours some of this molecular ion remained, but a significantly more abundant new quasimolecular ion was present a hexose lower at m/z 704 (FIG. 3b). In a parallel experiment an equivalent amount of trisaccharide was treated with coffee bean α-galactosidase and no digestion was observed (FIG. 3c). Finally, the products of 48-hour digestion with *C. lampas* β-galactosidase were further reacted with coffee bean α-galactosidase, which resulted in loss of the disaccharide peak at m/z 704 concomitant with retention of the trisaccharide peak at m/z 1001 (FIG. 3d). Taken together these data are consistent with the structure Gal β1–4 Gal α1–3 X, where X is 2,4-diacetamido-2,4,6-trideoxyhexose (FIG. 4).

DISCUSSION

Previous studies to establish the molecular basis of the apparent correlation between functional variation of meningococcal pilins and differences in their apparent M_r led to the postulation that pilin may undergo posttranslational modification; in particular, they may be glycosylated.[3] The presence of glycans was suggested by direct detection of carbohydrate moieties on pilins by biotin hydrazide labeling and by chemical deglycosylation which increased the apparent migration of pilins. In recent studies we showed that the tryptic/V8 protease peptide spanning residues 50–73 in the NH_2-terminal semiconserved-conserved region has extensive post-translation modifications. Pilins of variants 3 and 16 contain a covalently linked trisaccharide of structure Gal β1–4 Gal α1–3 X, where X is a 2,4-diacetamido-2,4,6-trideoxyhexose; *galE* mutants lack the digalactosyl moiety but retain the 2,4-diacetamido-2,4,6-trideoxyhexose substitution. The trisaccharide (or monosaccharide in the case of the *galE* mutants) can be released by reductive elimination and may therefore be attached to Ser or Thr. Two domains for potential *O*-glycosylation occur within the tryptic/V8 protease peptide spanning residues 50–73, namely, residues 62 and 63 which are within the consensus sequences for putative *N*-glycosylation of asparagine residues 60 and 61 and a tandem repeat cluster further downstream (see FIG. 2). Recent structural studies on gonococcal pilin[7] have identified Ser_{63} as a modified amino acid, and it is likely that it is also the site of modification in *N. meningitidis* pili of Class I (which are homologous to gonococcal pili).

Prokaryotes are capable of producing a wide variety of sugar structures. Among the rarest of these are diamino sugars, the first of which to be isolated was 4-acetamido-2-amino-2,4,6-trideoxyglucose (*N*-acetylbacillosamine).[8,9] Since then, several diamino sugar residues, including diacetamidotrideoxyhexoses, have been found to be constituents of polysaccharides isolated from *Pseudomonas aeruginosa, Vibrio cholerae, Escherichia coli,* and *Thiobacillus.*[10–13] However, to our knowledge, diacetamidotrideoxyhexoses have not previously been found as constituents of glycoproteins. The 2,4-diacetamido-2,4,6-trideoxyhexose sugar found in *N. meningitidis* is especially interesting as a novel linkage sugar because of its rarity in glycoconjugates.

In prokaryotes, glycosylation is uncommon, but it has been reported in archebacterial and eubacterial S layer proteins,[14] in mycobacterial 19 kD antigen,[15] and in bacterial cellulases.[16] Recently, glycosylation of *P. aeruginosa* pilin[17] as well as *Azospirillum brasilense* flagellin[18] has also been described.

Studies on purified pili of *N. gonorrhoeae* have recorded about 1.3% (w/w) of galactose per pilin subunit.[19] Whether this was covalently linked was not described. Later studies by Gubish *et al.*[20] indicated that beta-galactosidase affected adherence properties of a cyanogen bromide fragment (CNBr1: residues 8–102) derived from *N. gonorrhoeae* pilin. These regions of *N. gonorrhoeae* and *N. meningitidis* Class I pilins are highly homologous,[21] and our studies on *N. meningitidis* strain C311 also show that galactose is present in this region. However, by contrast to those of *N. gonorrhoeae* F62, Gal^- pili of *N. meningitidis* C311 clone 3 are as effective as fully glycosylated pili in mediating host cell interactions.[5]

The importance of the NH_2-terminal semiconserved pilus region in neisserial interactions has also been described by Rothbard *et al.,*[22] and antibodies against pilin peptides spanning regions 41–50 and 69–84 inhibited attachment of piliated *N. gonorrhoeae* to human endometrial cells. This would be consistent with our observations that Asp_{60} to Asn_{60} substitution affects epithelial interactions of *N. meningitidis* strain MC58.[2,3] However, variant gonococcal pili that do not show major changes in these regions[23] apparently interact to variable extents with host epithelial cells, and homologous inhibition was readily obtained with polyclonal antisera that failed to inhibit heterologous strains.[24] In addition, type-specific antigonococcal pilin monoclonal antibodies (mAbs), inhibit *N. gonorrhoeae* adhesion to epithelial cells, whereas mAb SM1, which reacts with the conserved pilus epitope $^{49}EYYLN^{53}$, is ineffective.[25] Taken together these data suggest that the spatial arrangement of pilin epitopes may be critical in determining the different roles of common and variable regions on pilin and that both may contribute to domains that interact directly or indirectly with receptors on host cells. The degree to which individual components of distinct pilins, with or without posttranslational modifications, participate in receptor interaction remains to be defined.

Glycosylation may alter the function of both eukaryotic and prokaryotic proteins.[16,26] However, in the present study, removal of galactose from pili of variant 3 did not affect adhesion to endothelial or epithelial cells. This, however, does not rule out the possibility that glycosyl residues may be important in adhesion in other strains or in as yet unknown or unexamined functions of pili. Whether 2,4-diacetamido-2,4,6-trideoxyhexose plays a role in adherence remains to be investigated. Glycosylation of bacterial cellulases is known to increase resistance to proteolytic degradation of these proteins[27] and to maintain conformational stability of others.[26,28] Pilin appears to be the only significant protein that is glycosylated on the surface, or even in extracts, of meningococci.[3] This suggests that pilin glycosylation may have some

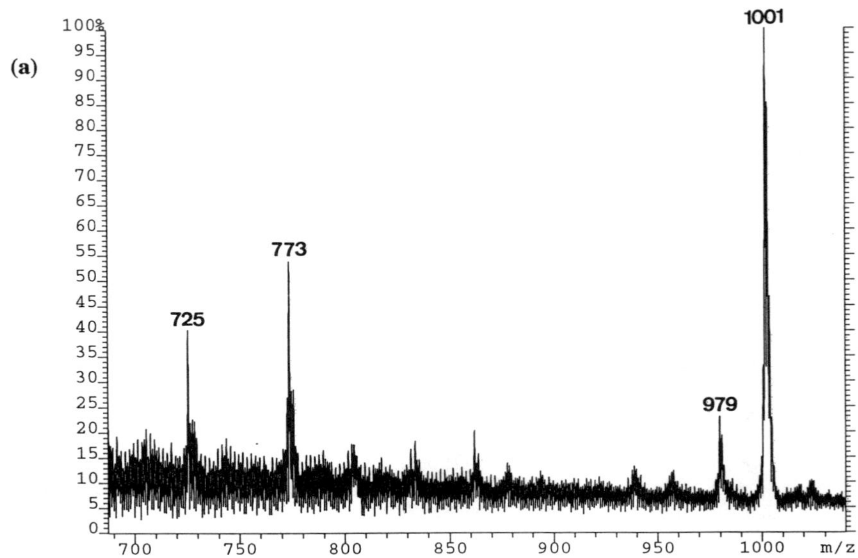

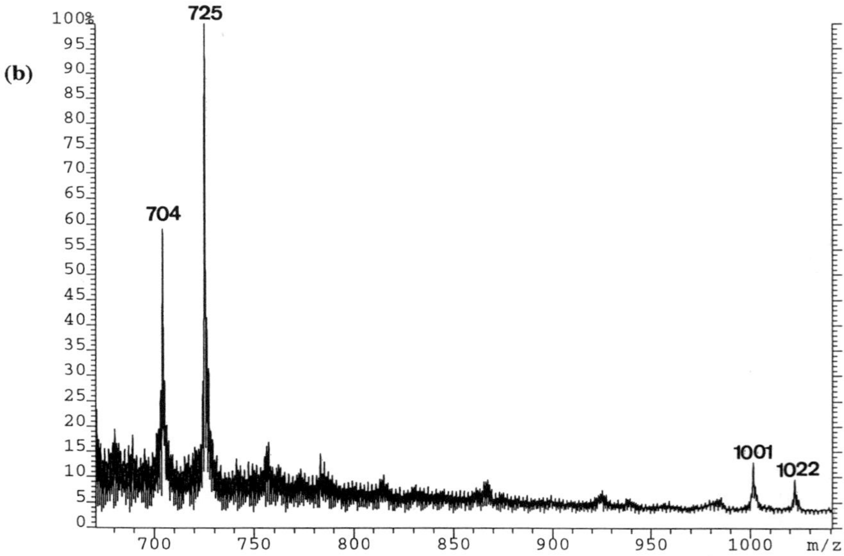

FIGURE 3a and b. *Choronia lampas* β-galactosidase treated perdeuteroacetylated saccharides deuterium labeled by NaBD$_4$ during reductive cleavage from the peptide [45]S-K[73] of variant 16. Partial FAB spectra at 0 minutes giving [M + H]$^+$ and [M + Na]$^+$ signals for the trisaccharide at m/z 979 and m/z 1001, respectively **(a)** and at 48 hours (as described in the text) **(b)**, are shown. Additional signals are attributable to hexose oligomers: signals at m/z 725 [M + Na]$^+$ and m/z 773 [M + Na]$^+$ correspond to nonreduced and deuterium-labeled reduced hexose dimers, respectively, whereas the signal at m/z 1022 [M + Na]$^+$ corresponds to a nonreduced hexose trimer. These signals are likely to be derived from contaminants.

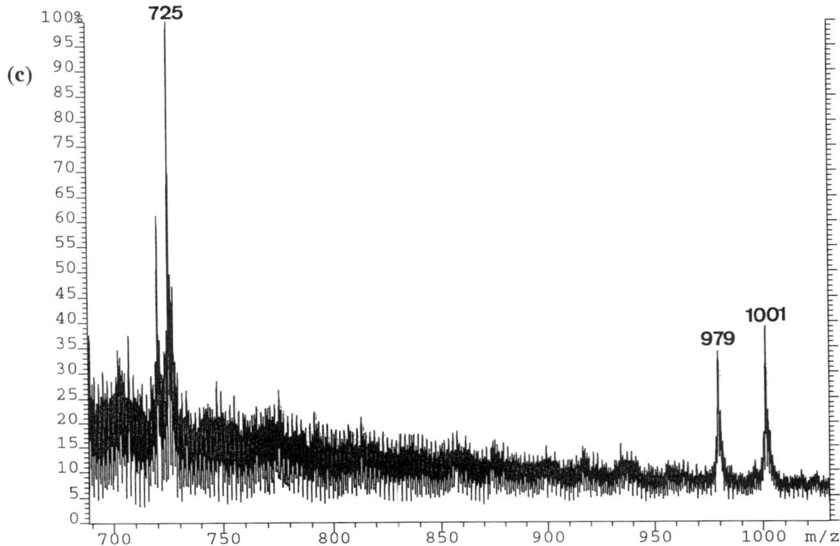

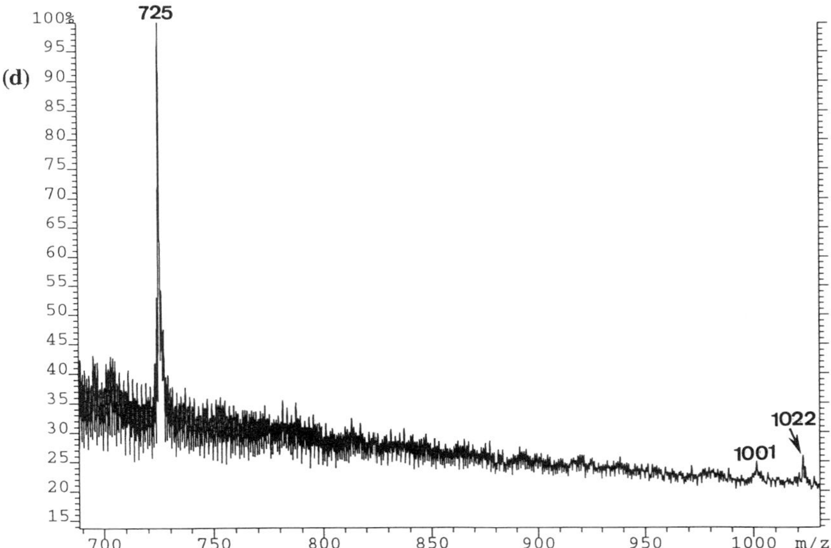

FIGURE 3c and d. (c) Partial FAB spectrum of a coffee bean α-galactosidase-treated perdeuteroacetylated saccharides deuterium labeled by $NaBD_4$ during reductive cleavage from peptide [45]S-K[73] of variant 16, affording $[M + H]^+$ and $[M + Na]^+$ signals for the undigested trisaccharide at m/z 979 and m/z 1001, respectively. No signal at m/z 704 is observed. (d) Partial FAB spectrum of the deuteroacetylated products of the *C. lampas* β-galactosidase digest after treatment with coffee bean α-galactosidase, resulting in loss of the signal at m/z 704. Additional signals at m/z 725 and m/z 1022 correspond to sodium adduct ions of nonreduced hexose dimers and trimers, respectively.

direct functional consequences in pathogenesis. One potential effect of the presence of terminal galactose may be that pili could become sialylated, a process that, when it occurs on gonococcal LPS, results in increased resistance to complement-mediated killing.[29] Moreover, normal human serum contains antibodies (anti-Gal) that react with terminal galactose structures on bacteria, including those on meningococcal pili.[6] Epitopes recognized by anti-Gal are also present on brain glycoproteins in man.[30] It is possible, therefore, that structural similarities between pili and brain tissue enable meningococci to be localized to the central nervous tissue by bridging via anti-Gal.

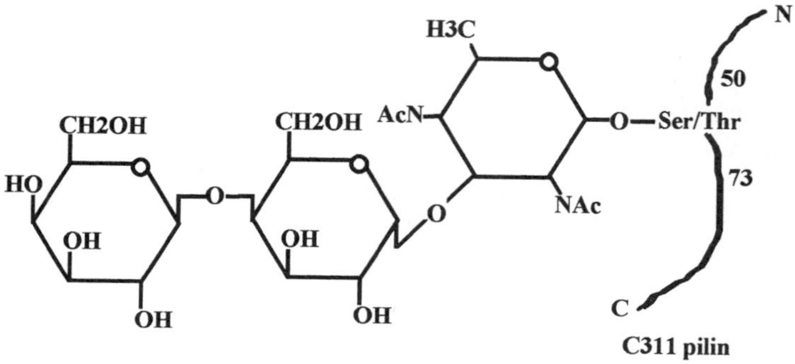

FIGURE 4. Proposed structure of the trisaccharide covalently attached to the tryptic peptide [50]Y-K[73] derived from pilins of strain C311. The stereochemistry of the 2,4-diacetamido-2,4,6-trideoxyhexose is not known.

EXPERIMENTAL PROCEDURES

Bacteria and Growth Conditions

Sources of *N. meningitidis* strains and growth conditions were described fully in a previous publication.[2] C311 is a serogroup B strain and produces Class I pili which react with the mAb SM1. Isolation of hyperadherence variants of C311 has been reported.[3] The piliated parental cultures were designated #3 (parental phenotype) or #16 (hyperadherent phenotype), and are referred to as 3 and 16 in this paper.

Construction of Nonreverting Insertion-Deletion Mutants in N. meningitidis galE

The preparation of *galE* constructs with kanamycin resistance (Kan[r]) cassettes has been described previously.[31] The construct was used to transform piliated variants 3 and 16, and mutants were selected on agar plates supplemented with 100 μg/ml kanamycin.[5]

Characterization of LPS of *galE* mutants: (a) Colony blotting: Previous studies have shown that mutation in the *galE* gene of strain MC58 resulted in the loss of reactivity of the bacteria with anti-LPS mAb SM82. This mAb was used to confirm the loss of the epitope from strain C311 on introduction of the *galE* mutation. (b) Migration on SDS-PAGE: LPS of the mutants migrated further than parental LPS

(FIG. 1), suggesting that galactose-containing units were lost from these macromolecules.

Characterization of Mutants and Variants of Meningococcal Strains: Immunochemical Methods

Expression of the major outer membrane antigens by C311 derivatives was determined by immunodot blotting, colony blotting, Western blotting, and electron microscopy (for piliation) as described previously.[2,32]

Sequence Analysis of Variant Pilins

The *pilE* sequences from variants of strain C311 were determined by direct sequencing following PCR amplification. Primary amplification, asymmetric amplification to produce single-stranded template, and the sequencing reactions per se were carried out as described previously.[3] Sequence analysis and alignments were performed using the PILEUP and TRANSLATE programs from the GCG suite of programs[33] running on SEQNET at the Daresbury Laboratories.

Purification of Pili

Pili from agar-grown variants and mutants of strain C311 were purified essentially as described for *N. gonorrhoeae*[34] by ethanolamine solubilization and ammonium sulfate precipitation.

Tryptic Digestion of N. meningitidis Strain C311 Pilin Proteins Isolated from Variants 3, 16, and Their galE Mutants

Porcine trypsin was purchased from Sigma. All other reagents, including deuterated reagents, were purchased from Aldrich, unless otherwise stated. *N. meningitidis* pilin protein samples were dialyzed in 50 mM ammonium bicarbonate buffer (pH 8.4) and directly freeze dried. Dry samples were then redissolved in 200 μl of 4 M urea (pH 8.4), and the appropriate amount of porcine trypsin (1:50, w:w, ratio of enzyme to protein) was added and incubated for 8 hours at 37°C. Digestion was terminated by direct freeze drying.

Reverse-Phase HPLC

Partial separation of tryptically digested peptides and glycopeptides was effected using an ultrasphere ODS HPLC column (25 cm × 4.6 mm, Beckman) fitted onto a Kontron HPLC system (Datasystem 450, HPLC pump 420, Detector 430 and Mixer M800). Samples were loaded in 0.1% trifluoro acetic acid (TFA) in milli-Q water and eluted with a solvent system of A = aqueous 0.1% TFA and B = a mixture of acetonitrile (Rathburns) and 0.1% aqueous TFA, 9:1, v:v at a flow rate of 1 ml/min. The column was eluted with a linear gradient from 100% A to 100% B over 60 minutes. Elution was monitored at 214 and 280 nm, and 1-ml fractions were collected. Dried fractions were redissolved in 5% acetic acid, and an aliquot of each was screened by FAB-MS and ES-MS.

FAB-MS, ES-MS, EI-MS

Detailed methodology for mass spectrometry was described by Dell[35] and in our recent publication.[5]

SUMMARY

Neisseria meningitidis pili are filamentous protein structures that are essential adhesins in capsulate bacteria. Pili of adhesion variants of meningococcal strain C311 contain glycosyl residues on pilin (PilE), their major structural subunit. Recent studies have shown that a novel *O*-linked trisaccharide substituent, not previously found as a constituent of glycoproteins, is present within a peptide spanning amino acid residues 50 to 73 of the PilE molecule. The structure was shown to be Gal β1–4 Gal α1–3 diacetamidotrideoxyhexose which is directly attached to pilin. Pilins derived from galactose epimerase (*galE*) mutants lack the digalactosyl moiety, but retain the diacetamidotrideoxyhexose substitution. These studies confirm our previous observations that meningococcal pili are glycosylated and provide the first structural evidence for the presence of covalently linked carbohydrate on pili. We have identified a completely novel protein/carbohydrate linkage on a multimeric protein that is an essential virulence determinant in *N. meningitidis*.

ACKNOWLEDGMENTS

We would like to thank Stephanie Barker, Maria Panico, and Ian Blench for technical assistance and Dr. Michael P. Jennings for the *galE* construct.

REFERENCES

1. VIRJI, M., H. KAYHTY, D. J. P. FERGUSON, C. ALEXANDRESCU, J. E. HECKELS & E. R. MOXON. 1991. The role of pili in the interactions of pathogenic *Neisseria* with cultured human endothelial cells. Mol. Microbiol. **5:** 1831–1841.
2. VIRJI, M., C. ALEXANDRESCU, D. J. P. FERGUSON, J. R. SAUNDERS & E. R. MOXON. 1992. Variations in the expression of pili: The effect on adherence of *Neisseria meningitidis* to human epithelial and endothelial cells. Mol. Microbiol. **6:** 1271–1279.
3. VIRJI, M., J. R. SAUNDERS, G. SIMS, K. MAKEPEACE, D. MASKELL & J. P. FERGUSON. 1993. Pilus-facilitated adherence of *Neisseria meningitidis* to human epithelial and endothelial cells: Modulation of adherence phenotype occurs concurrently with changes in amino acid sequence and the glycosylation status of pilin. Mol. Microbiol. **10:** 1013–1028.
4. DUNN, K. L. R., M. VIRJI & E. R. MOXON. 1995. Investigations into the molecular basis of meningococcal toxicity for human endothelial and epithelial cells: The synergistic effect of LPS and pili. Microb. Pathogen. **18:** 81–96.
5. STIMSON, E., M. VIRJI, K. MAKEPEACE, A. DELL, H. R. MORRIS, G. PAYNE, J. R. SAUNDERS, M. P. JENNINGS, S. BARKER, M. PANICO, I. BLENCH & E. R. MOXON. 1995. Meningococcal pilin: A glycoprotein substituted with digalactosyl 2,4-diacetamido-2,4,6-trideoxyhexose. Mol. Microbiol. **17:** 1201–1214.
6. HAMADEH, R. M., G. A. JARVIS, M. ESTABROOK & J. McL. GRIFFISS. 1994. Anti-Gal binds to pilus of *Neisseria meningitidis:* The Iga isotype blocks complement-mediatede killing. *In* Neisseria 94. J. S. Evans, S. E. Yost, M. C. J. Maiden & I. M. Feavers, Eds.: 132–133. Meriuex UK Ltd.
7. PARGE, H. E., K. T. FOREST, M. J. HICKEY, D. A. CHRISTENSEN, E. D. GETZOFF & J. A.

TAINER. 1995. Structure of the fibre-forming protein pilin at a 2.6 A resolution. Nature **378:** 32–38.

8. SHARON, N. & R. W. JEANLOZ. 1960. The diaminohexose component of a polysaccharide isolated from *Bacillus subtilis.* J. Biol. Chem. **235:** 1–5.

9. ZEHAVI, U. & N. SHARON. 1973. Structural studies of 4-acetamido-2-amino-2,4,6-trideoxy-D-glucose (*N*-Acetylbacillosamine), the *N*-acetyl-diamino sugar of *Bacillus licheniformis.* J. Biol. Chem. **248:** 433–438.

10. TAHARA, Y. & S. G. WILKINSON. 1983. The lipopolysaccharide from *Pseudomonas aeruginosa* NCTC 8505. Structure of the *O*-specific polysaccharide. Eur. J. Biochem. **134:** 299–304.

11. HERMANSSON, K., P. JANSSON, T. HOLME & B. GUSTAVSSON. 1993. Structural studies of the *Vibrio cholerae* O:4 O-antigen polysaccharide. Carbohydr. Res. **248:** 199–211.

12. WHITTAKER, D. V., L. A. S. PAROLIS & H. PAROLIS. 1994. *Escherichia coli* K48 capsular polysaccharide: A glycan containing a novel diacetamido sugar. Carbohydr. Res. **256:** 289–301.

13. SHASHKOV, A. S., S. CAMPOS-PORTUGUEZ, H. KOCHANOWSKI, A. YOKOTA & H. MAYER. 1995. The structure of the *O*-specific polysaccharide from *Thiobacillus* sp. IFO 14570, with three different diaminopyranoses forming the repeating unit. Carbohydr. Res. **269:** 157–166.

14. MESSNER, P. & U. B. SLEYTR. 1991. Bacterial surface layer glycoproteins. Glycobiology **1:** 545–551.

15. GARBE, T., D. HARRIS, M. VORDERMEIER, R. LATHIGRA, J. IVANYI & D. YOUNG. 1993. Expression of the *Mycobacterium tuberculosis* 19-kilodalton antigen in *Mycobacterium smegmatis:* Immunological analysis and evidence of glycosylation. Infect. Immun. **61:** 260–267.

16. BISARIA, V. X. & S. MISHRA. 1989. Regulatory aspects of cellulase biosynthesis and secretion. Crit. Revs. Biotech. **9:** 61–104.

17. CASTRIC, P. 1995. PilO, a gene required for glycosylation of *Pseudomonas aeruginosa* 1244 pilin. Microbiology **141:** 1247–1254.

18. MOENS, S., K. MICHIELS & J. VANDERLEYDEN. 1995. Glycosylation of the flagellin of the polar flagellum of *Azospirillum brasilense,* a Gram-negative nitrogen-fixing bacterium. Microbiology **141:** 2651–2657.

19. ROBERTSON, J. N., P. VINCENT & M. E. WARD. 1977. The preparation and properties of gonococcal pili. J. Gen. Microbiol. **102:** 169–177.

20. GUBISH, E. R., JR., K. C. S. CHEN & T. M. BUCHANAN. 1982. Attachment of gonococcal pili to lectin-resistant clones of Chinese hamster ovary cells. Infect. Immun. **37:** 189–194.

21. POTTS, W. J. & J. R. SAUNDERS. 1988. Nucleotide sequence of the structural gene for class I pilin from *Neisseria meningitidis:* Homologies with the *pilE* locus of *Neisseria gonorrhoeae.* Mol. Microbiol. **2:** 647–653.

22. ROTHBARD, J. B., R. FERNANDEZ, L. WANG, N. N. H. TENG & G. K. SCHOOLNIK. 1985. Antibodies to peptides corresponding to a conserved sequence of gonococcal pilins block bacterial adhesion. Proc. Natl. Acad. Sci. USA **82:** 915–919.

23. NICOLSON, I. J., A. C. F. PERRY, M. VIRJI, J. E. HECKELS & J. R. SAUNDERS. 1987. Localization of antibody-binding sites by sequence analysis of cloned pilin genes from *Neisseria gonorrhoeae.* J. Gen. Microbiol. **133:** 825–833.

24. VIRJI, M., J. S. EVERSON & P. R. LAMBDEN. 1982. Effect of anti-pilus antisera on virulence of variants of *Neisseria gonorrhoeae* for cultured epithelial-cells. J. Gen. Microbiol. **128:** 1095–1100.

25. VIRJI, M. & J. E. HECKELS. 1984. The role of common and type-specific pilus antigenic domains in adhesion and virulence of gonococci for human epithelial-cells. J. Gen. Microbiol. **130:** 1089–1095.

26. FUKUDA, M. & O. HINDSGAUL, EDS. 1994. Molecular Glycobiology: Frontiers in Molecular Biology. Oxford University Press.

27. LANGSFORD, M. I., N. R. GILKES, B. SINGH, B. MOSER, R. C. MILLER, R. A. J. WARREN & D. G. KILBURN. 1987. Glycosylation of bacterial cellulases prevents proteolytic cleavage between functional domains. FEBS Lett. **225:** 163–167.

28. BERG-FUSSMAN, A., M. E. GRACE, Y. IOANNOU & G. A. GRABOWSKI. 1993. Human acid

beta-glucosidase. *N*-glycosylation site occupancy and the effect of glycosylation on enzymatic activity. J. Biol. Chem. **268:** 14861–14866.

29. SMITH, H., J. A. COLE & N. J. PARSONS. 1992. The sialyation of gonococcal lipopolysaccharide by host factors: A major impact on pathogenicity. FEMS Microbiol. Lett. **100:** 287–292.

30. JAISON, P. L., V. M. KANNAN, M. GEETHA & P. S. APPUKUTTAN. 1993. Epitopes recognised by serum anti-α-galactoside antibody are present on brain glycoproteins in man. J. Biosci. **18:** 187–193.

31. JENNINGS, M. P., P. VAN DER LEY, K. E. WILKS, D. J. MASKELL, J. T. POOLMAN & E. R. MOXON. 1993. Cloning and molecular analysis of the *galE* gene of *Neisseria meningitidis* and its role in lipoplysaccharide biosynthesis. Mol. Microbiol. **10:** 361–369.

32. VIRJI, M., K. MAKEPEACE, D. J. P. FERGUSON, M. ACHTMAN, J. SARKARI & E. R. MOXON. 1992. Expression of the Opc protein correlates with invasion of epithelial and endothelial cells by *Neisseria meningitidis*. Mol. Microbiol. **6:** 2785–2795.

33. DEVEREUX, J., P. HAEBERLI & O. SMITHIES. 1984. A comprehensive set of sequence-analysis programs for the VAX. Nucl. Acid Res. **12:** 387–395.

34. HECKELS, J. E. & M. VIRJI. 1988. Preparation, characterisation and immunochemistry of pili and fimbriae. *In* Bacterial Cell Surface Techniques. I. C. Hancock & I. Poxton, Eds.: 67–72. John Wiley & Sons Ltd. London.

35. DELL, A. 1990. Preparation and description mass spectrometry of permethyl and peracetyl derivatives of oligosaccharides. Methods Enzymol. **193:** 647–660.

Genetic Analysis of the *Bordetella*-Host Interaction[a]

PEGGY A. COTTER[b] AND JEFF F. MILLER[b,c]

Department of Microbiology and Immunology
School of Medicine[b] and
Molecular Biology Institute[c]
University of California
Los Angeles, California 90095

Bordetellae are small gram-negative bacteria that cause respiratory tract infections in humans and other animals. *Bordetella pertussis* infects only humans and causes whooping cough or pertussis. This highly infectious disease continues to be a significant cause of morbidity and mortality in young children throughout the world.[1] *Bordetella bronchiseptica,* which is also highly infectious, displays a much broader host range, infecting a variety of mammals other than humans.[2] Although asymptomatic colonization of the respiratory tract is the most common result of bordetellosis, *B. bronchiseptica* can cause atrophic rhinitis in pigs, kennel cough in dogs, snuffles in rabbits, and bronchopneumonia in guinea pigs.[2]

B. pertussis and *B. bronchiseptica* synthesize a nearly identical set of virulence factors that are positively regulated by the BvgAS signal transduction system. Putative adhesins that allow the bacteria to adhere specifically to ciliated epithelial cells of the respiratory tract include filamentous hemagglutinin (FHA), a large rod-shaped protein that is both secreted and cell-associated[3–6]; fimbriae[7–9]; and a 69-kD outer membrane protein called pertactin.[10–12] A tracheal colonization factor, designated *tcfA,* has recently been described in *B. pertussis.*[13] Both *B. pertussis* and *B. bronchiseptica* synthesize a bifunctional adenylate cyclase/hemolysin,[6,14,15] whereas only *B. pertussis* synthesizes pertussis toxin.[16,17] Other Bvg-activated factors include a capsule, a dermonecrotic toxin, and a serum resistance factor.[18–20] Although adherent and/or toxic functions have been demonstrated for many of these factors *in vitro,* in no case has a function been definitively demonstrated *in vivo.*

In its active form, BvgAS also exerts negative control over genes required for the synthesis of flagella and the phenotype of motility in *B. bronchiseptica.*[21,22] Bvg control of motility is mediated by repression of a locus called *frlAB,* whose products form a transcriptional activator situated at the top of the motility regulatory hierarchy.[23] The *flaA* gene of *B. bronchiseptica,* situated at the bottom of the motility regulon, encodes the flagellin subunits that form the flagellar filament.[22]

While *frlAB* and *flaA* loci are present in *B. pertussis,* they are not expressed and *B. pertussis* is nonmotile.[22] However, Bvg-repressed genes, designated *vrg*s, have been identified in *B. pertussis* using Tn*phoA* mutagenesis.[24] Bvg-mediated repression of several *vrg*s was recently shown to involve a locus-designated *bvgR.*[25]

[a] Our work is supported by National Institutes of Health grants AI31548 and AI38417. P.A.C. was supported by National Institutes of Health postdoctoral fellowship grant AIO8747. J.F.M. is a Pew Scholar in the Biomedical Sciences.

[b] Address for correspondence: Department of Microbiology and Immunology, UCLA School of Medicine, 10833 LeConte Ave., Los Angeles, CA 90095. Tel: 310/206–7926; fax: 310/206–3865.

Bvg is inactivated by certain environmental signals, which in the laboratory include the presence of high concentrations of $MgSO_4$, nicotinic acid, or growth at low temperature.[26,27] Under these conditions, virulence factors are not expressed, and repression of motility genes in *B. bronchiseptica* and *vrg* expression in *B. pertussis* is relieved.[21,24,28] Thus, Bvg mediates a biphasic transition between two distinct phenotypic phases; the Bvg^+ phase, in which the various adhesins and toxins are expressed, and the Bvg^- phase, characterized by motility in *B. bronchiseptica* and *vrg* expression in *B. pertussis*. The switch from the Bvg^+ phase to the Bvg^- phase is commonly referred to as phenotypic modulation.

THE BVGAS SIGNAL TRANSDUCTION SYSTEM

The BvgAS signal transduction system is comprised of two proteins, BvgA and BvgS. BvgS resides in the cytoplasmic membrane and its periplasmic domain is thought to be involved in signal recognition.[29] The cytoplasmically located portion of BvgS consists of three distinct domains involved in transducing environmental signals to BvgA, a cytoplasmically located transcriptional regulator.[29,30] A region called the linker connects the membrane portion of BvgS to the cytoplasmically located signaling domains and is the site of mutations that lock BvgS in its active form.[31] This class of mutation has provided us with valuable tools for investigating the role of Bvg-mediated signal transduction in *Bordetella* pathogenesis.

BvgA and the cytoplasmic portion of BvgS ('BvgS) have been purified, and this complex signal transduction pathway has been reconstituted *in vitro*.[30,32] A combination of genetic and biochemical analyses have led to the model presented in FIGURE 1.[30,32] Under nonmodulating or Bvg^+ phase conditions, BvgS autophosphorylates at a conserved histidine residue in the transmitter domain. Phosphorylation of an aspartic acid residue in the receiver domain occurs next, followed by phosphorylation of a histidine residue in the C-terminal domain. The phosphorylated C-terminal domain appears to function as the substrate for phosphotransfer to BvgA, because the phosphorylated C-terminal domain alone can phosphorylate BvgA *in vitro*.[32] BvgA-phosphate is then capable of activating transcription of virulence gene expression and repressing *vrg* expression in *B. pertussis* and genes required for motility in *B. bronchiseptica*.

When modulating signals such as nicotinic acid or $MgSO_4$ are present, the phosphorelay cascade does not occur and BvgA remains inactive. Under these conditions virulence factors are not expressed and Bvg-repressed loci are expressed, resulting in the Bvg^- phase phenotype.

WHAT IS THE ROLE OF BVG-MEDIATED SIGNAL TRANSDUCTION IN THE *BORDETELLA* LIFE CYCLE?

The ability of *Bordetellae* to switch between distinct phenotypic phases has been recognized for many years, and considerable progress has been made in understanding how this switch occurs at the molecular level. Yet, the selective advantage provided by this ability and the role of Bvg-mediated signal transduction in pathogenesis are unknown. Speculation as to where or when this switch occurs is additionally hampered by the fact that despite rigorous examination of the signals to which Bvg responds in the laboratory, the true signals that are sensed in nature are also unknown. The approach we took to investigate the roles of the Bvg^+ and Bvg^- phases and the importance of Bvg-mediated signal transduction *in vivo* was to study respiratory infection in an animal model using *Bordetella* strains that are isogenic except for characterized mutations that specifically affect signal transduction. Because *B. pertussis* infects only humans, we focused on the interaction between *B. bronchiseptica* and two of its natural hosts, rabbits and rats.

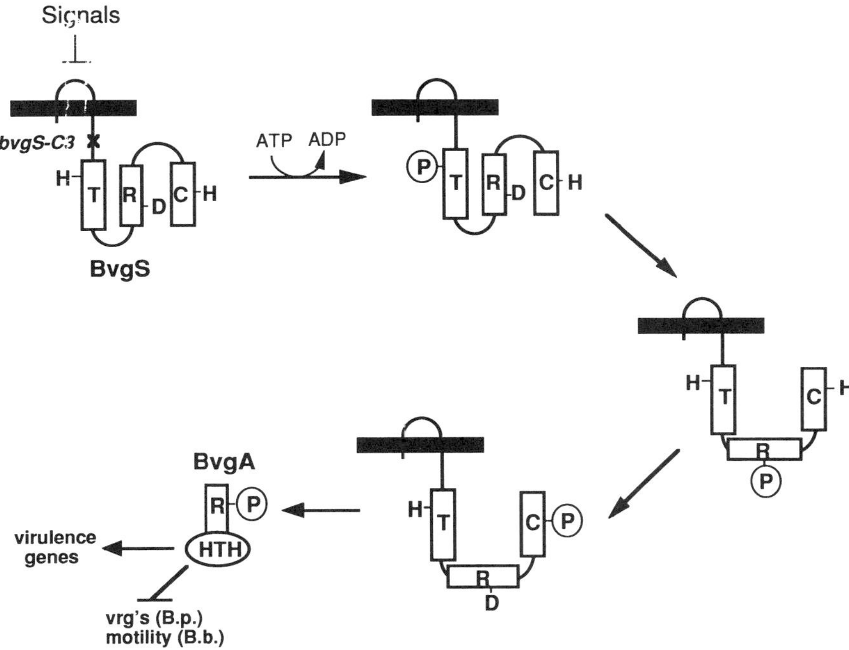

FIGURE 1. Model of BvgAS signal transduction. Proposed steps in the phosphorelay cascade leading to activation and repression of gene expression. Domains are abbreviated as follows: T = transmitter; R = receiver; C = COOH-terminal domain; HTH = helix-turn-helix motif. The *gray bar* represents the cytoplasmic membrane with the periplasmic domain of BvgS extending above it. The phosphoryl group is denoted by an encircled P. The location of the *bvgS*-C3 mutation is noted.

IS PHENOTYPIC MODULATION IMPORTANT DURING INFECTION?

We reasoned that if the ability to alternate between the Bvg$^+$ and the Bvg$^-$ phases was important *in vivo,* then mutants locked into one phase or the other would be altered in their ability to cause infection. A Bvg$^+$ phase locked derivative of our wild-type *B. bronchiseptica* strain, RB50, was constructed by transferring the *bvgS*-C3 allele,[31] which locks BvgS in its active form, to the chromosome of RB50 using an allelic exchange system that we developed for use in *B. bronchiseptica.*[23,33] We constructed a Bvg$^-$ phase locked derivative of RB50 by deleting *bvgS* sequences that code for the transmitter domain and most of the receiver domain.[33] By all criteria that we could use to test these strains *in vitro,* they displayed only Bvg$^+$ or Bvg$^-$ phase phenotypes, respectively, regardless of environmental conditions.[33]

Infection of New Zealand White (NZW) rabbits by *B. bronchiseptica* is typically asymptomatic. Bacteria efficiently colonize the entire respiratory tract and persist there despite the production of high titers of *Bordetella*-specific serum antibodies. We anticipated that if factors specific to the Bvg$^-$ phase are important for the initial interaction of the bacterium with the host, then the Bvg$^+$ phase locked mutant either would be unable to establish infection or would do so with a higher ID$_{50}$ than wild type. Alternatively, if modulation to the Bvg$^-$ phase, and thus downregulation of potentially antigenic Bvg$^+$ phase adhesins and toxins, is important either for evasion of host defenses or for limiting destruction to host tissues, then the Bvg$^+$ phase locked mutant would be expected to show either decreased persistence or increased disease compared to the wild type.

Groups of six NZW rabbits were inoculated with 10^2, 10^3, or 10^4 colony-forming units (cfu) of the wild-type strain or the Bvg$^+$ phase locked mutant, and two rabbits were inoculated with 10^6 cfu of the Bvg$^-$ phase locked mutant. Infections were followed for 3 weeks and colonization levels at various sites in the respiratory tract determined. The wild-type strain efficiently established infection with an ID$_{50}$ of about 100 cfu, as about half the animals in this group became infected (FIG. 2). All animals given larger doses became infected, and in all animals the level of colonization in the trachea and other sites was similar regardless of the inoculating dose. In contrast, the Bvg$^-$ phase locked mutant was unable to establish infection, even at a dose of 10^6 cfu. This result demonstrates that the Bvg$^+$ phase is required to establish infection and is consistent with the observation that most virulence factors identified so far are Bvg$^+$ phase specific. Surprisingly, however, the Bvg$^+$ phase locked mutant was indistinguishable from the wild type in its ability to establish infection. As with the wild-type strain, about half the animals given 100 cfu of the Bvg$^+$ phase locked strain became infected and all of the animals given larger doses became infected (FIG. 2). Colonization levels at all sites examined were similar, independent of the inoculating dose.

Clinically, all animals appeared healthy throughout the course of the experiment; there were no outward signs of respiratory disease and no pathology to respiratory tissue was observed either macroscopically or microscopically.

Western blots were used to obtain a qualitative assessment of the humoral immune response to infection by our wild-type and mutant strains. Whole cell extracts and outer membrane fractions were probed with serum obtained 3 weeks after inoculation. Serum from rabbits infected with the wild-type strain and the Bvg$^+$ phase locked mutant reacted similarly, recognizing many Bvg$^+$ phase-specific polypeptides as well as some antigens common to both phases (data not shown). No reactivity against polypeptides specific to the Bvg$^-$ phase was observed, and serum from uninfected animals was unreactive.

ELISAs were developed to quantiatively assess the immune response to specific Bvg$^+$ and Bvg$^-$ phase factors. All infected animals generated similar, high titers of serum antibody that recognized FHA regardless of the infecting strain or dose (FIG. 3). By contrast, none of the sera recognized purified flagellar filaments, and the lack of response against flagella was confirmed by immunoelectron microscopy (data not shown).

These results indicate that the Bvg$^+$ phase is both necessary and sufficient for establishment of respiratory tract infection in rabbits, and because antibodies against Bvg$^-$ phase-specific factors were not detected, we are tempted to conclude that the switch to the Bvg$^-$ phase does not even occur *in vivo.*

IS BVG-MEDIATED REPRESSION OF GENE EXPRESSION IMPORTANT DURING INFECTION?

The data presented above clearly show that the Bvg$^+$ phase is required during infection. Since Bvg simultaneously activates virulence gene expression and represses genes and operons required for motility in *B. bronchiseptica,* the Bvg$^+$ phase is characterized by the presence of Bvg$^+$ phase-specific adhesins and toxins as well as the absence of Bvg$^-$ phase-specific factors such as a rotating flagellar filament.

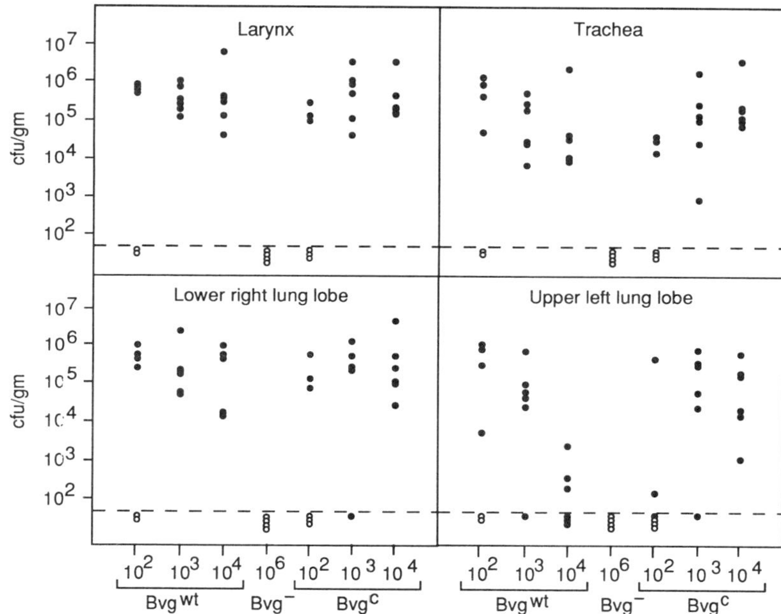

FIGURE 2. Scatter plots showing colonization levels in the larynx, trachea, and upper left and lower right lung lobes. Rabbits were inoculated with the wild-type (Bvg^{wt}), Bvg$^+$ phase-locked strain (Bvg^c), or Bvg$^-$ phase-locked strain (Bvg$^-$) at the doses (in cfu) indicated and sacrificed 3 weeks later. Colony-forming units (cfu) per gram of tissue are shown. *Open circles* represent uncolonized animals and *solid circles* represent infected animals. The lower limit of detection was 50 cfu/g, as represented by the *dashed line.*

Sequence similarity between *frlAB* and *flhDC* from *Escherichia coli* suggested that the *frlAB* gene products function as a transcriptional control factor situated at the top of the motility regulatory hierarchy,[23] thus representing the control point at which Bvg regulates this phenotype. To test this hypothesis a Bvg-activated promoter, that of the *fhaB* gene which encodes FHA, was inserted between the −10 and −35 sites in the *frlAB* promoter.[23] Insertion at this site is predicted to simultaneously disrupt the native promoter and provide a Bvg-activated promoter, thus reversing the expression pattern of this operon. The resulting strain, called Frl-reverse (Frl^r), synthesizes flagella and is motile only under Bvg$^+$ phase conditions and not under Bvg$^-$ phase conditions as assessed by motility assays, western blot and ELISA analyses, and immunoelectron microscopy (data not shown).[23]

These results confirm that repression of *frlAB* expression is the control point at which Bvg regulates the phenotype of motility. Perhaps even more importantly however, these experiments provided us with a strain for asking about the role of Bvg-mediated repression of gene expression in pathogenesis. In the Frl[r] strain the ability of Bvg to repress motility has been abrogated, and flagella are expressed ectopically in the Bvg[+] phase. We compared the Frl[r] strain with wild type in our rat model to determine if Bvg-mediated repression of motility is important for the development of infection.

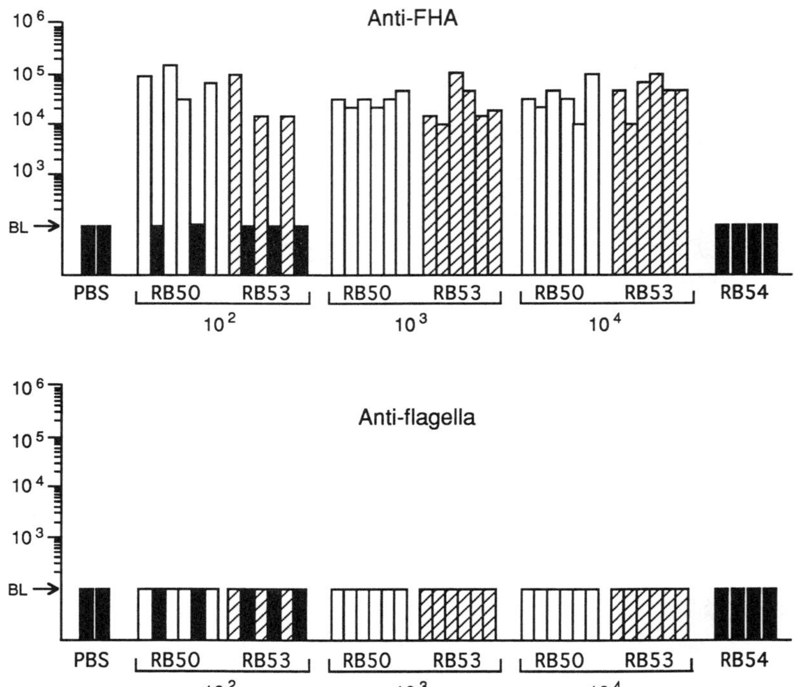

FIGURE 3. Antibody titers against purified FHA or purified flagellar filaments as determined by ELISA. Sera used were those obtained at sacrifice for each animal. The strains and doses (in cfu) used to infect each rabbit are indicated below the graph. *Solid bars* represent animals that did not become infected with *B. bronchiseptica, open bars* designate animals infected with the wild-type strain, and *hatched bars* designate animals infected with the Bvg[+] phase-locked mutant. Background levels of reactivity (BL) are indicated (*arrows*).

Rats are also natural hosts for *B. bronchiseptica,* and the infections established experimentally by our wild-type strain resemble very closely those established in rabbits, that is, bacteria colonize the respiratory tract asymptomatically and persist despite the production of high titers of anti-*Bordetella* antibodies.[23] When 3-week-old, female Wistar rats were inoculated with 10^3 cfu of the wild-type strain,

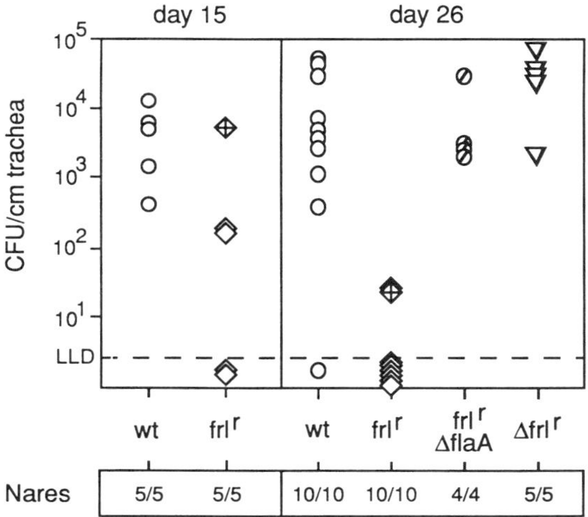

FIGURE 4. Scatter plots showing colonization levels in the trachea. Rats were inoculated with 10^3 cfu of the strains indicated and sacrificed after 15 or 26 days as indicated. cfu/cm trachea are shown. *Diamonds with a cross* in them designate the presence of motility-minus variants. Colonization of the nasal cavity (nares) is scored as plus or minus, and the number of animals that were positive over the number of animals inoculated per group are shown.

colonization levels in the trachea reached 10^3 to 10^4 cfu/cm trachea by day 15 postinoculation and remained at that level at least until day 26 postinoculation (FIG. 4). In contrast, the Frl-reverse strain was severely defective in its ability to colonize the trachea. At 15 days postinoculation, bacteria were recovered from the tracheas of

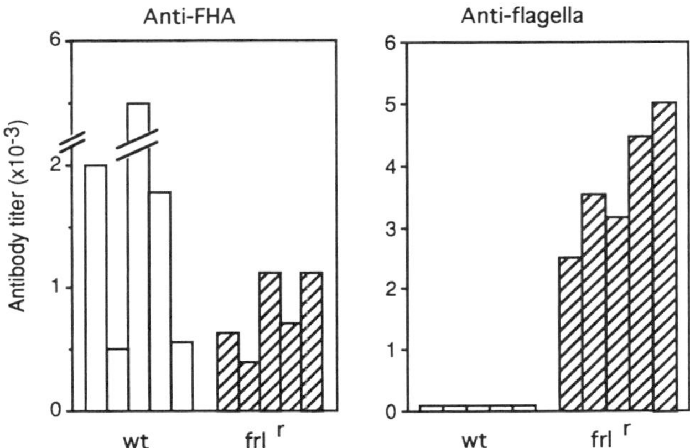

FIGURE 5. Antibody titers against purified FHA or purified flagellar filaments as determined by ELISA. Sera used were those obtained at the time of sacrifice (26 days postinoculation). *Open bars* represent sera from rats infected with the wild-type strain, and *hatched bars* designate sera from rats infected with the Frl[r] strain.

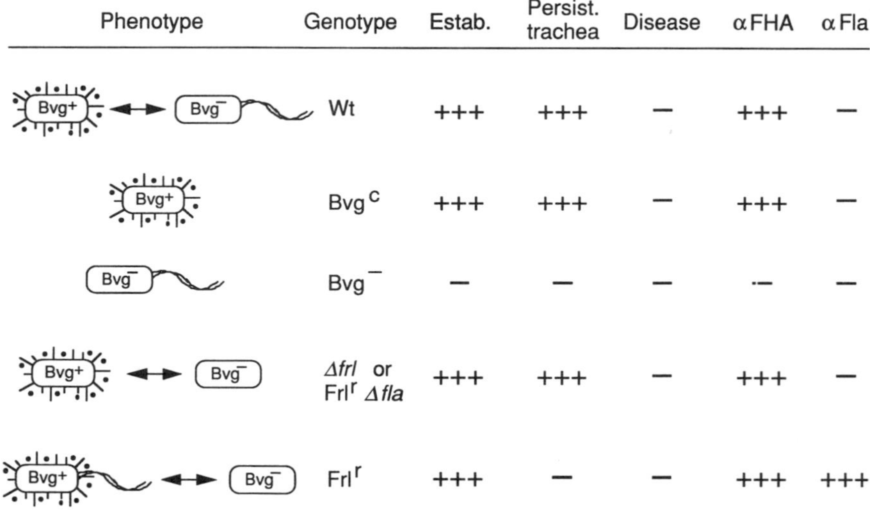

Phenotype	Genotype	Estab.	Persist. trachea	Disease	αFHA	αFla
	Wt	+++	+++	−	+++	−
	Bvg^C	+++	+++	−	+++	−
	Bvg⁻	−	−	−	−	−
	Δfrl or Frl^r Δfla	+++	+++	−	+++	−
	Frl^r	+++	−	−	+++	+++

FIGURE 6. Summary of phenotypes of the various mutant strains. Phenotypes with respect to virulence factor production and flagella synthesis are shown on the left. Estab. and Persist. trachea refer to the ability of each strain to establish infection (as assessed by the ability to colonize the nasal cavity) or to persist in the trachea (as assessed by recovery of bacteria from the trachea after 3 weeks). Disease is assessed by observing the animals for signs of respiratory distress as well as macroscopic and microscopic examination of respiratory tissue upon necropsy. αFHA and αFla refer to the induction of serum antibodies against FHA and flagella, respectively.

only three of five animals. In two of the animals the levels reached only about 10^2 cfu/cm trachea, and in the single animal in which higher levels were obtained the bacteria recovered were motility-minus variants. At day 26 low numbers of bacteria were recovered from the trachea in only 2 of 10 animals, and those were also shown to be motility-minus variants. The Frl^r strain was not defective in its ability to colonize the nasal cavity, however, as infection by the Frl^r strain was indistinguishable from wild type at this site and motility-minus variants were not recovered.

To determine if the defect in tracheal colonization in the Frl^r mutant is due to expression of flagella in the Bvg⁺ phase, an *flaA* deletion mutation was introduced into the Frl^r strain. This mutant was indistinguishable from wild type in its ability to colonize the trachea (FIG. 4).

These results indicate that inappropriate expression of flagella in the Bvg⁺ phase was detrimental to the infectious process and underscore the importance of Bvg-mediated repression *in vivo*. Thus, it appears to be just as important to turn some things off as it is to turn other things on.

When we examined the antibody response in animals infected with the Frl^r strain, we found that in contrast to animals infected with wild type, high titers of antiflagellar antibodies were produced, indicating that *B. bronchiseptica* flagella are indeed antigenic when expressed *in vivo* (FIG. 5). This result supports the conclusion that the switch to the Bvg⁻ phase may not even occur during infection.

FIGURE 6 summarizes the *in vivo* phenotypes of the various mutants. While both the wild-type and Bvg⁺ phase locked strains are capable of establishing persistent, asymptomatic respiratory tract infections, the Bvg⁻ phase locked strain is not, indicating that the Bvg⁺ phase is both necessary and sufficient for infection. The Frl^r strain is defective for colonization of the trachea, demonstrating the importance of Bvg-mediated repression of gene expression during infection. The fact that animals infected with the Frl^r strain produced antiflagellar antibodies whereas those infected with wild type did not indicates that the switch to the Bvg⁻ phase may not even occur *in vivo.*

IS PHENOTYPIC MODULATION IMPORTANT FOR SURVIVAL IN THE ENVIRONMENT?

If the ability to undergo phenotypic modulation is not required *in vivo,* then what is the role of the Bvg⁻ phase? *B. bronchiseptica* is reported to be capable of surviving and multiplying under conditions of severe nutrient limitation, and it has been suggested that these nutrient poor conditions may reflect those encountered outside the host.[34,35] This ability could contribute to the organism's ability to be transmitted from host to host, as transmission can be conceptually divided into three steps:

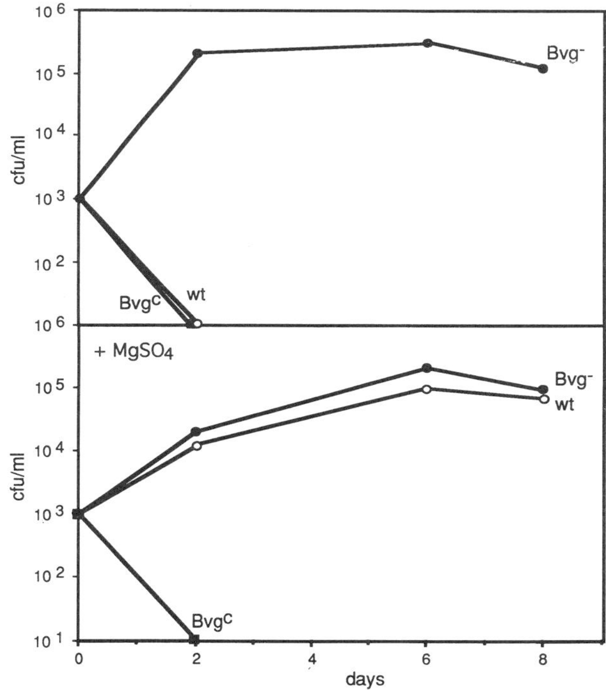

FIGURE 7. Growth and/or survival of wild-type and mutant strains in phosphate-buffered saline solution (PBS) with or without the addition of 40 mM MgSO₄. Strains were inoculated at 10^3 cfu/ml and incubated with shaking at 37°C. Graphs show data from one representative experiment that has been repeated several times with similar results.

release of the bacterium from an infected host, survival in the environment between hosts, and the initial interaction with a new, susceptible host. To determine if Bvg-mediated signal transduction is required for surviving nutrient depletion, we tested the ability of our wild-type and phase-locked strains to survive in phosphate-buffered saline (PBS). When cultures of PBS were started at 10^3 cfu/ml, the wild-type and Bvg$^+$ phase-locked strains were unrecoverable after 2 days, whereas the Bvg$^-$ phase-locked mutant had increased in number to about 10^5 cfu/ml (FIG. 7). If MgSO$_4$ was added to the cultures, the wild-type strain was also capable of surviving and multiplying, presumably due to MgSO$_4$ inducing a switch to the Bvg$^-$ phase. The Bvg$^-$ phase is therefore both necessary and sufficient for survival under nutrient-limiting conditions. These results are exactly the opposite of what we observed *in*

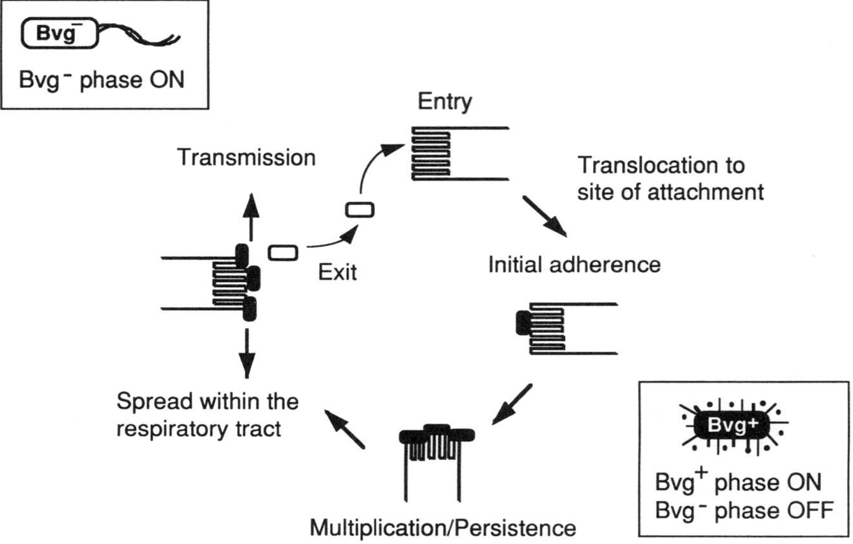

FIGURE 8. Model of the proposed life cycle for *B. bronchiseptica*. Bvg$^+$ phase bacteria are shown in *black* and Bvg$^-$ phase bacteria in *white*. We propose that the bacteria remain in the Bvg$^+$ phase while inside a mammalian host and switch to the Bvg$^-$ phase during transmission.

vivo, and we suspect that this ability may allow the organism to survive during transmission from one mammalian host to the next.

CONCLUSION

FIGURE 8 depicts our current view of the *Bordetella* life cycle. The bacteria enter the respiratory tract, probably by aerosol droplets, attach specifically to ciliated epithelial cells where they multiply, synthesize toxins and other factors, and spread further throughout the respiratory tract. The Bvg$^+$ phase appears to be necessary and sufficient for the *in vivo* part of the life cycle, because the data indicate that the Bvg$^+$ phase is required during infection, the switch to the Bvg$^-$ phase is not required for infection, and at least certain aspects of the Bvg⁻ phase must be turned off during infection. At some point at least some of the bacteria leave the infected host and are transmitted to a new, susceptible host. We speculate that the Bvg⁻ phase is required during this part of the cycle, and we are currently setting up transmission models to test this hypothesis.

REFERENCES

1. THE UNICEF REPORT. 1994. The state of the world's children 1994. U.S. Committee for UNICEF. New York.
2. GOODNOW, R. A. 1980. Biology of *Bordetella bronchiseptica*. Microbiol. Rev. **44:** 722–738.
3. RELMAN, D. A., M. DOMENGHINI, E. TUOMANEN, R. RAPPUOLI & S. FALKOW. 1989. Filamentous hemagglutinin of *Bordetella pertussis:* Nucleotide sequence and crucial role in adherence. Proc. Natl. Acad. Sci. USA **86:** 2637–2641.
4. TUOMANEN, E. & A. A. WEISS. 1985. Characterization of two adhesins of *Bordetella pertussis* for human ciliated respiratory epithelial cells. J. Infect. Dis. **152:** 118–125.
5. TUOMANEN, E., H. TOWBIN & G. ROSENFELDER. 1988. Receptor analogs and monoclonal antibodies that inhibit adherence of *Bordetella pertussis* for human ciliated respiratory epithelial cells. J. Exp. Med. **168:** 267–277.
6. ROOP, R. M., H. P. VEIT & R. J. SINSKY. 1987. Virulence factors of *Bordetella bronchiseptica* associated with the production of infectious atrophic rhinitis and pneumonia in experimentally infected neonatal swine. Infect. Immun. **55:** 217–222.
7. MOOI, F. R., W. H. JANSEN, H. BRUNINGS *et al.* 1992. Construction and analysis of *Bordetella pertussis* mutants defective in the production of fimbriae. Microb. Pathog. **12:** 127–135.
8. BLOM, J., J. A. HANSEN & F. M. POULSON. 1983. Morphology of cells and hemagglutinogens of *Bordetella* species: Resolution of substructural units in fimbriae of *Bordetella pertussis.* Infect. Immun. **42:** 308–317.
9. WILLEMS, R., A. PAUL, H. G. VAN DER HEIDE, A. R. TER AVEST & F. R. MOOI. 1990. Fimbrial phase variation in *Bordetella pertussis:* A novel mechanism for transcriptional regulation. EMBO **9:** 2803–2809.
10. CHARLES, I. G., G. DOUGAN, D. PICKARD, S. CHATFIELD, M. SMITH, P. NOVOTNY, P. MORISSEY & N. F. FAIRWEATHER. 1989. Molecular cloning and characterization of protective outer membrane protein P.69 from *Bordetella pertussis.* Proc. Natl. Acad. Sci. USA **86:** 3554–3558.
11. ROBERTS, M., N. F. FAIRWEATHER & E. LEININGER. 1991. Construction and characterization of *Bordetella pertussis* mutants lacking the *vir*-regulated P.69 outer membrane protein. Molec. Microbiol. **5:** 1393–1404.
12. LEININGER, E., M. ROBERTS, J. G. KENIMER *et al.* 1991. Pertactin, an Arg-Gly-Asp-containing *Bordetella pertussis* surface protein that promotes adherence of mammalian cells. Proc. Natl. Acad. Sci. USA **88:** 345–349.
13. FINN, T. M. & L. A. STEVENS. 1995. Mol. Microbiol. **16:** 625–634.
14. ENDOH, M., T. TAKEZAWA & Y. NAKASE. 1980. Adenylate cyclase activity of *Bordetella* organisms. Its production in liquid medium. Microbiol. Immunol. **24:** 95–104.
15. GLASER, P., D. LADANT, O. SEZER, F. PICHOT, A. ULLMANN & A. DANCHIN. 1988. The calmodulin-sensitive adenylate cyclase of *Bordetella pertussis:* Cloning and expression in *Escherichia coli.* Mol. Microbiol. **2:** 19–30.
16. ARICO, B. & R. RAPPUOLI. 1987. *Bordetella parapertussis* and *Bordetella bronchiseptica* contain transcriptionally silent pertussis toxin genes. J. Bacteriol. **169:** 2847–2853.
17. MILLER, J. F., J. J. MEKALANOS & S. FALKOW. 1989. Coordinate regulation and sensory transduction in the control of bacterial virulence. Science **243:** 916–922.
18. WEISS, A. A. & E. L. HEWLETT. 1986. Virulence factors of *Bordetella pertussis.* Annu. Rev. Microbiol. **40:** 661–686.
19. WALKER, K. E. & A. A. WEISS. 1994. Characterization of the dermonectrotic toxin in members of the genus *Bordetella.* Infect. Immun. **62:** 3817–3828.

20. FERNANDEZ, R. C. & A. A. WEISS. 1994. Cloning and sequencing of a *Bordetella pertussis* serum resistance locus. Infect. Immun. **62:** 4727–4738.
21. AKERLEY, B. J., D. M. MONACK, S. FALKOW & J. F. MILLER. 1992. Role of the *bvgAS* locus in negative control of motility and flagella synthesis by *Bordetella bronchiseptica*. J. Bacteriol. **174:** 980–990.
22. AKERLEY, B. J. & J. F. MILLER. 1993. Flagellin transcription in *Bordetella bronchiseptica* is regulated by the BvgAS virulence control system. J. Bacteriol. **175:** 3468–3479.
23. AKERLEY, B. J., P. A. COTTER & J. F. MILLER. 1995. Ectopic expression of the flagellar regulon alters the development of the Bordetella-host interaction. Cell **80:** 611–620.
24. KNAPP, S. & J. J. MEKALANOS. 1990. Two trans-acting regulatory genes (*vir* and *mod*) control antigenic modulation in *Bordetella pertussis*. J. Bacteriol. **170:** 5059–5066.
25. MERKEL, T. & S. STIBITZ. 1995. Identification of a locus required for the regulation of *bvg*-repressed gene in *Bordetella pertussis*. J. Bacteriol. **177:** 2727–2736.
26. LACEY, B. W. 1960. Antigenic modulation of *Bordetella pertussis*. J. Hyg. **58:** 57–93.
27. MELTON, A. R. & A. A. WEISS. 1989. Environmental regulation of expression of virulence determinants in *Bordetella pertussis*. J. Bacteriol. **171:** 6206–6212.
28. WEISS, A. A. & S. FALKOW. 1984. Genetic analysis of phase variation in *Bordetella pertussis*. Infect. Immun. **43:** 263–269.
29. STIBITZ, S. & M. S. YANG. 1991. Subcellular localization and immunological detection of proteins encoded by the *vir* locus of *Bordetella pertussis*. J. Bacteriol. **173:** 4288–4296.
30. UHL, M. A. & J. F. MILLER. 1994. Autophosphorylation and phosphotransfer in the *Bordetella pertussis* BvgAS signal transduction cascade. Proc. Natl. Acad. Sci. USA **91:** 1163–1167.
31. MILLER, J. F., S. A. JOHNSON, W. J. BLACK, D. T. BEATTIE, J. J. MEKALANOS & S. FALKOW. 1992. Isolation and analysis of constitutive sensory transduction mutations in the *Bordetella pertussis bvgS* gene. J. Bacteriol. **174:** 970–979.
32. UHL, M. A. & J. F. MILLER. 1996. Integration of multiple domains in a two-component sensor protein: the Bordetella pertussis BvgAS phosphorelay. EMBO **15:** 1028–1036.
33. COTTER, P. A. & J. F. MILLER. 1994. BvgAS mediated signal transduction: Analysis of phase-locked regulatory mutants of *Bordetella bronchiseptica* in a rabbit model. Infect. Immun. **62:** 3381–3390.
34. PORTER, J. F., R. PARTON & A. C. WARDLAW. 1991. Growth and survival of *Bordetella bronchiseptica* in natural waters and in buffered saline without added nutrients. Appl. Env. Microbiol. **57:** 1202–1206.
35. PORTER, J. F. & A. C. WARDLAW. 1993. Long-term survival of *Bordetella bronchiseptica* in lake water and in buffered saline without added nutrients. FEMS. Microb. Letts. **110:** 33–36.

What Happens *in Vivo* to Bacterial Pathogens?

HARRY SMITH[a]

The Medical School
University of Birmingham
Edgbaston
Birmingham B15 2TT, UK

It is now widely accepted that bacterial behavior *in vivo* can be different from that *in vitro* and should come under scrutiny in any serious study of pathogenicity. This was not always so. In the 1950s, after the anthrax toxin had been demonstrated for the first time in the plasma of infected guinea pigs,[1] I advocated this approach,[2] but it failed to catch on. At that time, pathogenicity was not a popular subject. Also, separating organisms grown *in vivo* in the large quantities then needed for meaningful examination of their properties was inconvenient and sometimes dangerous. It was far easier to work with organisms grown *in vitro,* and there was much to be learned from them. Organisms grown *in vivo* were not studied much until the 1980s. By then, pathogenicity had become a popular area, and techniques (notably sodium dodecyl sulfate polyacrylamide gel electrophoresis [SDS-PAGE] and western blotting) had become available for analyzing components of the small numbers of organisms that could be obtained relatively easily from infected animals. The effectiveness of this approach in confirming or disproving putative virulence determinants indicated by studies *in vitro* and in revealing differences between *in vivo* and *in vitro* organisms that might be related to virulence soon became apparent.[3,4] More recently, there has been an additional impetus. Regulation of virulence gene expression and the influence on it of environmental conditions *in vitro* are popular subjects.[5] This has encouraged speculation on what might happen *in vivo*[5–7] where environmental conditions are not only different from those *in vitro* but change as the infection progresses. This paper attempts to channel current interest in what *might* happen *in vivo* into effort to find out what *does* happen. It updates previous reviews of papers up to 1990.[3,4]

The environment *in vivo* influences bacterial pathogenicity not only by affecting production of virulence determinants but also by controlling growth rate. Intense interest in the first overshadows consideration of the second, although it is equally important in pathogenicity. The neglected area is considered first.

LACK OF KNOWLEDGE OF GROWTH RATES *IN VIVO* AND THE FACTORS THAT CONTROL THEM

Bacterial growth *in vivo* is essential for pathogenicity. Rapid multiplication is needed for acute disease to overwhelm initial defenses and cause sickness before the immune response can be effective. A slow growth rate might lead to less stimulation of host defenses in chronic disease.[8] In carrier states the pathogen may enter a resistant, stationary phase.[9] Growth rates *in vivo* will be determined largely by

[a] Tel: 0121-414-6920; fax: 0121-414-5925.

temperature, osmolarity, pH, Eh, and nutrient availability in different tissues. However, a pathogen may adapt to prevailing conditions and multiply at a rate most suited to the stage of disease.

It is frustrating that we know so little about the growth rates of pathogens during infection. Increases or decreases in bacterial population in blood, lymph nodes, and spleen are recorded frequently, such as for mutants of salmonellae in mice,[10] but they are the results of bacterial multiplication and destruction by host defenses. Rapidly increasing populations means that doubling times are short. The problem arises when populations increase or decrease slowly. True multiplication rates, which may be high but disguised by a high death rate due to efficient host defenses, are unknown. A stationary population does not necessarily mean that the pathogen is in a stationary state. The position over growth rates has not changed since it was last reviewed.[3,4] Briefly, bacterial doubling times *in vivo* can be measured by using either the proportion of organisms containing a genetic marker that distributes at each division into only one of two daughter cells or the increase in ratios of wild-type organisms to nongrowing temperature-sensitive mutants. These methods have been used only for infections with *Escherichia coli, Salmonella typhimurium,* and *Pseudomonas aeruginosa.*[3,6]

Equally frustrating is the position of studies on nutrients and metabolism that underpin bacterial growth *in vivo*. Only mechanisms of overcoming iron restriction have received adequate attention. Most pathogens have been investigated in this respect and many strategies studied at the molecular level. The subject progresses constantly.[11–13] Its erudition contrasts starkly with the dearth of knowledge on the use of other nutrients *in vivo*. For example, the vast knowledge about the nutrition and metabolism of *E. coli in vitro* has not yet been applied to growth *in vivo* of pathogenic strains.[14] The same applies to other pathogens. In the past it was shown that local concentrations of preferred nutrients could determine the tissue specificity of pathogens, such as urea in human kidney for *Proteus mirabilis* and erythritol in fetal tissues of domestic animals for brucellae.[3,6] These promising leads were never extended. In a nutshell, the host and bacterial determinants of growth *in vivo* are largely unknown.

The holdup in this area is not due to lack of experimental approaches. As already stated, growth rates *in vivo* can be measured[3,6,15] and stationary states could be detected by similar methods. The effects of nutrients such as $PO_4^{3/4-}$, Mg^{2+}, Zn^{2+}, amino acids, sugars, and vitamins could be examined by modifications of the methods used for iron, which began with the effects of iron salts on growth in serum-containing media and virulence in animal models.[3] Observations on auxotrophic mutants would indicate the availability of particular nutrients *in vivo,* such as leucine auxotrophs of mycobacteria, in contrast to the wild types, failed to grow in mice.[16] As described in a later section, techniques for measuring environmental parameters *in vivo,* such as the use of reporter genes,[17] might indicate concentrations of nutrients in various tissues. Then, growth rates *in vivo* could be compared with those seen *in vitro* under conditions similar to those *in vivo*.

The brakes on progress are the need for animal experiments and the lack of interest in microbial physiology. Animal experiments are more difficult, more expensive, and less repeatable than are those *in vitro*. These experiments have already demonstrated the effects of iron limitation *in vivo,* so work on this topic can proceed *in vitro* on the reasonable assumption that it is relevent *in vivo*. This stage has not been reached for other nutrients; the initial animal experiments must be carried out. Microbial physiology is not as popular as it was before the impact of genetics and molecular biology. Physiologists that are available have to be persuaded that work on the nutrition and metabolism of pathogens could be rewarding. Overall, with the exception of studies on iron limitation, the prospect for progress in this important aspect of pathogenicity is not good.

EFFECT OF THE ENVIRONMENT *IN VIVO* ON PRODUCTION OF VIRULENCE DETERMINANTS

In diseased animals bacterial pathogens produce all the determinants necessary for the manifestations of virulence. Environmental conditions *in vivo* (osmolarity, pH, Eh, and nutrient availability) are different from those in laboratory cultures. They not only are more complex, but also change as infection proceeds because of inflammatory influxes, tissue breakdown, and spread from one anatomic site to another. When pathogens are moved from animals to laboratory cultures and vice versa, phenotypic change and selection of genotypes occur.[3,4] Similar changes in phenotypes and genotypes will also happen *in vivo* as the environment varies with progress of infection.[6,7] These facts have three implications for studies of pathogenicity. Putative determinants of virulence indicated by experiments with organisms grown *in vitro* may not be formed *in vivo*. One or more of the full armory of virulence determinants that are formed *in vivo* may not be produced under arbitrarily chosen conditions of growth *in vitro*. All members of the armory are not necessarily produced *in vivo* at the same time or place; the complement could vary with the phase of infection and the anatomic site. The first two implications have been heeded in studies of pathogenicity over the last 10 years, but attention to the third is generally yet to come.

Confirmation That Putative Virulence Determinants Detected in Vitro *Are Produced* in Vivo *and Contribute to Virulence*

Increasingly, confirmation of *in vivo* production of putative determinants is being adopted as good practice. Bacteria obtained from patients or infected animals are examined for putative determinants by SDS-PAGE and immunoblotting. Convalescent sera are probed for appropriate antibodies. TABLE 1 lists a few of numerous recent examples. However, some surprising gaps still exist. Antibodies to invasion proteins Ipa B, C, and D of *Shigella flexneri* have been detected in patients[3,7] as have those against the internalin of *Listeria monocytogenes* (M. Juvin and J. L. Gaillard, personal communication). However, I am not aware of this having been done for the product of the *act*A gene of *L. monocytogenes,* the invasin of *Yersinia enterocolitica* and *Y. pseudotuberculosis,* or the products of the cell-invasion genes of *S. typhimurium.*

Ensuring that the putative determinants contribute to the virulence, by comparing in appropriate animal models the wild types with specifically deficient mutants,[32] is also becoming standard practice. Proof of the relevance of listerolysin O to mouse virulence is a typical example.[33] Sometimes production of a putative virulence determinant *in vivo* does not correlate with virulence. The 17-kD product of the *ail* gene of *Y. enterocolitica* is formed in Peyer's Patches of infected mice, but observations on a deficient mutant indicated that it was not required for either initial invasion or establishing systemic infection.[34] The invasin of *Y. enterocolitica* is involved in invasion of Peyer's Patches but not in establishing systemic infection.[35] The type 1 fimbriae of *E. coli* F-18 are produced in abundance in mice, but observations on mutants show that they are not important in virulence.[36]

TABLE 1. Confirmation That Putative Virulence Determinants Detected *in Vitro* Are Produced *in Vivo*

Bacterial Species	Host	Site of Recognition	Putative Determinant Demonstrated *in Vivo* (and/or Its Antibody)	Reference
Proteus mirabilis	Man	Urine	IgA protease	18
Vibrio cholerae	Rabbit	Intestine	Toxin-coregulated-pili	19
Bordetella pertussis	Man	Blood	Adenylate cyclase	20
Pseudomonas aeruginosa	Man	Sputum	Alginate	21
Streptococcus pneumoniae	Man	Urine	Capsular polysaccharide Type-specific polysaccharide	22
	Man	Serum	Pneumolysin	26
	Mice	Lung, spleen	Pneumolysin	26
Pasteurella hemolytica AI	Goat	Blood	Neuraminidase	23
Listeria monocytogenes	Man	Serum	Listeriolysin O	24
		CSF	Listeriolysin O	25
Escherchia coli	Man	Serum	Verotoxin I	27
Yersinia spp.	Man Rabbit Mice	Serum	YadA YopE, YopH, and others	28, 29, 30
Bacteriodes fragilis	Man	Serum	Iron-regulated OMP	31

Another healthy sign is that behavior in tests *in vitro* is being compared with the pathology of disease. Studies on intestinal invasion by *S. flexneri* are a good example.[37–39] Using Hela cells, the role of plasmid gene products IpaB, IpaC, IpaD, and IcsB to entry, intracellular movement, and transfer between cells was established. However, the situation *in vivo* is different because colonic enterocytes, unlike Hela cells, have a brush border and shigellae cannot penetrate it. The pathology of infections in primates and rabbit intestinal loops suggests that shigellae invade the colonic mucosa initially by a nonspecific mechanism, that is, ingestion by M cells of lymphoid follicles and delivery to antigen processing macrophages in the lamina propria. Macrophage apoptosis and inflammation follow, leading to disruption of the epithelial cell layer. Shigellae can then invade through the sides and bases of cells using the determinants recognized by the Hela cell studies. Other intestinal pathogens such as *L. monocytogenes, Yersinia* spp., and *Salmonella* spp. also seem to invade via M cells, so the relevence *in vivo* of determinants indicated by their invasion of cell lines *in vitro* is coming under scrutiny.[40] It is a trend to be encouraged in other areas of pathogenicity.

Comparison of In Vivo *and* In Vitro *Grown Bacteria to Reveal Previously Unknown Virulence Determinants*

Increasingly, bacteria grown *in vivo* are being compared with those grown *in vitro* by SDS-PAGE and sometimes in biologic tests. Bacterial components formed *in vivo* and not or less so *in vitro* are frequently demonstrated. Repression *in vivo* of components formed *in vitro* is also detected. TABLE 2 lists some of many recent examples. These studies are undertaken to recognize bacterial constituents that may be important for diagnosis and vaccination as well as to reveal virulence determinants.

With regard to the latter, recognizing a previously unknown component is only the first step. It must be shown to be responsible for a biologic property related to pathogenicity (such as interference with phagocytosis) and to contribute to virulence *in vivo*.[6,7] Experiments with determinant deficient mutants are important.[6,7] Unfortunately, this essential follow-up is not as popular as the original revelation by SDS-PAGE. I shall return to this point.

TABLE 2. Differences between Bacteria Grown *in Vivo* and *in Vitro* That Are Possibly Important in Pathogenicity

Species	Host	Site of Bacteria	Different Property of *in Vivo* Organisms	Reference
Staphylococcus aureus	Rabbit	Heart	More type 8 capsular poly-saccharide	41
	Guinea pig	Peritoneal chambers	Greater amount of TSST-1	42
S. epidermidis	Guinea pig	Peritoneal chambers	2 Iron-regulated proteins formed and 4 proteins repressed	43
	Pigs	Peritoneal chambers	2 Proteins not seen *in vitro* and many proteins repressed	44
Pasteurella haemolytica	Rabbit	Peritoneal chambers	3 Iron-regulated proteins (antibodies to them in bovine serum)	45
	Cattle	Peritoneal chambers	1 Protein not seen *in vitro*, 3 iron-regulated proteins, several proteins repressed	46
Campylobacter jejuni	Rabbit	Lung Intestinal loops	Several proteins not seen *in vitro* (antibodies to 2 in human serum)	47
Yersinia enterocolitica	Mice	Intestinal loops Peyer's Patches	1 Protein not seen *in vitro* 3 Proteins not seen *in vitro*, several proteins repressed	48
Bacteriodes fragilis	Mice	Peritoneal chambers	Protein profiles; iron-regulated proteins not induced	49
Borrelia burgdorferi	Mice	Skin infection	Outer surface protein A down-regulated	50
Haemophilus somnus	Calves	Lung at intervals	Composition and antigenicity of LPS change	51
Neisseria meningitidis	Man	Cerebrospinal fluid	Lower expression of class 3 epitope on OMP	52
Aeromonas salmonicida	Trout	Peritoneal chambers	Increased pathogenicity and resistance to bactericidins and phagocytes, several proteins and antigens not seen *in vitro*, LPS change, acid poly-saccharide capsule	53 54
Legionella pneumophila	Guinea pig Man Mice	Macrophages	4 Proteins not seen *in vitro*	55
Salmonella typhimurium	Mice	Macrophages	Several stress proteins	56

Identification of Virulence Determinants Produced at Successive Stages in the Disease Process and the Host Factors Involved

In the experiments just described, the multiple influences of the undefined conditions *in vivo* are accepted as a whole. Furthermore, bacteria grown *in vivo* are collected from the most convenient and prolific source. Differences in the complement of virulence determinants between bacteria harvested at different stages of infection and at different anatomic sites are largely disregarded. The future goal should be to identify bacterial virulence determinants throughout the infection process and the host factors that induce them, a formidable task. Current interest in environmental regulation of virulence genes, however, might be channeled in this direction. A summary of this subject follows.

Present Studies on Regulation of Virulence Determinant Production in Vitro: *Their Relevance to What Happens* in Vivo

Soon after it was known that bacteria possess global regulatory networks which induce or repress diverse and unlinked genes in response to environmental signals,[57] coordinate regulation of production of virulence determinants was demonstrated, such as the *tox*R gene system of *Vibrio cholerae.*[58]

Global regulation of gene expression[59] usually involves a hierarchical network of regulons. These are groups of genes controlled by a common regulator, usually a DNA-binding protein that recognizes control regions of its subservient genes. "Ground level" regulons are under control of higher regulons and so on, with DNA supercoiling and DNA-associated proteins influencing some of the top members of the hierarchy. Some regulators have two components. One protein senses the environmental parameter (e.g., osmolarity, phosphate concentration) and the other exercises regulatory function. In the histidine protein kinase response family, a phosphorylation reaction passes the information from the first protein to the second. Cross-talking between regulators can occur, that is, sensor molecules from one pathway affect response regulators from another. The EnvZ-OmpR and PhoP-PhoQ systems are members of the histidine kinase family. They respond to osmotic and phosphate signals, respectively, and regulate many cellular processes of both pathogens and nonpathogens.[59] It is not surprising that these regulons affect virulence, for example, mutations in *S. typhimurium* that turn off the EnvZ-OmpR and PhoP-PhoQ systems reduce virulence for mice.[59] Investigating these systems is extremely popular. To me, however, studying the higher regulons because they affect virulence carries a danger of becoming involved in ever more complex systems that control bacterial metabolism as a whole. For those interested in bacterial pathogenicity, effort should perhaps be concentrated on "ground level" regulons that are more immediately concerned with virulence determinants.

Several regulons of this nature have been studied *in vitro*. The *tox*R system[60] regulates production of both components of cholera toxin, an adhesin, synthesis of some OMPs, and the property of serum resistance.[60] It is modulated by temperature, osmolarity, pH, oxygen status, and availability of amino acids.[60] *Bordetella pertussis* forms the *bvg* (originally called *vir*) system which regulates production of adenylate cyclase, filamentous hemagglutinin, toxin, and hemolysin and is affected by temperature, $MgSO_4$, and nicotinamide.[61] *Yersinia* spp. have two known independent regulatory networks.[29] One responds to temperature and regulates production of enterotoxin, invasins, adhesins, lipopolysaccharides, and *Yersinia* OMPs (Yops). The other responds to Ca^{2+} and regulates only Yop production.[29,30,62] *Yersinia* spp. grow well at

37°C provided Ca^{2+} is present, but Yop production is low. Reducing Ca^{2+} restricts growth, but Yop production increases. The *vir*R regulon of *S. flexneri* responds to temperature and causes production at 37°C of invasion plasmid virulence determinants.[63] The *fur* regulon in *E. coli* and other pathogens responds to iron concentrations and regulates production of siderophores, OMPs concerned with iron uptake, and some toxins.[64] The *atx*A gene of *Bacillus anthracis* regulates transcription of the three anthrax toxin genes, *pag*, *lef*, and *cya*, under the influence of bicarbonate concentration and probably temperature.[65]

The presence *in vivo* of virulence determinants whose production *in vitro* is controlled by a certain regulon does not necessarily mean that the regulon itself operates identically *in vivo*. Unknown factors may affect it, or a different regulatory system may be involved. However, the designated regulon is probably playing some role if deletion of the regulon genes affects virulence and the environmental factors that affect the regulon *in vitro* are present *in vivo*. The *tox*R system operates in humans, because a deletion mutant produced less colonization and diarrhea in volunteers than did the wild type.[66] However, the influence of environmental conditions is confusing. In cultures, *V. cholerae* produces more toxin, at low temperature rather than at 37°C, under aerobic rather than anaerobic conditions, and at low rather than high pH.[67] Yet, it produces toxin and other *tox*R-regulated gene products in the human intestine which is at 37°C, anaerobic, and at alkaline pH.[67] The *bvg* regulon of *B. pertussis* seems to act in mice, because mutants deficient in genes controlled by *bvg* were less virulent.[61,68] It probably also functions in patients, but apart from the permissive temperature (37°C), the modulators of its action *in vivo* are unknown.[69] Neither is its role in phase variation *in vivo*[70] clear. Ca^{2+} regulation of Yop production by *Yersinia* spp. almost certainly does not occur *in vivo*[29,30,62] where Yop formation occurs freely at high Ca^{2+} concentrations that are nonpermissive *in vitro*.[29,30,62] The mechanisms operating *in vivo* are not yet clear, but studies with Hela cells suggest that contact with phagocytes may be the key.[30] Mutants deficient in the *vir* regulon of *S. flexneri* failed to invade the conjunctiva of guinea pigs,[63] but virulence tests in rabbit loops or primates, as far as I am aware, have not been recorded. It probably functions in patients because it is permissive at 37°C. I could not find reports of comparisons of *fur* regulon-deficient mutants of *E. coli* with wild types in virulence tests in animals, but recently a *fur*-deficient mutant of *P. aeruginosa* was found less able than the wild type to produce corneal infections of mice.[71] It is known that iron supplies are limited *in vivo*.[3,64] The *atx*A-regulating gene of *B. anthracis* functions *in vivo*, because *atx*A-deficient mutants infect but do not kill mice, and antibody response to all three toxin components is decreased.[65] Also, *lac*Z fusions to each of the three toxin genes showed them all to be expressed in infections of peritoneal chambers in guinea pigs (Jean-Claude Sirard, personal communication). Furthermore, concentrations of bicarbonate (about 20 mM) and CO_2 (about 40 mm Hg) in humans are similar to those that activate toxin production *in vitro*.

In summary, most but not all virulence determinant regulons investigated *in vitro* appear to function *in vivo*, but the environmental modulators of their action at different stages of infection are often not clear.

How to Gain More Information on What Happens in Vivo

The first step is to recognize the virulence genes that are expressed at progressive stages of infection and in different anatomic sites. The second is to detect differences in environmental parameters (temperature, osmolarity, pH, oxygen status, ion concentration, and nutrient and substrate availability) that might be responsible for any changes detected in expression of virulence genes. The third is to try to relate the two and identify the regulon involved.

Recognition of Virulence Genes Expressed in Vivo. As described already, the "classic" way is to examine organisms obtained directly from infected animals for the products of these genes. Again, I stress that demonstration of differences between *in vivo* and *in vitro* grown organisms is only the beginning. A previously unknown bacterial component must be proved to be the determinant of a relevant biologic property and to contribute to virulence *in vivo*. So often this is not done. An example, which deals with gene expression at progressive stages of infection, is as follows. In the intestinal lumen of mice, *Y. enterocolitica* produced a plasmid-mediated OMP (23 kD) not seen in cultures *in vitro*. On invasion of Peyer's patches, this and two further novel proteins (210 and 240 kD) were produced.[48] There the matter lies. The possible function of these novel OMPs in initial invasion has not been investigated. Occasionally, original observations are taken through to the ultimate goal (see later).

Recently the "classic" procedure has been supplemented by new methods for identifying gene expression *in vivo*. The *in vivo* expression technology (IVET) has three variations. The first used auxotrophic mutants as a selection system.[72] DNA segments from a wild-type *S. typhimurium* were attached to a synthetic operon so that they could provide promoters to a promoterless *pur*A gene and a promoterless *lac*Z operon. The resulting genes were introduced into a *pur*A auxotrophic mutant of *S. typhimurium* which, unless complemented, does not grow *in vivo*. In mice, some bacteria grew in the spleen, indicating *pur*A expression by the synthetic gene due to activity of promoters provided by the wild-type genes, that is, those expressed *in vivo*. Bacteria with genes not expressed *in vivo* were virtually eliminated. Plating the bacterial population recovered from the spleen on McConkey lactose agar distinguished members with genes expressed *in vitro* as well as *in vivo* (red colonies, Lac$^+$ and Pur$^+$, 95%) and those having genes expressed only *in vivo* (white colonies, Lac$^-$ and Pur$^-$, 5%).[72] The genes concerned had been termed *ivi* ("*in vivo* induced") genes.[72] Sequence analysis of some of the Lac$^-$ strains indicated that five different operons were expressed *in vivo* and three resided in genes of as yet unknown function.[72,73]

The second IVET system was similar to the first but used antibiotic resistance for selection.[73,74] The promoterless *pur*A gene was replaced by a promoterless chloramphenicol acetyltransferase (*cat*) gene and the mice were dosed with choloramphenicol. Again, plating on McConkey lactose agar distinguished between organisms containing genes expressed *in vivo* and *in vitro* (red colonies; 95% for *S. typhimurium*) and those containing genes expressed only *in vivo* (white colonies; 5%). Genetic and sequence analysis showed one of the *ivi* of genes of *S. typhimurium* was *fad*B which encodes an enzyme involved in fatty acid oxidation.[74]

The third IVET system used genetic recombination to report gene expression.[75] A resolvase was produced from a promoterless copy of the *tnp*R gene of the transposable element γδ under the influence of promoters provided by the genes expressed by the pathogen (e.g., *V. cholerae*) *in vivo*. The resolvase excised a chloramphenicol resistance reporter gene, making the organisms antibotic sensitive. Bacteria in tissue homogenates were replica plated on medium alone and medium with chloramphenicol. Colonies sensitive to chloramphenicol contained organisms whose genes were expressed *in vivo*. This system cannot distinguish genes expressed only *in vivo* from those expressed *in vivo* and *in vitro*, but it can be used for relatively few organisms, in different tissues, and at different stages of infection. Furthermore, it is adaptable to many pathogens, because *tnp*R requires only Mg^{2+} and negatively supercoiled DNA as substrates.[67] The method has revealed over 20 *ivi* genes in *V. cholerae*.[67]

Recently,[76] a method for demonstrating genes expressed *in vivo* was devised for bacteria that do not form auxotrophs and for which gene transfer systems are not available. The proteins coded by gene expression libraries were separated by SDS-PAGE and immunoblotted with sera obtained from live infected animals (that is, antibodies to gene products expressed *in vivo*) and with antisera against heat-killed bacteria (that is, antibodies to gene products expressed *in vitro*). Comparisons of the immunoblots indicate products formed only *in vivo*. It has been used for *Borrelia burgdorferi* infections in mice with expression libraries prepared by ligating DNA fragments to a phage which was then grown in *E. coli*. Six genes expressed only *in vivo* were demonstrated, and one, *p21*, coded for a new 20-kD protein.[76] The method only detects genes whose products are antigenic.

Another method,[77] used for *Mycobacterium tuberculosis,* was to restore a virulence characteristic (ability to grow fast in the spleen and lungs of mice) to an avirulent strain (H37Ra) by complementation with a gene library from a virulent strain (H37Rv). The gene library was constructed in an integrating cosmid vector pYUB178 and electroporated into H37Ra. Repeated infection of mice and recovery from the spleens and lungs selected individual faster growing members from the pool of recombinants. The H37Rv DNA inserts was then retrieved. A 23-kb DNA fragment, *ivg,* which provides growth advantage *in vivo* was identified.[77]

Finally, transposons carrying unique, detectable sequences were used to tag and inactivate particular genes in a population of *S. typhimurium* that was inoculated into mice.[78] Bacteria recovered from the spleens of the mice and those in the inoculum were compared to determine which of the tagged genes the members carried. The tagged genes that were present in members of the inoculum but not in the recovered bacteria were those whose inactivation had led to loss in virulence, that is, the virulence genes. Some of the virulence genes identified by this reverse selection were known, but nine were different.

Most bacterial pathogens should be amenable to one or another of these new systems for recognizing gene expression *in vivo*. As for the "classic" system, however, this is only the start. The expressed gene must be shown to contribute to virulence and its product and biologic function identified. Such studies are in progress. Mutations in the *ivi* genes of *S. typhimurium,* detected by the auxotrophic IVET system, reduced virulence for mice.[72] The *ivi* gene of *S. typhimurium* demonstrated by the antibiotic selection system *fad*B encodes an enzyme that may inhibit host defenses by oxidizing fatty acids such as arachidonic acid, which are either bactericidal themselves or stimulate local antibacterial inflammatory responses.[74] The roles in virulence of the *ivi* genes of *V. cholerae* identified by the recombinant system and the *p21* gene of *B. burgdorferi* demonstrated by the antibody system are not yet clear. Certainly, the 25-kb DNA fragment, *ivg,* of *M. tuberculosis* is involved in virulence, because the method of selection is in fact a virulence test.[77]

Some studies have been conducted with macrophages in culture to indicate genes involved in intracellular growth. Application of the antibiotic selection system to cultured macrophages infected with *S. typhimurium* revealed *ivi* fusions that grew far better in macrophages than did nonselected control strains; these genes have yet to be characterized.[74] In macrophages derived from human blood, most mRNAs formed by *M. avium* were like those produced in cultures, but one was different.[79] The use of mRNAs in this way is still another system for recognizing genes expressed *in vivo*. The gene concerned, its product and function have not yet been identified.

Clearly, it is now possible to identify virulence genes at progressive stages of infection and in different anatomic sites.

Measurement of Environmental Parameters That Might be Responsible for Changes in Expression of Virulence Genes. Geigy Scientific Tables[80–82] contain much information on temperature, osmolarity, oxygen status, cations, anions, amino acids, sugars, and other compounds in blood, saliva, gastric juices, bile, intestinal juices, urine, vaginal secretions, lung secretions, cerebrospinal fluid, synovial fluid, brain, kidney, and liver. Also, factors at potential sites of infection can be measured by standard physiologic and pathologic procedures.[80–82] Elements present in body fluids, cells, or subcellular particles *in situ* can be measured by X-ray microanalysis[83] during electron microscopy as for intestinal cells of mice infected with rotavirus.[84] Quantitative fluorescence microscopy of carriers of dyes that react to environmental parameters have been used to indicate, for example, the pH in the phagolysosomes of macrophages.[85] Also, *lacZ* fusions to genes whose expression levels respond to such parameters have been used to estimate Ca^{2+} levels in human macrophages containing *Y. pestis*[86] and levels of oxygen, pH, Fe, Mg, glucose, and mannose in tissue culture cells infected with *S. typhimurium.*[17] Both techniques could be used on specimens taken from infected animals. In short, information on the environment *in vivo* is either already available or can be gained, if the will is there.

Relating Environmental Parameters to Virulence Determinant Production. There are two levels of investigation. First, differences between the environment *in vivo* and that *in vitro* should be related to the production *in vivo* of virulence determinants not formed under the conditions *in vitro.* Second, differences occurring at progressive stages of infection in various anatomic sites should be related to changes in virulence gene expression. In both cases, consideration should be given to the possible operation *in vivo* of any regulons identified *in vitro.* The mixed environmental parameters *in vivo* could be simulated *in vitro* and production of relevant virulence determinants monitored. Studies on the operation of the *bvg* regulon of *B. pertussis* under different concentrations of $MgSO_4$ and nicotinic acid derivatives[69] are along these lines. Also, an acid pH *in vitro* and in the phagolysosomes of mouse macrophages has been shown to induce PhoP-PhoQ transcription by *S. typhimurium* and hence the *pag* gene essential for intracellular growth.[85] If such simulation studies fail, identifying the additional environmental factors acting *in vivo* might be difficult. However, experiments suggested by studies *in vitro* such as contact of yersinae with phagocytes (see above) could be tried. Also, if differences in virulence determinant production are detected at progressive stages of infection in various anatomic sites, concomitant changes in environment may be crucial for the virulence determinants that have either appeared or disappeared. Finally, it should be remembered that density-dependent interbacterial signaling may change gene expression when bacteria reach a certain concentration in the tissues.

The IVET system has already demonstrated virulence gene expression *in vivo* that is unexpected from experience with *in vitro* cultures. Both the antibiotic and recombinant selection systems have shown that *V. cholerae* expresses many *ivi* genes in the intestines of orally infected mice, but none are *tox*R regulated.[67,72] Toxin, however, is produced in the intestine because diarrhea is apparent. Is it possible that toxin production *in vivo* is controlled by another regulon? Another surprise is that the recombinant IVET system showed that although the *irg*A gene of *V. cholerae* was expressed as expected in iron-limiting media and in mouse peritoneal cavities, this was not so in the disease relevant sites, mouse intestine and rabbit ileal loops.[67,72,74] Either iron is readily available in the intestine or in this site regulation of the *irg*A gene is different from that in the peritoneal cavity.

The message of this section is clear. There is a lot we do not know about how bacterial pathogens react to the environment of the host, but we have the tools to find out and are beginning to learn.

SIALYLATION OF GONOCOCCAL LIPOPOLYSACCHARIDES BY HOST FACTORS: A MAJOR INFLUENCE ON PATHOGENICITY REVEALED BY STUDYING ORGANISMS GROWN *IN VIVO*

Gonococci in urethral exudates from patients are resistant to complement-mediated killing by human serum, but in most cases the resistance is lost on one subculture *in vitro*.[87] A vigorous follow-up of this observation had the following results. Serum resistance *in vivo* is due to sialylation of high M_r LPS components by a gonococcal sialyltransferase. The substrate for the bacterial enzyme is host cytidine 5'-monophospho-*N*-acetyl neuraminic acid (CMP-NANA), and the sialylation is enhanced by host lactic acid.[87,88] Prompted by this work, other groups have shown that LPS sialylation affects many different facets of gonococcal pathogenicity including overall virulence in humans.[87] Furthermore, it led to demonstration that LPS sialylation occurs in meningococci and affects their pathogenicity in several ways. These combined results are an example of the rewards that can stem from in-depth analysis of original observations of differences between pathogenic bacteria grown *in vivo* and those grown *in vitro*. The work was reviewed recently.[87] It is summarized here; only references not given in the review[87] are quoted.

Lipopolysaccharide Sialylation and Serum Resistance in Vivo

The loss of serum resistance of urethral exudate gonococci on subculture *in vitro* was restored by incubation for 2–3 hours with genital secretions, serum, or extracts of red and white blood cells. Fractionation of blood cell sonicates using a biologic assay for resistance-inducing activity produced active material in diffusates from high M_r fractions which was identified by mass spectrometry as CMP-NANA. Incubation of gonococci with synthetic CMP-NANA induced serum resistance.

Sialylation of LPS components by CMP-NANA was demonstrated by using CMP-^{14}CNANA and autoradiography of LPS bands separated by SDS-PAGE, as well as the shift of those bands to higher M_r. Gonococci form many LPS components, but not all are sialylated. Mostly, components of high M_r are affected, and one main recipient (4.5 kD) has a side chain, Galβ1-4GlcNAcβ1-3Galβ1-4Glc-, in which the terminal galactose is sialylated. Other components, however, can be sialylated and sometimes more than one in a single strain. Electron microscopy of ruthenium red-stained organisms shows the sialylated LPS as an irregular surface coat.

A sialyltransferase indicated for the first time by the sialylation experiments with gonococci was detected in Triton × 100 extracts of strain F62 and then demonstrated in all gonococcal and meningococcal strains examined.

The fact that LPS sialylation is responsible for serum resistance was shown by serum resistance accompanying sialylation by CMP-NANA, by CMP preventing both sialylation and resistance induction, and by restoration of serum susceptibility when sialyl groups were removed by neuraminidase. The sialylated components, however, must be of high M_r (>4.2 kD). The mechanism of serum resistance is not clear, but interference with the action of both natural antibody and complement has been noted. A minority of gonococcal strains are serum resistant without LPS sialylation, but the determinants are not clear.

Most gonococci *in vivo* contain sialylated LPS components, and treatment with neuraminidase removes both sialyl groups and serum resistance. Thus, the serum resistance of gonococci in 15 of 18 urethral exudates was reduced by neuraminidase treatment and the surface structure stainable by ruthenium red disappeared. In another study, gonococci in seven different samples of exudate reacted minimally in immunogold labeling with a monoclonal antibody that binds to the site on the conserved 4.5-kD component which can be sialylated by CMP-NANA. After treatment with neuraminidase, however, the gonococci in all samples reacted strongly.

A second host factor enhances the action of CMP-NANA. Like CMP-NANA, it was present in diffusate from high M_r fractions of blood cell sonicates. It enabled gonococci just emerging from lag phase to fix up to twofold more radiolabel on their LPS than did controls during incubation with CMP-^{14}CNANA.[87] Furthermore, when separated from CMP-NANA by high pressure liquid chromatography, it increased the serum resistance-inducing activity of CMP-NANA.[88] It was purified from diffusates of blood cell sonicates dialyzed at 18–20°C by gel exclusion and identified as lactic acid by magnetic resonance spectroscopy and gas chromatography/mass spectrometry.[88] Nanogram quantities of authentic lithium L-lactate enhanced LPS sialylation by CMP-NANA and increased its resistance-inducing activity to the same extent as shown by the preparations from blood.[88] No other blood cell fraction had enhancer activity. The mechanism of action of lactic acid is not yet known.

Confirmation of the essential points of these studies came from the properties of a mutant (JBI) deficient in sialyltransferase activity.[89] It was isolated by insertion mutagenesis of strain F62 with transposon Tn1545Δ 3 and screening for unlabeled colonies after incubation with CMP-^{14}CNANA. In contrast to the wild type, extracts of the mutant did not catalyze sialylation of LPS. In SDS-PAGE, the mutant had the same five LPS components as did the wild type, but two were in different amounts. The same three components of both strains reacted with the monoclonal antibody that detects the sialylatable Galβ1-4GlcNAc group, but only those of the wild type shifted to higher M_r on incubation with CMP-NANA. In contrast to the wild type, the mutant was unable to become serum resistant when incubated with CMP-NANA, blood cell sonicates, or their diffusates.[89] This not only confirms that LPS sialylation is responsible for serum resistance but also shows that blood cells do not contain a mechanism for sialylating gonococcal LPS which is independent of CMP-NANA, such as direct transfer of sialyl groups from sialylated glycoproteins and glycolipids as happens for *Trypanasoma cruzi.*[90]

Lipopolysaccharides Sialylation and Other Aspects of Pathogenicity

The heavy surface accumulation of sialylated LPS would be expected to affect facets of pathogenicity in addition to serum resistance. Several groups[87] have shown this to be so. Sialylation of LPS by CMP-NANA interferes with entry to epithelial cells, killing by neutrophils in opsonophagocytosis tests with normal human serum, the bactericidal and opsonophagocytosis action of antisera against gonococcal proteins, and stimulation of the immune system.[87] Infection experiments with volunteers were consistent with these results. After inoculation of volunteers with a strain whose LPS could not be sialylated, a variant was recovered from the volunteers. The LPS of this variant could be sialylated, and in subsequent volunteer experiments it was more virulent than the parent strain provided that the variant was inoculated intraurethrally after being grown in a medium without CMP-NANA (i.e., its LPS was not sialylated). If the inoculum was grown with CMP-NANA, it was not so infective which is consistent with LPS sialylation-inhibiting ability to invade epithelial cells.

Availability of CMP-NANA and Lactic Acid to Gonococci in Vivo *and Their Significance in Pathogenicity*

This section discusses the work on gonococci in the context of a main point of this paper, the importance of relating environmental parameters *in vivo* to production of virulence determinants. There is no doubt that most gonococci *in vivo* have some LPS components sialylated, that this sialylation profoundly affects various facets of pathogenicity, and that the gonococcal determinants concerned are: (1) LPS components capable of sialylation, and (2) the sialyltransferase. Also, the host factors responsible, CMP-NANA and lactic acid, are available in sites relevant to disease. CMP-NANA occurs in human cells including those of the blood and cervical epithelium.[87] It will be readily available to gonococci within phagocytes and epithelial cells, but normally only minute amounts are found extracellularly.[87] Lactic acid is present in vaginal secretions, ejaculate, urine, aqueous humor, blood, cerebrospinal fluid, neutrophils, and monocytes. Both CMP-NANA and lactic acid would be released to extracellular gonococci from dying epithelial cells and phagocytes during inflammation that occurs in gonorrhea. Certainly, resistance-inducing activity has been demonstrated in genital secretions.[87] Furthermore, conditions *in vivo* are often anaerobic, and gonococci form lactic acid from glucose under these conditions.[88] Interestingly, when anaerobically grown gonococci were incubated with CMP-NANA, they incorporated more sialic acid into their LPS than did aerobically grown gonococci and were converted to serum resistance two to three times faster.[88]

Interaction between lactic acid and CMP-NANA may be especially important early in infection. The tests for enhancement by lactic acid of LPS sialylation and resistance induction by CMP-NANA involved small numbers of gonococci just emerging from lag phase, and in both cases, enhancement was up to twofold. In the primary lodgment phase of infection,[6] relatively few organisms, either moving out of lag phase or growing slowly, have to resist the humoral and cellular components of massive inflammation. Survival is essential for disease to ensue, and the chance will be better if CMP-NANA induction of gonococcal resistance to killing by serum and phagocytes is both increased and accelerated.

Extension of the Studies to Meningococci

Some meningococci contain LPS components that either are endogenously sialylated (sero groups B, C, W, and Y) or can be sialylated by exogenous CMP-NANA (groups A and 29E).[87] They also contain the LPS sialyltransferase.[87] Pathogenicity is affected by LPS sialylation but not as profoundly as for gonococci because of another powerful virulence determinant, capsular polysaccharide. LPS sialylation appears to interfere with: adhesion and invasion of epithelial cells by noncapsulated strains, serum killing of most strains, and killing of some strains in opsonophagocytosis tests.[87] In an outbreak of group B infection, an immunotype capable of LPS sialylation was associated with invasive disease and an immunotype incapable of LPS sialylation with the carrier state.[87] Capsulation was the major virulence determinant in an intranasal infant mouse model of infection, but capability of LPS sialylation was also significant.[87]

CONCLUSIONS

In most cases we do not know in precise terms what happens to bacterial pathogens *in vivo*. This applies particularly to rates of growth and the underpinning nutrition and metabolism. The subject is neglected, and there is little chance of its revival in the near future. Turning to production of virulence determinants, it is now accepted as good practice to confirm that virulence determinants indicated by studies *in vitro* are produced *in vivo* and contribute to virulence. Furthermore, comparisons of organisms grown *in vivo* and *in vitro* to recognize bacterial components induced by the environment *in vivo* are increasing. In most cases, however, these studies are not followed up to prove that the previously unknown components are virulence determinants. As regards the influence of changing environmental conditions *in vivo* on virulence determinant production at different stages of infection, current studies *in vitro* have evoked speculation on what might happen *in vivo* but provide little specific information. Recently, methods were evolved for finding out what happens *in vivo,* and a few bright spots in current studies should encourage more people to try.

ACKNOWLEDGMENTS

The author's thanks are due to Dr. C. W. Penn and Dr. N. J. Parsons for critical reading of this manuscript and helpful suggestions.

REFERENCES

1. SMITH, H. & J. KEPPIE. 1954. Nature **173:** 869–870.
2. SMITH, H. 1958. Ann. Rev. Microbiol. **12:** 77–102.
3. SMITH, H. 1990. J. Gen. Microbiol. **136:** 377–393.
4. SMITH, H. 1991. Proc. Roy. Soc. (Lond.) B **246:** 97–105.
5. HORMAECHE, C. E., C. W. PENN & C. J. SMYTH. 1992. Molecular Biology of Bacterial Infection. Cambridge University Press. Cambridge.
6. SMITH, H. 1995. Biol. Rev. **70:** 277–316.
7. SMITH, H. 1995. *In* Virulence Mechanisms of Bacterial Pathogens, 2nd Ed., J. A. Roth, C. A. Bolen, K. A. Brogden, F. C. Minion & M. J. Wannemuehler, Eds. :335–357. ASM Press. Washington, DC.
8. PENN, C. W. 1992. Symp. Soc. Gen. Microbiol. **49:** 107–125.
9. KOLTER, R., D. A. SIEGELE & A. TORMO. 1993. Ann. Rev. Microbiol. **47:** 855–874.
10. CHATFIELD, S., J. L. LI, M. SYDENHAM, G. DOUCE & G. DOUGAN. 1992. Symp. Soc. Gen. Microbiol. **49:** 299–312.
11. WOOLDRIDGE, K. G. & P. H. WILLIAAMS. 1993. FEMS Microbiol. Rev. **12:** 325–348.
12. CORNELISSEN, C. N. & P. F. SPARLING. 1994. Microb. Pathog. **14:** 843–850.
13. WEINBERG, E. D. 1995. *In* Virulence Mechanisms of Bacterial Pathogens, 2nd Ed. J. A. Roth, C. A. Bolen, K. A. Brogden, F. C. Minion & M. J. Wannemuehler, Eds. :79–93. ASM Press. Washington, DC.
14. SMITH, H. 1992. Canad. J. Microbiol. **38:** 747–752.
15. GULIG, P. A. & T. J. DOYLE. 1993. Infect. Immun. **61:** 504–511.
16. McADAM, R. A., T. R. WEISBROD, J. MARTIN, J. D. SCUDIRE, A. M. BROWN, J. D. CIRILLO, B. R. BLOOM & W. R. JACOBS. 1995. Infect. Immun. **63:** 1004–1012.
17. GARCIA DEL PORTILLO, F., J. W. FOSTER, M. E. MAGUIRE & B. B. FINLAY. 1992. Molec. Microbiol. **6:** 3289–3297.
18. SENIOR, B. W., L. M. LOOMS & M. A. KERR. 1991. J. Med. Microbiol. **35:** 203–207.
19. JONSON, G., J. HOLMGREN & A. M. SEVENNERHOLME. 1992. Infect. Immun. **60:** 4278–4284.
20. FARFEL, Z., S. KONEN, E. WIERTZ, R. KLAPMUTS, P. A. K. ADDEY & E. HANSKI. 1990. J. Med. Microbiol. **32:** 173–177.

21. PEDERSON, S. S., A. KHARAAMI, F. ESPERSEN & N. HØIBY. 1990. Infect. Immun. **58:** 3363–3368.
22. BROMBERG, K., G. TANNIS & A. RODGERS. 1990. Med. Microbiol. Immunol. **179:** 335–338.
23. STRAUSS, D. C. & C. W. PURDY. 1994. Infect. Immun. **62:** 4675–4678.
24. BERCHE, P., K. A. REICH, M. BONNICHON, J. L. BERETTI, C. GEOFROY, J. RAVENEAU, P. COSSART, J. L. GAILLARD, P. GESLIN, H. KREIS & M. VERON. 1990. Lancet **335:** 624–627.
25. GAILLARD, J. L., J. L. BERETTI, M. BOULOT-TOLLE, J. M. WILHEIM, J. L. BERTRAND, T. HERBELLEAU & P. BERCHE. 1992. Lancet **340:** 560.
26. BOULNOIS, G. J. 1992. J. Gen. Microbiol. **138:** 249–259.
27. KARMALI, M. A., M. PETRIC, M. WINKLER, M. BIELASZEWSKA, J. BRUNTON, N. VAN DE KAR, T. MOROOKA, G. BALAKRISHNANAIR, S. E. RICHARDSON & G. S. ARBUS. 1994. J. Clin. Microbiol. **32:** 1457–1463.
28. POERREGAARD, A. 1992. Dan. Med. Bull. **39:** 155–172.
29. CORNELIS, G. R. 1992. Symp. Soc. Gen. Microbiol. **49:** 231–265.
30. FORSBERG, A., R. ROSQVIST & H. WOLF-WATZ. 1994. Trends Microbiol. **2:** 14–19.
31. OTTO, B. R., W. R. VERWEIJ, M. SPARRIUS, A. M. I. J. VERWEIJ-VAN-VWIGHT, C. E. NORD & D. M. MACLAREN. 1991. Infect. Immun. **59:** 2999–3300.
32. FOSTER, T. J. 1992. Symp. Soc. Gen. Microbiol. **49:** 173–191.
33. PORTNAY, D. A., P. S. JACKS & D. J. HINRICKS. 1988. J. Exp. Med. **167:** 1459–1471.
34. WACHTEL, M. R. & V. L. MILLER. 1995. Infect. Immun. **63:** 2541–2548.
35. PEPE, J. C. & V. L. MILLER. 1993. Proc. Natl. Acad. Sci. USA **90:** 6473–6477.
36. KROGFELT, K. A., B. A. MCCORMICK, R. L. BURGHOFF, D. C. LAUX & P. S. COHEN. 1991. Infect. Immun. **59:** 1567–1568.
37. GOLDBERG, M. B. & P. J. SANSONETTI. 1993. Infect. Immun. **61:** 4941–4946.
38. PERDOMO, O. J. J., J. M. CAVAILON, M. HUERRE, H. OHAYAN, P. GOUNON & P. J. SANSONETTI. 1994. J. Exp. Med. **180:** 1307–1319.
39. ZYCHLINSKY, A., B. KENNEY, R. MENARD, M. C. PREVOST, I. B. HOLLAND & P. J. SANSONETTI. 1994. Molec. Microbiol. **11:** 619–628.
40. FINLAY, B. B. & A. SIEBERS. 1995. *In* Virulence Mechanisms of Bacterial Pathogens, 2nd Ed. J. A. Roth, C. A. Bolen, K. A. Brogden, F. C. Minion & M. J. Wannemuehler, Eds. :33–45. ASM Press. Washington, DC.
41. LEE, J. C., S. TAKEDA, P. J. LIVOLSI & L. C. PAOLETTI. 1993. Infect. Immun. **61:** 1853–1855.
42. PIKE, W. J., A. COCKAYNE, C. A. WEBSTER, R. C. B. SLACK, A. P. SHELTON & J. P. ARBUTHNOTT. 1991. Microb. Pathog. **10:** 443–450.
43. MODUN, B., P. WILLIAMS, W. J. PIKE, A. COCKAYNE, J. P. ARBUTHNOTT, R. FINCH & S. P. DENYER. 1992. Infect. Immun. **60:** 2551–2553.
44. MCDERMID, K. P., D. W. MORCK, M. E. OLSON, M. K. DASGUPTA & J. W. COSTERTON. 1993. Infect. Immun. **61:** 1743–1749.
45. MORCK, D. W., B. D. ELLIS, P. A. G. DOMINGUE, M. E. OLSON & J. W. COSTERTON. 1991. Microbial Pathogen. **11:** 373–378.
46. DAVIES, R. L., J. MCCLUSKEY, H. A. GIBBS, J. G. COOTE, J. H. FREER & R. PARTON. 1994. Microbiology **140:** 3293–3300.
47. PANIGRAHI, P., G. LOSENSKY, L. J. DETOLLA & J. G. MORRIS, JR. 1992. Infect. Immun. **60:** 4938–4944.
48. NAUMANN, M., C. HANSKI & E. O. REICHEN. 1991. J. Med. Microbiol. **35:** 257–263.
49. PATRICK, S. & D. A. LUTTON. 1990. FEMS Microbiol. Lett. **71:** 1–4.
50. BARTHOLD, S. W., E. FIKRIG, L. K. BOCKENSTEDT & D. H. PERSING. 1995. Infect. Immun. **63:** 2255–2261.
51. INZANA, T. J., R. P. GOGLEWSKI & L. B. CORBEIL. 1992. Infect. Immun. **60:** 2943–2951.
52. WALL, R. A., H. A. DAVIES & S. P. BORRIELLO. 1989. FEMS Microbiol. Lett. **65:** 129–136.
53. GARDUNO, R. A., J. C. THORNTON & W. W. KAY. 1993. Infect. Immun. **61:** 3854–3862.
54. THORNTON, J. C., R. A. GARDUNO, S. J. CARLOSS & W. W. KAY. 1993. Infect. Immun. **61:** 4582–4589.
55. MIYAMOTO, H., S. I. YASHIDA, H. TANIGUCHI, M. H. QIN, H. FUJUO & Y. MIZUGUCHI. 1993. Microbiol Pathogen. **15:** 469–484.
56. BUCHMEIER, N. A. & F. HEFFRON. 1990. Science **248:** 730–732.

57. GOTTESMAN, S. 1984. Annu. Rev. Genet. **18:** 415–441.
58. MILLER, J. F., J. J. MEKALANOS & S. FALKOW. 1989. Science **243:** 916–922.
59. DORMAN, C. J. & H. N. N. BHRIAIN. 1992. Symp. Soc. Gen. Microbiol. **49:** 193–230.
60. DI RITA, V. J. 1992. Molec. Microbiol. **6:** 451–458.
61. MELTON, A. R. & A. A. WEISS. 1989. J. Bacteriol. **171:** 6206–6212.
62. STRALEY, S. C., G. V. PIANO, E. SKRZPEK, P. L. HADDIX & K. A. FIELDS. 1993. Molec. Microbiol. **8:** 1005–1010.
63. MAURELLI, A. T. & P. J. SANSONETTI. 1988. Proc. Natl. Acad. Sci. USA **85:** 2820–2824.
64. LITWIN, C. M. & S. B. CALDERWOOD. 1993. Clin. Microb. Rev. **6:** 137–149.
65. DAI, Z., J. C. SIRARD, M. MOCK & T. M. KOEHLER. 1995. Molec. Microbiol. **16:** 1171–1181.
66. HERRINGTON, D. A., R. H. HALL, G. LOSONSKY, J. J. MEKALANOS, R. K. TAYLOR, & M. M. LEVINE. 1988. J. Exp. Med. **168:** 1487–1492.
67. MEKALANOS, J. J. 1995. Harvey Lectures. **89:** 1–13. Wiley-Liss Inc.
68. BEATTIE, D. T., R. SHAHIN & J. J. MEKALANOS. 1992. Infect. Immun. **60:** 571–577.
69. MELTON, A. R. & A. A. WEISS. 1993. Infect. Immun. **61:** 807–815.
70. LACEY, B. W. 1960. J. Hyg. **58:** 57–93.
71. PRESTON, M. J., S. M. J. FLEISZIG, T. S. ZAIDI, J. B. GOLDBERG, V. D. SHORTRIDGE, M. L. VASIL & G. B. PIER. 1995. Infect. Immun. **63:** 3497–3501.
72. MAHAN, M. J., J. M. SLAUCH & J. J. MEKALANOS. 1993. Science **259:** 686–688.
73. MAHAN, M. J., J. M. SLAUCH, P. C. HANNA, A. CAMILLI, J. W. TOBIAS, M. K. WALDER & J. J. MEKALANOS. 1994. Infect. Agent. Dis. **2:** 263–268.
74. MAHAN, M. J., J. W. TOBIAS, J. M. SLAUCH, P. C. HANNA, R. J. COLLIER & J. J. MEKALANOS. 1995. Proc. Natl. Acad. Sci. USA **92:** 669–673.
75. CAMILLI, A., D. T. BEATTIE, & J. J. MEKALANOS. 1994. Proc. Natl. Acad. Sci. USA **91:** 2634–2638.
76. SUK, K., S. DAS, W. SUN, B. JWANG, S. W. BARTHOLD, R. A. FLAVELL & E. FIKRIG. 1995. Proc. Natl. Acad. Sci. USA **92:** 4269–4273.
77. PASCOPELLA, L., F. M. COLLINS, J. M. MARTIN, M. H. LEE, G. F. HATFULL, C. K. STOVER, B. R. BLOOM & W. R. JACOBS. 1994. Infect. Immun. **62:** 1313–1319.
78. HENSEL, M., J. E. SHEA, C. GLEESON, M. D. JONES, E. DALTON & D. W. HOLDEN. 1995. Science **269:** 400–403.
79. PLUM, G. & J. W. CLARKE-CURTISS. 1994. Infect. Immun. **62:** 476–483.
80. LENTNER, C. 1981. Geigy Scientific Tables. Vol. 1. Units of Measurement, Body Fluids, Composition of the Body, Nutrition. Ciba Geigy. Basel.
81. LENTNER, C. 1984. Geigy Scientific Tables. Vol. 3. Physical Chemistry, Composition of Blood, Hemotology, Somatometric Data. Ciba Geigy. Basel.
82. LENTNER, C. 1990. Geigy Scientific Tables. Vol. 5. Heart and Circulation. Ciba Geigy. Basel.
83. MORGAN, A. J. 1985. X-ray Micro-analysis: Electron Microscopy for Biologists. Oxford University Press. Oxford.
84. SPENCER, A. J., M. P. OSBOURNE, S. T. HADDON, J. COLLINS, W. G. STARKEY, D. C. A. CANDY & J. STEPHEN. 1990. J. Pediatr. Gastroenterol. Nutr. **10:** 516–529.
85. ARANDA, C. M. A., J. A. SWANSON, W. P. LOOMES & S. I. MILLER. 1992. Proc. Natl. Acad. Sci. USA **89:** 10079–10083.
86. POLLACK, C., S. C. STRALEY & M. S. KLEMPNER. 1986. Nature **322:** 834–836.
87. SMITH, H., N. J. PARSONS & J. A. COLE. 1995. Microb. Pathog. **18:** 365–377.
88. PARSONS, N. J. G. BOONS, P. R. ASHTON, P. B. REDFERN, P. QUIRK, Y. GAO, C. CONSTANTINIDOU, J. PATEL, J. BRAMLEY, J. A. COLE & H. SMITH. 1996. Microb. Pathog. **20:** 87–100.
89. BRAMLEY, J., R. DEMARCO DE HORMAECHE, C. CONSTANTINIDOU, X. NASSIF, N. J. PARSONS, P. JONES, H. SMITH & J. A. COLE. 1995. Microb. Pathog. **18:** 187–195.
90. SCHENKMAN, R. P. F., F. VANDEKERCKHOVE & S. SCHENKMAN. 1993. Infect. Immun. **61:** 898–902.

Integrins: Role in Cell Adhesion
and Communication

JENS GILLE AND ROBERT A. SWERLICK

Department of Dermatology
Emory University School of Medicine
Atlanta, Georgia 30322

The function of cell adhesion molecules has been a dominant focus of scientific interest over the last 20 years.[1-4] Research has been greatly facilitated by the development and refinement of specific investigative tools including affinity chromatography, monoclonal antibody technology, and molecular cloning techniques. These tools have allowed us to define specific families of cell adhesion proteins and to examine their roles in normal and pathologic processes.[5] The major families of cell adhesion molecules include integrins, immunoglobulin gene superfamily, selectins, cadherins, cartilage-link proteins, and cell surface mucins which serve as ligands for selectins. This review focuses on integrin receptors and their biologic functions in adhesive interactions, in the organization of the actin-based cytoskeleton, and in adhesion-dependent signaling events.

INTEGRINS: A HISTORICAL PERSPECTIVE

The term integrin was coined almost a decade ago to describe cell surface receptors that linked and integrated extracellular matrix proteins to the cell cytoskeleton.[6,7] Much of this work followed the development of two monoclonal antibodies directed against an avian adhesion molecule complex known as CSAT.[8] Subsequently, the employment of antibodies directed against CSAT led to identification of multifunctional adhesion complexes on mammalian cell types as well, including fibroblasts, myocytes, and neuronal cells. Antibodies to CSAT were able to localize to adhesion complexes and to inhibit their function. Unbeknown to investigators examining cell-matrix interactions, additional areas of research would ultimately converge on integrin biology from different foci. Studies of platelet function had focused on a protein complex on the surface of platelets, referred to as the GPIIb/IIIa complex.[9-12] Interaction of soluble and bound extracellular matrix proteins with the GPIIb/IIIa complex was found to be critical for platelet activation. This receptor was promiscuous in that it could interact with different extracellular matrix proteins. The description of individuals with a deficiency of leukocyte adhesion associated with absence of specific cell surface glycoproteins marked the beginning of studies that linked integrin function to control of immunity and inflammation.[13] These patients were subsequently found to lack expression of a specific integrin β chain (β_2) which leads to the inability of leukocytes to exit the vasculature and to migrate into tissues.[14] Thereafter, the very late antigens (VLA) identified on the cell surface of T cells were found to be members of integrin receptor family as well.[15] Thus, studies that previously focused on the diverse topics of cell-matrix interactions, leukocyte-endothelial cell binding, T-cell activation, and platelet aggregation finally converged on the common theme of integrin expression and function.

93

INTEGRIN STRUCTURE

All integrins are composed of noncovalently associated α and β chains which form heterodimeric receptor complexes.[7,16,17] The α and β subunits contain a large extracellular domain, a short transmembrane domain, and an intracytoplasmic carboxy-terminal domain of variable length. The extracellular domains of both the α and β chains form the ligand binding domain. At least 17 α and 8 β chains may heterodimerize to produce more than 20 different receptors (FIG. 1). Alternatively spliced variants of α and β subunits may contribute to an even greater degree of diversity and complexity in integrin receptor structure.[18,19]

The eight identified β chains share about 40–48% amino acid sequence homology.[16,20] Except for the β4 integrin chain, which is nearly twice as large because of an extremely large intracytoplasmic domain,[21] the β subunits vary minimally in size (between 90 and 110 kD). Each of the β chains contains a characteristic fourfold repeat of cysteine-rich segments and a highly conserved region in the cytoplasmic domain (FIG. 2). The conserved region contains a DXSXS (X representing any

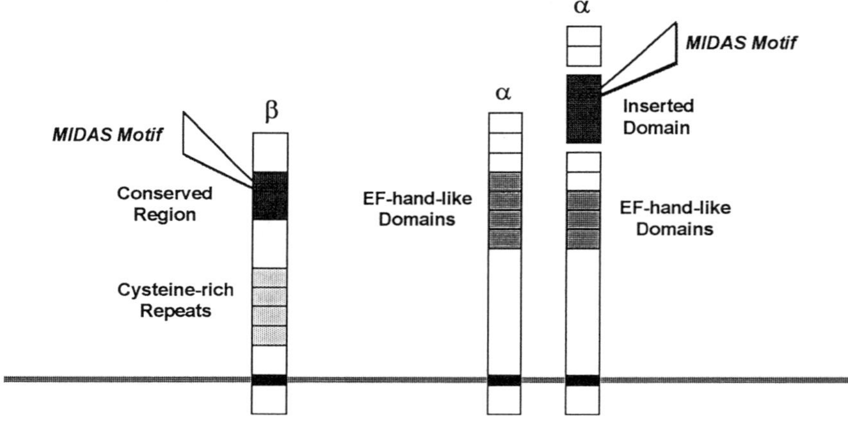

FIGURE 1. Structural domains of integrin heterodimers.

amino acid), which has been implicated in cation-dependent ligand binding and is also referred to as metal ion-dependent adhesion site or MIDAS motif.[22,23] The cytoplasmic tail sequences of the integrin β chains appear to be important in connecting to both the cytoskeletal and the signaling complex (to be discussed).[24–27]

The 17 different integrin α chains (FIG. 1) display more extended structural heterogeneity than do the β subunits.[16,20,27] Some α subunits consist of two chains, a heavy and a light chain, which are disulfide-linked in the extracellular domains (α3, α5, and α6). However, each α subunit is composed of a sevenfold repeat of homologous domains, of which three or four in each α unit contain divalent cation-binding EF-handlike domains with a conserved DXDXDXXXDXXX motif (X representing any amino acid; FIG. 2).[20] These sequences were shown to be involved in cation-dependent ligand binding to integrin receptors. The α_1, α_2, and α_E chains as well as the α subunits of all β_2 heterodimers contain an additional residue sequence which is inserted between the second and third repeat of the homologous

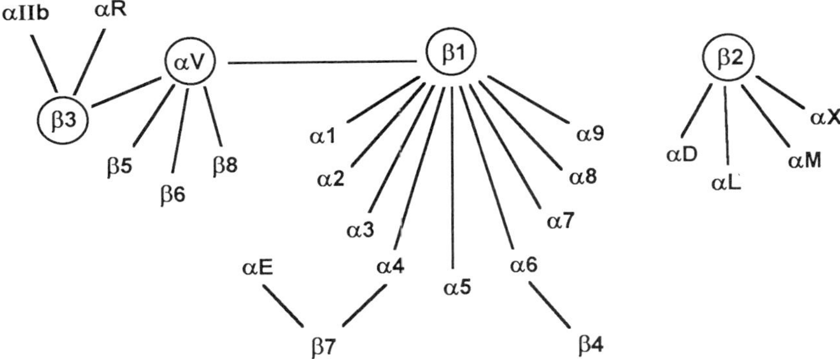

FIGURE 2. $\alpha\beta$ pairings of integrin receptors.

domain. Interestingly, this inserted domain (I domain), which shares significant homology with the collagen-binding domain of the von Willebrand factor, also contains the consensus DXSXS motif, providing these α chains with an additional potential binding site for cation-dependent integrin-ligand interactions.[23]

THE INTEGRIN FAMILY TREE

Although the possible number combinations of the different α and β chains exceeds 100, a much more limited set of heterodimers actually forms (FIG. 1). Most of these combinations can be arranged in three basic groups based on sharing common chains and/or recognizing similar matrix proteins or adhesion motifs (TABLES 1–4). These groups include integrins that contain the β_1, β_2, and β_3 or α_v chains and three complexes that fall outside the previous groups.

The largest group consists of integrins that contain the β_1 integrin chain. β_1 integrins are ubiquitously distributed on nucleated cells as well as platelets[28] (TABLE

TABLE 1. β_1 Integrin Ligands and Distribution[a]

	Ligands	Motifs	Distribution
$\alpha_1\beta_1$	Col, Lm		EC, SMC, TC, Monos
$\alpha_2\beta_1$	Col, Fn, Lm, Echovirus 1	DGEA	Plt, EC, Fb, SMC, TC, EPC
$\alpha_3\beta_1$	Col, Epiligrin, Fn, Lm, Invasin	RGD	EC, TC, EPC, Fb
$\alpha_4\beta_1$	Fn, Invasin, VCAM-1	EILDV (Fn)	TC, Monos, Eos, LC, ER
		QIDSPL (VCAM-1)	
$\alpha_5\beta_1$	Fn, Invasin	RGD	Fb, EC, Monos, TC, Plt
$\alpha_6\beta_1$	Lm, Invasin		Plts, TC, EC, EPC
$\alpha_7\beta_1$	Lm		Myocytes
$\alpha_8\beta_1$			SMC
$\alpha_9\beta_1$	Col, Lm, Tenascin	RGD	EPC, Myocytes
$\alpha_v\beta_1$	Fn, Vn	RGD	Fb

[a]Abbreviations: Fn = fibronectin, Lm = laminin, Col = collagen, EC = endothelial cells, SMC = smooth muscle cells, TC = T cells, Plt = platelets, Fb = fibroblasts, EPC = epithelial cells, Monos = monocytes, Eos = eosinophils.

TABLE 2. αv and β_3 Integrins—Ligands and Distribution[a]

	Ligands	Motifs	Distribution
$\alpha_v\beta_1$	Fn, Vn	RGD	Fb
$\alpha_v\beta_5$	Vn, HIV Tat, Adenovirus	RGD	EC, EPC, Fb, Tumors
$\alpha_v\beta_6$	Fn, Tenascin	RGD	EPC
$\alpha_v\beta_3$	Vn	RGD	Melanoma
$\alpha_v\beta_3$	Col, Fib, Fn, Lm, Opn, Pn, TSP, Vn, vWf, HIV Tat, Tenascin, Adeno-virus	RGD	EC, FB, Monos, SMC, OC, Plt, Tumors
$\alpha_{IIB}\beta_3$	Col, Fib, Fn, TSP, Vn, vWf, *Borrelia burgdorferi*	KQAGDV RGD	Plt, Mega
$\alpha_R\beta_3$	Fib, Fn, Vn, vWf	RGD	PMN

[a]Abbreviations: Col = collagen, EC = endothelial cells, Eos = eosinophils, EPC = epithelial cells, Fib = fibrinogen, Fb = fibroblasts, Fn = fibronectin, Lm = laminin, Mega = megakaryocytes, Monos = monocytes, OPN = Osteopontin, Plt = platelets, PMN = neutrophils, SMC = smooth muscle cells, TC = T cells, TSP = thrombospondin, Vn = vitronectin, vWf = von Willebrand disease.

1). With the exception of the $\alpha_4\beta_1$ complex, β_1 integrins are generally unrestricted in their expression to any given cell lineage. Because of the substantial overlap in ligand binding among β_1 integrin receptors, evaluation of the functional role of a given complex in adhesive interactions within a cellular context may not be feasible. β_1 integrin receptors generally mediate adhesion of mesenchymal and epithelial cells to matrix proteins. The $\alpha_4\beta_1$ integrin is unique in that it may mediate both cell-cell and cell-matrix binding. It is expressed on bone marrow-derived cells[15] (except for neutrophils), on certain tumor cells,[29] and in muscle development.[30] $\alpha_4\beta_1$ mediates cell-cell interactions by binding to vascular cell adhesion molecule 1 (VCAM-1) and also binds to alternatively spliced fibronectin (CS-1 region) by an RGD-independent mechanism.[31,32] Remarkably, $\alpha_4\beta_1$ may also mediate cell binding under flow conditions, a property initially found to be specific for selectins.[33,34]

A second major group of integrins shares either the $\beta3$ or the α_v integrin chain (TABLE 2). The best characterized receptors, the $\alpha_{IIB}\beta_3$ (platelet glycoprotein IIb/IIIa) and the closely related receptor $\alpha_v\beta_3$, are promiscuous in their ligand recognition. Unlike $\alpha_v\beta_3$, the $\alpha_{IIB}\beta_3$ complex on platelets requires an activation signal to mediate binding (see below). α_v is the most indiscriminate α chain, and in many respects behaves like an integrin β chain. It may form dimers with at least five different β chains, including the β_1 chain. Each of these β_3 or α_v integrin chain containing complexes recognizes RGD domains in extracellular matrix proteins and may bind to vitronectin (except for $\alpha_v\beta_6$).[35–38]

TABLE 3. β_2 Integrins—Ligands and Distribution[a]

	Ligand	Motif	Distribution
$\alpha_L\beta_2$	ICAMs (1–3)		TC, BC, LGL, Monos, PMN, Eos
$\alpha_M\beta_2$	Fib, Fn, Factor X, ICAM-1, iC3b		PMN, Monos, Macros, LGL
$\alpha_X\beta_2$	Fib, iC3b	GPRP	Monos, Macros, PMN
$\alpha_D\beta_2$			TC, Macros

[a]Abbreviations: BC = B cells, EC = endothelial cells, Eos = eosinophils, EPC = epithelial cells, FIB = fibrinogen, LGL = large granular lymphocytes, Macros = macrophages, Monos = monocytes, Plt = platelets, PMN = neutrophils, TC = T cells, iC3b = inactivated component of complement.

The third group of integrins share the β_2 integrin chain (TABLE 3). The expression of β_2 integrins is restricted to leukocytes.[39] These receptors are important for leukocyte transmigration from blood vessels. $\alpha_L\beta_2$ (LFA-1) is expressed on virtually all leukocytes and can recognize multiple members of the ICAM family of adhesion proteins. The expression of $\alpha_M\beta_2$ and $\alpha_X\beta_2$ is restricted to monocytes, macrophages, and granulocytes. These complexes may also recognize fibrinogen and inactivated C3b and are important for phagocytosis of opsonized particles and bacteria.[40]

Three complexes do not fit orderly into any of the previous groups (TABLE 4). The α_4 subunit also forms receptor complexes with the β_7 integrin chain.[41–43] Like $\alpha_4\beta_1$, this complex can bind to VCAM-1 or the CS-1 region of fibronectin. In addition, the $\alpha_4\beta_7$ integrin may serve as a ligand for the mucosal leukocyte addressin MAdCAM. The β_7 subunit also dimerizes with the α_E chain to form the leukocyte-specific integrin $\alpha_E\beta_7$. This complex is expressed on T lymphocytes associated with epithelial cells in the gut and skin.[44,45] Binding of $\alpha_E\beta_7$-containing T cells to a member of the cadherin family of adhesion molecules, E-cadherin, may represent a mechanism by which these lymphocytes remain in their respective epithelial tissues.[46] The α_6 subunit can form integrin complexes with both the β_1 and the β_4 integrin chain.[47,48] Although initially restricted to epithelial tissues, it has also been observed on endothelial cells and Schwann cells.[49]

TABLE 4. Other Integrins—Ligands and Distribution[a]

	Ligands	Motif	Distribution
$\alpha_6\beta_4$	Lm		EC, EPC, Schwann Cells
$\alpha_4\beta_7$	Fn, MAdCAM, VCAM-1	EILDV (Fn)	Gut homing TC
$\alpha_E\beta_7$	E-Cadherin		Epithelial TC

[a]Abbreviations: Lm = laminin, EC = endothelial cells, TC = T cells, Plt = platelets, EPC = epithelial cells.

INTEGRIN FUNCTION: BEYOND ADHESION

The biologic significance of integrin-mediated adhesive events goes beyond simple physical cellular linkages to matrix proteins or other cells. Adhesion was shown to be important for survival and proliferation of various cell types, and recent work has indicated that these signals are integrin mediated. Cell-matrix adhesive interactions via integrins result in a cascade of cellular responses, which ultimately not only promote cell binding but also lead to cell spreading.[50] Both integrin-mediated attachment and spreading are critical for cell survival, because cells that adhere but cannot spread may undergo programmed cell death.[50–53] In many respects, the survival signals transmitted by integrin receptors can mimic or augment signals induced by growth factors.[54] Thus, integrin receptor function not only mediates adhesive events, but also results in cell shape changes and activation of signal transduction pathways. Cell shape changes and altered transcription rates of specific genes as a consequence of integrin receptor engagement are exquisite examples indicating that adhesive interactions initiate a flow of information to regulate many fundamental cellular processes. Although adhesive functions were the first to be described and characterized, examination of integrin-dependent transduction of biochemical and mechanical signals has only recently become an active field of research, leading to rapid identification of involved molecules and proteins. A simplified view of integrin biology may distinguish between three overlapping and interacting functional complexes: the well-characterized adhesive complex, the signaling complex, and the cytoskeletal complex (FIG. 3).

INTEGRIN FUNCTION: THE ADHESIVE COMPLEX

Integrin receptors mediate adhesion to recognition sites of extracellular matrix (ECM) proteins, to cellular counterreceptors, and to soluble factors (e.g., microbial pathogens, plasma proteins, and antibodies). The combination of these adhesive interactions allows for distinct modes of integrin binding. Integrin-mediated cell-matrix interactions may result in stable adherence, as at basement membrane sites, or may exhibit a transient character to facilitate cell locomotion and migration. Many of the known integrin receptors exert competing and overlapping binding affinities for different ECM proteins (TABLES 1–4). A common motif of integrin binding sites is the RGD peptide sequence that is present in a wide range of ECM proteins. Integrins also promote homo- or heterotypic cell-cell binding as well as cell adhesion to extracellular matrices. Integrin-dependent cell-cell binding is mediated by a more restricted set of integrins. Leukocytes mostly bind to other cells via β_1 or β_2 linkages. Integrin-mediated binding through multivalent proteins, such as fibrinogen, may result in higher order aggregates of indirect cell-cell and/or cell-matrix binding complexes. For example, integrin-dependent binding of multiple platelets to fibrinogen or vWf as well as their respective matrix proteins has been implicated in platelet aggregation.[9,28] Additionally, fibrinogen may serve as a link between ICAM-1 on endothelial cells and β_3 integrins on monocytes.[55] Similarly, cell surface receptors for thrombospondin on sickle red blood cells can mediate adhesion to immobilized matrix molecules on endothelial cells.[56] Therefore, the capability of integrin receptors to interconnect multiple cellular and/or extracellular compartments allows for indirect adhesive interactions as well.

The structural consensus motif critical for integrin-ligand contact is the DXSXS sequence in concert with two additional nonadjacent threonine and aspartate residues.[22,23] This sequence, also referred to as metal ion-dependent adhesion site or MIDAS motif (see above), is present in all integrin β chains and the inserted domains of the 7 I domain-containing α chains. Cross-linking studies with RGD

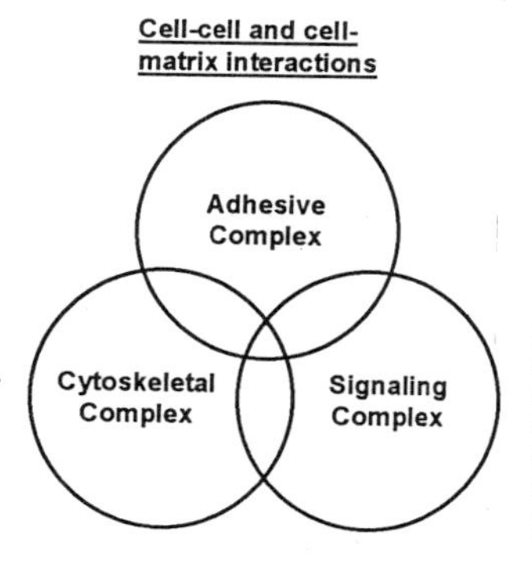

FIGURE 3. Schematic representation of the different functional integrin complexes.

TABLE 5. Factors Affecting Complexity and Specificity of Integrin Receptor Function

- Cell type-specific receptor distribution
- Level of cell surface receptor expression
- Receptor activation state, dependent upon:
  - ◇ Ligand binding of extracellular matrix (ECM) proteins, and/or of respective counter-receptors on circulating/migrating cells, and/or of soluble factors (e.g., fibrinogen, mAb)
  - ◇ Cytokines, chemokines, growth factors, hormones, divalent cations, etc.
  - ◇ Activation of other (also integrin) receptors distinct from the inactive/resting integrin receptors (e.g., T-cell receptor activation)
  - ◇ Physical stimuli (e.g., traction, hydrodynamic stress)
- Coexistence and cofunction with additional integrin and/or non-integrin receptors
- Cell type- and stimulus-dependent activation of signal transduction pathways
- Combinations of all factors within the context of space and time

peptide sequence have shown that this cation-binding MIDAS-like motif has been directly implicated in functional ligand binding to the β_3 subunit of the $\alpha_{IIB}\beta_3$ receptor.[57] Furthermore, mutations within the DXSXS motif of the β_1, β_2, and β_3 subunit have been demonstrated to prevent ligand binding, even in integrins with I region-containing α chains.[58,59] These observations would support a model in which at least one or two MIDAS motifs of the integrin receptor contributed to the cation-dependent functional ligand binding site. In regard to the α chains, additional motifs critical for ligand- and cation-binding have been observed as well.[60]

Several mechanisms may determine the quality and quantity of integrin-dependent binding events (TABLE 5). The structural properties of integrin receptor binding site and ligand, the level of receptor expression, as well as the activation state of both receptor and ligand fundamentally affect integrin adhesive function. Previously, growth factors were shown to increase the expression levels of integrin in a cell-specific context.[61] Although quiescent microvascular endothelial cells do not express $\alpha_v\beta_3$ *in vivo*, its expression is induced at sites of angiogenesis, which appears to be mediated in part by growth factors.[62] Stimulation of microvascular endothelial cells with angiogenetic factors *in vitro* resulted in comparable changes of integrin expression.[63] Additionally, the function of a given integrin complex may be altered by changes in the activation state rather than changes in gross expression. A variety of factors has been implicated in regulating receptor affinity characteristics (TABLE 5), including the membrane lipid composition,[64] the relative concentrations of divalent cations,[65–67] as well as the presence of activating cytokines or chemokines.[68,69] β_2 integrins on leukocytes are activated by proinflammatory cytokines or bacterial products, and leukocyte activation results in marked changes in receptor affinity without changes in receptor number.[39] The $\alpha_4\beta_1$ integrin complex changes binding affinity depending on the activation state. Whereas $\alpha_4\beta_1$ integrins on unactivated circulating T cells will bind the bacterial protein invasin, minimal activation of the $\alpha_4\beta_1$ receptor promotes adhesion to VCAM-1 on endothelial cells.[66] At higher levels of activation, $\alpha_4\beta_1$ will bind to the alternatively spliced forms of fibronectin via the CS-1 domain, and at even higher activation states, $\alpha_4\beta_1$ may adhere to the extracellular matrix protein thrombospondin.[70,71] Rapid changes in the activation state rather than increases in receptor expression levels are also critical for $\alpha_{IIB}\beta_3$ function on platelets in order to promote binding to fibrinogen and other ligands.[9,28,72]

INTEGRIN FUNCTION: THE CYTOSKELETAL COMPLEX

The engagement and aggregation of integrin adhesive complexes are frequently associated with the formation of so-called focal adhesions or focal contacts, in which clustered integrin receptors colocalize with intracellular cytoskeletal actin-based microfilaments. This assembly of adhesive and cytoskeletal protein complexes appears to be important in transient and stable adhesion, cell morphology, cell spreading, and cell mobility. Recent studies have established that the cytoplasmic domains of the β chain represent a key element in directing integrin receptors to focal adhesion contacts in a ligand-independent fashion, whereas the cytoplasmic tail of the α subunits sends the ligand-specific signal after integrin engagement.[24,73–75] Since integrin cytoplasmic domains lack intrinsic enzymatic activity, a model has been proposed in which physical interaction of the tail sequences with cytoskeletal proteins along with signaling molecules provides the information to regulate the assembly of the cytoskeleton. This model is supported by several studies showing accumulation and colocalization of several cytoskeletal proteins with the cytoplasmic tails of clustered integrin receptors.[27,76]

The nature of the integrin engagement appears to determine the quality and quantity of the actin-based microfilament organization.[76,77] Simple occupancy of certain integrins by monovalent ligand without induction of receptor aggregation does not lead to either protein phosphorylation (representing one of the earliest events in the signaling cascade) or accumulation of the cytoskeletal complex. A signal that induces integrin aggregation without occupying the receptor (e.g., primary antibodies linked to a clustering antibody) results in protein phosphorylation and activation of multiple signaling molecules, but it is not sufficient to induce complete accumulation of cytoskeletal proteins. Only ligand occupancy in concert with receptor aggregation induces complete accumulation of all cytoskeletal proteins. The enormous body of information on the molecular interactions of the adhesive, cytoskeletal, and signaling complex was recently arranged and reviewed in detail in excellent articles.[27,76,78]

INTEGRIN FUNCTION: THE SIGNALING COMPLEX

The signaling pathways activated by integrin receptor engagement are extensive and show considerable similarities to initiated pathways through growth factors.[54,79] The phosphorylation of distinct tyrosine residues has been shown to be an early and common event in integrin signaling. However, it has yet to be established how integrin engagement may activate tyrosine kinase activity, because the cytoplasmic integrin domains lack intrinsic enzymatic activity. An important substrate of tyrosine phosphorylation is the focal adhesion kinase (FAK),[80] which associates with a repertoire of additional kinases and signaling adapter proteins to activate various signaling pathways. The consequences of these linkages to other pathways are manifold. The induction of the RAS-MAP kinase pathway may lead to activation of transcription factors, such as NF-κB and c-Fos, thus serving as a link between integrin engagement and changes in gene transcription of affected genes.[27,81] MAP kinases can also activate latent cytoplasmic phospholipases, resulting in the release of a variety of lipid messengers. These include phospholipase A2 (PLA2), arachidonic acid, phospholipid kinases, and phospholipase C (PLC).[27,78] Activation of PLC results in the production of diacylglycerol (DAG) and inositol triphosphate, which are important mediators for the activation of multiple forms of protein kinase C.

Each of these elements appears to be important for focal adhesion formation and linkage to microfilament organization. Inhibitors of lipoxygenase or PKC may inhibit focal adhesion formation, whereas PKC stimulants may augment focal contacts assembly under certain circumstances.[27] Involvement of non-tyrosine kinase pathways in cytoskeleton formation is critical, because only a distinct subset of cytoskeletal protein requires tyrosine phosphorylation for accumulation at sites of integrin engagement.

INTEGRIN FUNCTION: COMPLEXITY VERSUS SPECIFICITY

Despite the fact that many integrins are exclusively expressed by specific cell types, a significant overlap and redundancy for binding of matrix proteins or cellular ligands exist. Various integrins recognize different ligands, which may also bind to additional integrin receptors (TABLES 1–4). The discrepancy between redundant adhesive pathways resulting in distinct responses may be explained on the basis of ligand-independent but integrin receptor-specific signaling. Several lines of evidence indicate that part of the specificity is conferred by integrin cytoplasmic domains that may transduce signals in a ligand-independent fashion.[82,83] Studies comparing the functions of a wild-type β_1 and a chimeric $\beta_{1/5}$ receptor, in which the cytoplasmic domain of β_1 was replaced with that of β_5, revealed dramatic differences in integrin-dependent proliferation and migration, but not adhesion.[83] Although the β_1 cytoplasmic tail selectively contributed to cell proliferation, the β_5 cytoplasmic domain more effectively promoted cell migration. These results support a model in which different integrin receptors utilize common mechanisms to control adhesive interactions, but translate similar adhesive information into contrasting postligand events, depending on the particular properties of the respective cytoplasmic domains.

It has also become apparent that signals generated by integrins are oftentimes similar regardless of the receptor-ligand interaction involved.[1] Therefore, it has been proposed that signal processing rather than signal generation may be critical in determining the specific responses to particular integrin interactions as well.[84] A study on extracellular matrix-dependent gene expression in epithelial cells that examined β-casein expression as a functional downstream event supports this model.[85] This study identifies at least two components of ECM-mediated signals required for β-casein expression. The first signal is a physical stimulus involving changes in cell shape, whereas the second represents a biochemical signal associated with β_1 integrin clustering and tyrosine phosphorylation. Although the biochemical stimulus (binding to laminin) resulted in signal generation (tyrosine phosphorylation) in both flat and rounded cells, only rounded cells promptly processed the signal and expressed β-casein.

An additional exciting area of distinctive integrin-specific signaling concerns cooperative effects on integrin-dependent gene expression.[86,87] Results of a recent study by Huhtala *et al.*[87] demonstrate that fibronectin-mediated signaling by the $\alpha_5\beta_1$ and the $\alpha_4\beta_1$ integrins, which recognize distinct domains on fibronectin, cooperatively regulate metalloproteinase (MMP) expression by synovial fibroblasts. Whereas engagement of the $\alpha_5\beta_1$ receptor markedly upregulates MMP expression, activation of both integrins results in considerable loss of expression. This study underscores the functional importance of coexisting neighboring receptors on the same cell, an additional putative mechanism by which specific integrin-signaling may be accomplished.

It has become evident that the nature of integrin-mediated adhesive interactions depends on numerous specific processes which ultimately result in a cascade of signaling events that determine whether cells remain stationary or migrate, grow and divide, or undergo programmed cell death or whether cells differentiate or remain undifferentiated. The understanding of how these pathways converge on physiologic and pathologic cell function will likely lead to novel therapeutic advances for the treatment of a wide variety of human diseases.

SUMMARY

Adhesive interactions are crucial for the integrity and function of all cells and tissues. As one of the major families of cell adhesion receptors, the integrins have been the focus of scientific interest for more than a decade. The resulting studies have tremendously enhanced the understanding of integrin-mediated adhesive interactions and have unveiled novel integrin functions in the cytoskeletal organization of microfilaments and in the activation of diverse signaling pathways. These functions are critically involved in the regulation of multiple processes, such as tissue development, inflammation, tumor cell growth and metastasis, and programmed cell death. The global view of integrin receptor biology has radically changed and has become much more subtle and elaborate. The enormous complexity of integrin function is determined by the heterodimeric formation of more than 20 functional integrin receptors, the cell type-specific distribution, the receptor activation state, the presence of different activation and deactivation signals, and the subsequent employment of distinct cytoskeletal and signaling complexes within a more dimensional network of time and space. This article summarizes the structural and functional properties of the integrin receptors and emphasizes some of the major achievements made in the past to enhance the understanding of integrin biology.

REFERENCES

1. JULIANO, R. L. & S. HASKILL. 1993. Signal transduction from the extracellular matrix. J. Cell Biol. **120:** 577–585.
2. GIANCOTTI, F. G. & F. MAINIERO. 1994. Integrin-mediated adhesion and signaling in tumorigenesis. Biochim. Biophys. Acta **1198:** 47–64.
3. SCHWARTZ, M. A. & D. E. INGBER. 1994. Integrating with integrins. Mol. Biol. Cell **5:** 389–393.
4. SHATTIL, S. J., M. H. GINSBERG & J. S. BRUGGE. 1994. Adhesive signaling in platelets. Curr. Opin. Cell Biol. **6:** 695–704.
5. HYNES, R. O. 1994. The impact of molecular biology on models for cell adhesion. Bioessays **16:** 663–669.
6. TAMKUN, J. W., D. W. DESIMONE, D. FONDA, R. S. PATEL, C. BUCK, A. F. HORWITZ & R. O. HYNES. 1986. Structure of integrin, a glycoprotein involved in the transmembrane linkage between fibronectin and actin. Cell **46:** 271–282.
7. RUOSLAHTI, E. & M. D. PIERSCHBACHER. 1987. New perspectives in cell adhesion: RGD and integrins. Science **238:** 491–497.
8. GREVE, J. M. & D. I. GOTTLIEB. 1982. Monoclonal antibodies which alter the morphogy of culture chick myogome cells. J. Cell Biochem. **18:** 221–230.
9. PHILLIPS, D. R., I. F. CHARO, L. V. PARISE & L. A. FITZGERALD. 1988. The platelet membrane glycoprotein GPIIb/IIIa complex. Blood **71:** 831.
10. PLOW, E. F., J. C. LOFTUS, E. G. LEVIN, D. S. FAIR, D. DIXON, J. FORSYTH & M. H. GINSBERG. 1986. Immunologic relationship between platelet membrane glycoprotein GPIIb/IIIa and cell surface molecules expressed by a variety of cells. Proc Natl. Acad. Sci. USA **83:** 376.

11. ZIMRIM, A. B., R. EISMAN, G. VILAIRE, E. SCHWARTZ, J. S. BENNETT & M. PONCZ. 1988. Structure of platelet glycoprotein IIIa. A common subunit for two different membrane receptors. J. Clin. Invest. **81:** 1470.

12. PERUTELLI, P. & P. G. MORI. 1992. The human platelet membrane glycoprotein IIb/IIIa complex: a multi functional adhesion receptor. Haematologica **77:** 162–168.

13. ANDERSON, D. C. & T. A. SPRINGER. 1989. Leukocyte adhesion deficiency: an inherited defect in the Mac-1, LFA-1, and the p150,95 glycoproteins. Annu. Rev. Med. **38:** 175–194.

14. KISHIMOTO, T. K., K. O'CONNOR, A. LEE, T. M. ROBERTS & T. A. SPRINGER. 1987. Cloning of the beta subunit of the leukocyte adhesion proteins: homology to an extracellular matrix receptor defines a novel supergene family. Cell **48:** 681–690.

15. HEMLER, M. E. 1990. VLA proteins in the integrin family: structures, functions, and their role on leukocytes. Annu. Rev. Immunol. **8:** 365–400.

16. LOFTUS, J. C., J. W. SMITH & M. H. GINSBERG. 1994. Integrin-mediated cell adhesion: the extracellular face. J. Biol. Chem. **269:** 25235–25238.

17. HYNES, R. O. 1987. Integrins: a family of cell surface receptors. Cell **48:** 549–552.

18. LANGUINO, L. R. & E. RUOSLAHTI. 1992. An alternative form of the integrin beta 1 subunit with a variant cytoplasmic domain. J. Biol. Chem. **267:** 7116–7120.

19. VAN KUPPEVELT, T. H., L. R. LANGUINO, J. O. GAILIT, S. SUZUKI & E. RUOSLAHTI. 1989. An alternative cytoplasmic domain of the integrin beta 3 subunit. Proc. Natl. Acad. Sci. USA **86:** 5415–5418.

20. HYNES, R. O. 1992. Integrins: versatility, modulation, and signalling in cell adhesion. Cell **69:** 11–25.

21. SUZUKI, S. & Y. NAITOH. 1990. Amino acid sequence of a novel integrin beta 4 subunit and primary expression of the mRNA in epithelial cells. EMBO J. **9:** 757–763.

22. LEE, J. O., P. RIEU, M. A. ARNAOUT & R. LIDDINGTON. 1995. Crystal structure of the A domain from the alpha subunit of integrin CR3 (CD11b/CD18). Cell **80:** 631–638.

23. BERGELSON, J. M. & M. E. HEMLER. 1995. Do integrins use a 'MIDAS touch' to grasp an Asp? Curr. Biol. **5:** 615–617.

24. SASTRY, S. K. & A. F. HORWITZ. 1993. Integrin cytoplasmic domains: mediators of cytoskeletal linkages and extra- and intracellular initiated transmembrane signaling. Curr. Opin. Cell Biol. **5:** 819–831.

25. YLANNE, J., Y. CHEN, T. E. O'TOOLE, J. C. LOFTUS, Y. TAKADA & M. H. GINSBERG. 1993. Distinct functions of integrin alpha and beta subunit cytoplasmic domains in cell spreading and formation of focal adhesions. J. Cell Biol. **122:** 223–233.

26. SHATTIL, S. J., B. HAIMOVICH, M. CUNNINGHAM, L. LIPFERT, J. T. PARSONS, M. H. GINSBERG & J. S. BRUGGE. 1994. Tyrosine phosphorylation of pp125FAK in platelets requires coordinated signaling through integrin and agonist receptors. J. Biol. Chem. **269:** 14738–14745.

27. CLARK, E. A. & J. S. BRUGGE. 1995. Integrins and signal transduction pathways: The road taken. Science **268:** 233–239.

28. GINSBERG, M. H., J. C. LOFTUS & E. F. PLOW. 1988. Cytoadhesins, integrins, and platelets. Thromb. Haemost. **59:** 1–6.

29. MOULD, A. P., J. A. ASKARI, S. E. CRAIG, A. N. GARRATT, J. CLEMENTS & M. J. HUMPHRIES. 1994. Integrin alpha 4 beta 1-mediated melanoma cell adhesion and migration on vascular cell adhesion molecule-1 (VCAM-1) and the alternatively spliced IIICS region of fibronectin. J. Biol. Chem. **269:** 27224–27230.

30. ROSEN, G. D., J. R. SANES, R. LACHANCE, J. M. CUNNINGHAM, J. ROMAN & D. C. DEAN. 1992. Roles for the integrin VLA-4 and its counter receptor VCAM-1 in myogenesis. Cell **69:** 1107–1119.

31. CHAN, B. M., M. J. ELICES, E. MURPHY & M. E. HEMLER. 1992. Adhesion to vascular cell adhesion molecule 1 and fibronectin. Comparison of alpha 4 beta 1 (VLA-4) and alpha 4 beta 7 on the human B cell line JY. J. Biol. Chem. **267:** 8366–8370.

32. ELICES, M. J., L. OSBORN, Y. TAKADA, C. CROUSE, S. LUHOWSKYJ, M. E. HEMLER & R. R. LOBB. 1990. VCAM-1 on activated endothelium interacts with the leukocyte integrin VLA-4 at a site distinct from the VLA-4/fibronectin binding site. Cell **60:** 577–584.

33. ALON, R., P. D. KASSNER, M. W. CARR, E. B. FINGER, M. E. HEMLER & T. A. SPRINGER.

1995. The integrin VLA-4 supports tethering and rolling in flow on VCAM-1. J. Cell Biol. **128:** 1243–1253.

34. SWERLICK, R. A., J. R. ECKMAN, A. KUMAR, M. JEITLER & T. M. WICK. 1993. Alpha 4 beta 1-integrin expression on sickle reticulocytes: Vascular cell adhesion molecule-1-dependent binding to endothelium. Blood **82:** 1891–1899.

35. NISHIMURA, S. L., D. SHEPPARD & R. PYTELA. 1994. Integrin alpha v beta 8. Interaction with vitronectin and functional divergence of the beta 8 cytoplasmic domain. J. Biol. Chem. **269:** 28708–28715.

36. MARSHALL, J. F., D. C. RUTHERFORD, A. C. MCCARTNEY, F. MITJANS, S. L. GOODMAN & I. R. HART. 1995. Alpha v beta 1 is a receptor for vitronectin and fibrinogen, and acts with alpha 5 beta 1 to mediate spreading on fibronectin. J. Cell Sci. **108:** 1227–1238.

37. WEINACKER, A., A. CHEN, M. AGREZ, R. I. CONE, S. NISHIMURA, E. WAYNER, R. PYTELA & D. SHEPPARD. 1994. Role of the integrin alpha v beta 6 in cell attachment to fibronectin. Heterologous expression of intact and secreted forms of the receptor. J. Biol. Chem. **269:** 6940–6948.

38. KIM, J. P., K. ZHANG, J. D. CHEN, R. H. KRAMER & D. T. WOODLEY. 1994. Vitronectin-driven human keratinocyte locomotion is mediated by the alpha v beta 5 integrin receptor. J. Biol. Chem. **269:** 26926–26932.

39. SPRINGER, T. A. 1990. Adhesion receptors of the immune system. Nature **346:** 425–434.

40. RELMAN, D., E. TUOMANEN, S. FALKOW, D. T. GOLENBOCK, K. SAUKKONEN & S. D. WRIGHT. 1990. Recognition of a bacterial adhesion by an integrin: macrophage CR3 (alpha M beta 2, CD11b/CD18) binds filamentous hemagglutinin of *Bordetella pertussis.* Cell **61:** 1375–1382.

41. YUAN, Q., W. M. JIANG, D. HOLLANDER, E. LEUNG, J. D. WATSON & G. W. KRISSANSEN. 1991. Identity between the novel integrin beta 7 subunit and an antigen found highly expressed on intraepithelial lymphocytes in the small intestine. Biochem. Biophys. Res. Commun. **176:** 1443–1449.

42. POSTIGO, A. A., P. SANCHEZ-MATEOS, A. I. LAZAROVITS, F. SANCHEZ-MADRID & M. O. DE LANDAZURI. 1993. Alpha 4 beta 7 integrin mediates B cell binding to fibronectin and vascular cell adhesion molecule-1. Expression and function of alpha 4 integrins on human B lymphocytes. J. Immunol. **151:** 2471–2483.

43. BERLIN, C., E. L. BERG, M. J. BRISKIN, D. P. ANDREW, P. J. KILSHAW, B. HOLZMANN, I. L. WEISSMAN, A. HAMANN & E. C. BUTCHER. 1993. Alpha 4 beta 7 integrin mediates lymphocyte binding to the mucosal vascular addressin MAdCAM-1. Cell **74:** 185.

44. RUSSELL, G. J., C. M. PARKER, K. L. CEPEK, D. A. MANDELBROT, A. SOOD, E. MIZOGUCHI, E. C. EBERT, M. B. BRENNER & A. K. BHAN. 1994. Distinct structural and functional epitopes of the alpha E beta 7 integrin. Eur. J. Immunol. **24:** 2832–2841.

45. CEPEK, K. L., C. M. PARKER, J. L. MADARA & M. B. BRENNER. 1993. Integrin alpha E beta 7 mediates adhesion of T lymphocytes to epithelial cells. J. Immunol. **150:** 3459–3470.

46. CEPEK, K. L., S. K. SHAW, C. M. PARKER, G. J. RUSSELL, J. S. MORROW, D. L. RIMM & M. B. BRENNER. 1994. Adhesion between epithelial cells and T lymphocytes mediated by E-cadherin and the alpha E beta 7 integrin. Nature **372:** 190–193.

47. NIESSEN, C. M., F. HOGERVORST, L. H. JASPARS, A. A. DE MELKER, G. O. DELWEL, E. H. HULSMAN, I. KUIKMAN & A. SONNENBERG. 1994. The alpha 6 beta 4 integrin is a receptor for both laminin and kalinin. Exp. Cell Res. **211:** 360–367.

48. LEE, E. C., M. M. LOTZ, G. D. STEELE, JR. & A. M. MERCURIO. 1992. The integrin alpha 6 beta 4 is a laminin receptor. J. Cell Biol. **117:** 671–678.

49. SEPP, N. T., L. A. CORNELIUS, N. ROMANI, L. J. LI, S. W. CAUGHMAN, T. J. LAWLEY & R. A. SWERLICK. 1995. Polarized expression and basic fibroblast growth factor-induced down-regulation of the alpha 6 beta 4 integrin complex on human microvascular endothelial cells. J. Invest. Dermatol. **104:** 266–270.

50. RUOSLAHTI, E. & J. C. REED. 1994. Anchorage dependence, integrins, and apoptosis. Cell **77:** 477–478.

51. BATES, R. C., A. BURET, D. F. VAN HELDEN, M. A. HORTON & G. F. BURNS. 1994. Apoptosis induced by inhibition of intercellular contact. J. Cell Biol. **125:** 403–415.

52. MEREDITH, J. E., JR., B. FAZELI & M. A. SCHWARTZ. 1993. The extracellular matrix as a cell survival factor. Mol. Biol. Cell **4:** 953–961.

53. RE, F., A. ZANETTI, M. SIRONI, N. POLENTARUTTI, L. LANFRANCONE, E. DEJANA & F. COLOTTA. 1994. Inhibition of anchorage-dependent cell spreading triggers apoptosis in cultured human endothelial cells. J. Cell Biol. **127:** 537–546.

54. ZACHARY, I. & E. ROSENGURT. 1992. Focal adhesion kinase (p125^{FAK}): A point of convergence in the action of neuropeptides, integrins, and oncogenes. Cell **71:** 891–894.

55. LANGUINO, L. R., J. PLESCIA, A. DUPERRAY, A. A. BRAIN, E. F. PLOW, J. E. GELTOSKY & D. C. ALTIERI. 1993. Fibrinogen mediates leukocyte adhesion to vascular endothelium through an ICAM-1 dependent pathway. Cell **73:** 1423–1434.

56. BRITTAIN, H. A., J. R. ECKMAN, R. A. SWERLICK, R. J. HOWARD & T. M. WICK. 1993. Thrombospondin from activated platelets promotes sickle erythrocyte adherence to human microvascular endothelium under physiologic flow: A potential role for platelet activation in sickle cell vaso-occlusion. Blood **81:** 2137–2143.

57. D'SOUZA, S. E., T. A. HAAS, R. S. PIOTROWICZ, V. BYERS-WARD, D. E. MCGRATH, H. R. SOULE, C. CIERNIEWSKI, E. F. PLOW & J. W. SMITH. 1994. Ligand and cation binding are dual functions of a discrete segment of the integrin beta 3 subunit: Cation displacement is involved in ligand binding. Cell **79:** 659–667.

58. BAJT, M. L., T. GOODMAN & S. L. MCGUIRE. 1995. Beta 2 (CD18) mutations abolish ligand recognition by I domain integrins LFA-1 (alpha L beta 2, CD11a/CD18) and MAC-1 (alpha M beta 2, CD11b/CD18). J. Biol. Chem. **270:** 94–98.

59. BAJT, M. L. & J. C. LOFTUS. 1994. Mutation of a ligand binding domain of beta 3 integrin. Integral role of oxygenated residues in alpha IIb beta 3 (GPIIb-IIIa) receptor function. J. Biol. Chem. **269:** 20913–20919.

60. HOGG, N., R. C. LANDIS, P. A. BATES, P. STANDLEY & A. M. RANDI. 1994. The sticking point: how integrins bind to their ligands. Trends Cell Biol. **4:** 379–382.

61. RIIKONEN, T., L. KOIVISTO, P. VIHINEN & J. HEINO. 1995. Transforming growth factor-beta regulates collagen gel contraction by increasing alpha 2 beta 1 integrin expression in osteogenic cells. J. Biol. Chem. **270:** 376–382.

62. BROOKS, P. C., R. A. CLARK & D. A. CHERESH. 1994. Requirement of vascular integrin alpha v beta 3 for angiogenesis. Science **264:** 569–571.

63. SWERLICK, R. A., E. J. BROWN, Y. XU, K. H. LEE, S. MANOS & T. J. LAWLEY. 1992. Expression and modulation of the vitronectin receptor on human dermal microvascular endothelial cells. J. Invest. Dermatol. **99:** 715–722.

64. CONFORTI, G., A. ZANETTI, I. PASQUALI-RONCHETTI, D. QUAGLINO, JR., P. NEYROZ & E. DEJANA. 1990. Modulation of vitronectin receptor binding by membrane lipid composition. J. Biol. Chem. **265:** 4011–4019.

65. HONDA, S., Y. TOMIYAMA, A. J. PELLETIER, D. ANNIS, Y. HONDA, R. ORCHEKOWSKI, Z. RUGGERI & T. J. KUNICKI. 1995. Topography of ligand-induced binding sites, including a novel cation-sensitive epitope (AP5) at the amino terminus, of the human integrin beta 3 subunit. J. Biol. Chem. **270:** 11947–11954.

66. SHIMIZU, Y. & J. L. MOBLEY. 1993. Distinct divalent cation requirements for integrin-mediated CD4+ T lymphocyte adhesion to ICAM-1, fibronectin, VCAM-1, and invasin. J. Immunol. **151:** 4106–4115.

67. KIRCHHOFER, D., J. GRZESIAK & M. D. PIERSCHBACHER. 1991. Calcium as a potential physiological regulator of integrin-mediated cell adhesion. J. Biol. Chem. **266:** 4471–4477.

68. PENBERTHY, T. W., Y. JIANG, F. W. LUSCINSKAS & D. T. GRAVES. 1995. MCP-1-stimulated monocytes preferentially utilize beta 2-integrins to migrate on laminin and fibronectin. Am. J. Physiol. **269:** C60–68.

69. LEVESQUE, J. P., D. I. LEAVESLEY, S. NIUTTA, M. VADAS & P. J. SIMMONS. 1995. Cytokines increase human hemopoietic cell adhesiveness by activation of very late antigen (VLA)-4 and VLA-5 integrins. J. Exp. Med. **181:** 1805–1815.

70. MASUMOTO, A. & M. E. HEMLER. 1993. Multiple activation states of VLA-4. Mechanistic differences between adhesion to CS1/fibronectin and to vascular cell adhesion molecule-1. J. Biol. Chem. **268:** 228–234.

71. YABKOWITZ, R., V. M. DIXIT, N. GUO, D. D. ROBERTS & Y. SHIMIZU. 1993. Activated T-cell adhesion to thrombospondin is mediated by the alpha 4 beta 1 (VLA-4) and alpha 5 beta 1 (VLA-5) integrins. J. Immunol. **151:** 149–158.

72. PHILLIPS, D. R., I. F. CHARO & R. M. SCARBOROUGH. 1991. GPIIb-IIIa: The responsive integrin. Cell **65:** 359–362.
73. KASSNER, P. D. & M. E. HEMLER. 1993. Interchangeable alpha chain cytoplasmic domains play a positive role in control of cell adhesion mediated by VLA-4, a beta 1 integrin. J. Exp. Med. **178:** 649–660.
74. KASSNER, P. D., S. KAWAGUCHI & M. E. HEMLER. 1994. Minimum alpha chain cytoplasmic tail sequence needed to support integrin-mediated adhesion. J. Biol. Chem. **269:** 19859–19867.
75. LAFLAMME, S. E., L. A. THOMAS, S. S. YAMADA & K. M. YAMADA. 1994. Single subunit chimeric integrins as mimics and inhibitors of endogenous integrin functions in receptor localization, cell spreading and migration, and matrix assembly. J. Cell Biol. **126:** 1287–1298.
76. YAMADA, K. M. & S. MIYAMOTO. 1995. Integrin transmembrane signaling and cytoskeletal control. Curr. Opin. Cell. Biol. **7:** 681–689.
77. MIYAMOTO, S., S. K. AKIYAMA & K. M. YAMADA. 1995. Synergistic roles for receptor occupancy and aggregation in integrin transmembrane function. Science **267:** 883–885.
78. SCHWARTZ, M. A. 1992. Transmembrane signalling by integrins. Trends Cell Biol. **2:** 304–308.
79. SCHLAEPFER, D. D., S. K. HANKS, T. HUNTER & P. VAN DER GEER. 1994. Integrin-mediated signal transduction linked to Ras pathway by GRB2 binding to focal adhesion kinase. Nature **372:** 786–791.
80. PARSONS, J. T., M. D. SCHALLER, J. HILDEBRAND, T. H. LEU, A. RICHARDSON & C. OTEY. 1994. Focal adhesion kinase: Structure and signalling. J. Cell Sci. Suppl. **18:** 109–113.
81. THOMAS, G. 1992. MAP kinase by any other name smells just as sweet. Cell **68:** 3–6.
82. AKIYAMA, S. K., S. S. YAMADA, K. M. YAMADA & S. E. LAFLAMME. 1994. Transmembrane signal transduction by integrin cytoplasmic domains expressed in single-subunit chimeras. J. Biol. Chem. **269:** 15961–15964.
83. PASQUALINI, R. & M. E. HEMLER. 1994. Contrasting roles for integrin beta 1 and beta 5 cytoplasmic domains in subcellular localization, cell proliferation, and cell migration. J. Cell Biol. **125:** 447–460.
84. ROSKELLEY, C. D., A. SREBROW & M. J. BISSELL. 1995. A hierarchy of ECM-mediated signalling responses regulates tissue-specific gene expression. Curr. Opin. Cell Biol. **7:** 736–747.
85. ROSKELLEY, C. D., P. Y. DESPREZ & M. J. BISSELL. 1994. Extracellular matrix-dependent tissue-specific gene expression in mammary epithelial cells requires both physical and biochemical signal transduction. Proc. Natl. Acad. Sci. USA **91:** 12378–12382.
86. BLYSTONE, S. D., I. L. GRAHAM, F. P. LINDBERG & E. J. BROWN. 1994. Integrin alpha v beta 3 differentially regulates adhesive and phagocytic functions of the fibronectin receptor alpha 5 beta 1. J. Cell Biol. **127:** 1129–1137.
87. HUHTALA, P., M. J. HUMPHRIES, J. B. MCCARTHY, P. M. TREMBLE, Z. WERB & C. H. DAMSKY. 1995. Cooperative signaling by alpha 5 beta 1 and alpha 4 beta 1 integrins regulates metalloproteinase gene expression in fibroblasts adhering to fibronectin. J. Cell Biol. **129:** 867–879.

Regulation of Chemokine Gene Expression in Human Endothelial Cells by Proinflammatory Cytokines and *Borrelia burgdorferi*

KLAUS EBNET,[a] MARKUS M. SIMON,[b]
AND STEPHEN SHAW

*Experimental Immunology Branch
National Cancer Institute
National Institutes of Health
Bethesda, Maryland 20892*

LEUKOCYTE ADHESION TO ENDOTHELIUM

Adhesion of leukocytes to microvascular endothelium is a prerequisite for their migration into tissues. This process occurs constantly in secondary lymphoid organs where naive lymphocytes migrate into distinct compartments where they meet and respond to antigen (immune surveillance). The binding of leukocytes to endothelial cells (EC) is also initiated in the course of inflammatory responses, leading to the recruitment of blood cells into the affected tissue. Therefore, adhesion of leukocytes to endothelium plays a central role in both physiologic and pathologic situations.

THE ADHESION CASCADE

Extensive studies in the past have led to the formulation of a model that describes the interaction between leukocytes and endothelium as a multistep process, the so-called "adhesion cascade."[1–4] The first step of the cascade, which can be visualized microscopically as the rolling of leukocytes along the endothelial surface, slows down the velocity of the rolling lymphocyte approximately 100-fold compared to the flow velocity of the blood[5] and provides close spatial proximity between the two cell types. In the second step, leukocytes are activated by signals present at the luminal surface of the endothelium. In the third step, leukocytes firmly adhere to the activated EC and finally extravasate into the affected tissue.

The molecules involved in the first and third steps of the cascade have been characterized in detail. It is generally accepted that tethering or primary adhesion is mediated by interaction between selectins and their carbohydrate ligands.[6] Firm adhesion involves the interaction between integrins on the leukocyte surface ("transformed" into the active conformation by the triggering step) and immunoglobulin (Ig)-superfamily members on the EC surface such as ICAM-1, VCAM-1, and MAdCAM-1.[1,2] Modifications of this model came recently from the observations that some integrins and their counterreceptors also support tethering and rolling.[7,8]

---

[a] Present address: Institute of Cell Biology, ZMBE, University of M=FCnster, Mendelstr. 11, D-48149 M=FCnster, Germany.
[b] Max-Planck-Institut fuer Immunbiologie, Stuebeweg 51, D-79108 Freiburg, Germany.

Primary candidates for the second step are chemoattractants including the classic chemoattractants and the recently described family of chemotactic cytokines, the so-called chemokines.[9] The model of chemokines as mediators of the triggering step is attractive for several reasons. First, they act via seven-transmembrane domain G-protein–coupled receptors which are used for other time-critical sensory functions.[10] Second, they are positively charged and can interact with negatively charged proteoglycans at the EC surface.[11] The resulting retention in the glycocalyx prevents washout by the blood flow. A role for chemokine immobilization in triggering strong adhesion was suggested for interleukin 8 (IL-8) and macrophage inflammatory protein (MIP)-1β.[12,13] Third, they exist in a large number with more than 25 chemokines described so far. Because the tissue- and lymphocyte subset-specific homing is assumed to result from the combination of at least one distinct receptor-ligand pair at each of the three steps, a large number of chemokines as potential triggering molecules increases the number of possible combinations and therefore contributes to specificity and diversity in lymphocyte homing.[1,4]

CHEMOKINE PRODUCTION BY ENDOTHELIAL CELLS

At least six of the chemokines described so far are produced by EC. Among these, monocyte chemotactic protein (MCP)-1 and IL-8 are most extensively analyzed and been described in both *in vivo* and *in vitro* model systems.[9,14] In addition, RANTES and IFN-γ-inducible protein 10 (IP-10) are produced by endothelium *in vivo*.[15,16] Gro-α expression is inducible by a variety of stimuli *in vitro*.[17,18] We recently found that monokine induced by gamma interferon (mig) is inducible in cultured endothelium by inflammatory stimuli and bacterial endotoxin (K. Ebnet, J. M. Farber, and S. Shaw, manuscript submitted).

Among the strongest inducers of chemokine production by EC are the classic proinflammatory cytokines tumor necrosis factor-alpha (TNF-α), IL-1, and gamma interferon (IFN-γ). Chemokine expression can be induced by other soluble factors like immune-derived cytokines such as IL-4 and IL-10[19,20] or histamine[21] and thrombin[22] but also by bacterial products such as lipopolysaccharides (LPS)[9] or capsular polysaccharides from the gram-positive *Staphylococcus aureus*.[23]

REGULATION OF CHEMOKINE PRODUCTION IN ENDOTHELIAL CELLS BY PROINFLAMMATORY CYTOKINES

In the first step, we analyzed how endothelial cells transform an inflammatory signal into a chemokine response. In particular, we were interested in the kinetics of EC activation and whether different stimulating agents lead to different patterns of the chemokine response. To this end, human cultured EC (SV-40 transformed microvascular-derived EC line HMEC-1[24] or human umbilical vein EC [HUVEC]) were stimulated with various proinflammatory cytokines and analyzed for the induction of chemokine mRNAs by a semiquantitative polymerase chain reaction (PCR) approach.

Six chemokine genes were found to be upregulated in HMEC-1 cells and HUVEC by a combination of TNF-α, IL-1β, and IFN-γ at 100 U/ml each, including the CC chemokines RANTES and MCP-1 and the CXC chemokines IL-8, gro-α, IP-10, and mig. On the other hand, MIP-1α and MIP-1β were not induced under these conditions (TABLE 1).

ENDOTHELIAL CELLS RAPIDLY UPREGULATE CHEMOKINE GENE EXPRESSION IN RESPONSE TO INFLAMMATORY CYTOKINES

To avoid extensive damage of host tissue by a pathogen, it is advantageous for the host to mount an inflammatory response as quickly as possible. If chemokines play a central role in the regulation of an inflammatory response, they are expected to be rapidly upregulated during inflammation. To analyze the kinetics of chemokine mRNA upregulation in response to inflammatory stimuli, HMEC-1 cells and HUVEC were stimulated for various time periods with a combination of TNF-α, IL-1β, and IFN-γ at 100 U/ml each. From the five chemokines tested, MCP-1, IL-8, and IP-10 were rapidly upregulated, reaching approximately 70% of the maximal response after 30 minutes (FIG. 1, data are shown for HMEC-1; similar results were obtained with HUVEC). Mig upregulation was somewhat slower with a half-maximal response after about 50 minutes. RANTES required about 2 hours to reach the half-maximal level. These data indicate that the endothelium can respond extremely

TABLE 1. Chemokine Gene Expression in Cultured Human Endothelial Cells[a]

		HMEC-1			HUVEC	
Chemokine	Class	Not Stim.	Mix (4 h)	LPS (4 h)	Not Stim.	Mix (4 h)
RANTES	CC	−	+	+	−	+
MIP-1α	CC	−	−	−	nd	nd
MIP-1β	CC	−	−	−	nd	nd
MCP-1	CC	+/−	++	++	+/−	++
IL-8	C × C	+/−	++	++	+/−	++
gro-α	C × C	−	++	++	−	++
IP-10	C × C	−	++	++	−	+
mig	C × C	−	++	++	−	+

[a]Human endothelial cells (HMEC-1, a human microvascular derived endothelial cell line, and HUVEC, human umbilical vein endothelial cells) were stimulated for 4 hours with a mix of proinflammatory cytokines (TNF-α, IL-1β, and IFN-γ, 100 U/ml each) or with bacterial lipopolysaccharide (LPS) (1 μg/ml). Chemokine gene expression was analyzed by RT-PCR. Symbols: − = negative; +/− = weak; + = strong; ++ = very strong. Abbreviations: nd = not done; not stim. = not stimulated.

fast to proinflammatory cytokines with chemokine upregulation. However, they also suggest that distinct chemokines are differentially regulated. As expected from their rapid induction, all chemokines were upregulated in the presence of the protein synthesis inhibitor cycloheximide (data not shown), indicating that new protein synthesis is not required.

ENDOTHELIAL CELLS RESPOND TO LOW DOSES OF PROINFLAMMATORY CYTOKINES

At the beginning of an infection, tissue-derived inflammatory signals might be limiting. However, it is at this stage that an effective immune response against the pathogen is required to limit replication of the pathogen. To analyze the potential of the endothelium to respond to low doses of inflammatory stimuli, HMEC-1 cells were stimulated with various doses of a mix of TNF-α, IL-1β, and IFN-γ and

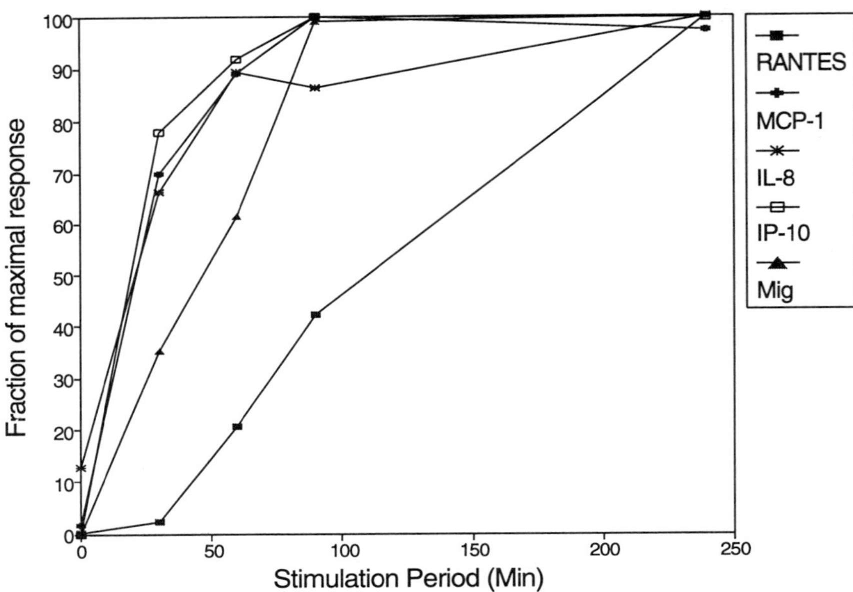

FIGURE 1. Kinetics of chemokine gene expression in HMEC-1 endothelial cells in response to proinflammatory cytokines. HMEC-1 cells were incubated with TNF-α, IL-1β, and IFN-γ (100 U/ml each) for 4 hours. Total RNA was reverse transcribed, and the cDNA was amplified by polymerase chain reaction (PCR) with primers specific for the various chemokine genes. The PCR products were hybridized with internal oligonucleotide probes using enhanced chemiluminescence. Signals were analyzed by laser densitometry and corrected for differences in the levels of the housekeeping gene glyceraldehyde phosphate dehydrogenase (GAPDH).

analyzed for the upregulation of chemokine mRNAs by RT-PCR. MCP-1 and IL-8 were significantly upregulated at a dose of 0.1 U/ml of the cytokine mix (FIG. 2; similar results were obtained with HUVEC). For RANTES, IP-10, and mig an increase in mRNA levels was observed at 1–10 U/ml of cytokine mix. These results indicate a high sensitivity of EC against inflammatory cytokines and suggest the potential of the endothelium to amplify a weak inflammatory cytokine signal into a strong chemokine signal.

DISTINCT STIMULI SYNERGIZE IN THE STIMULATION OF ENDOTHELIAL CELLS TO PRODUCE CHEMOKINES

Production of chemokines can be induced by a variety of stimuli, and two inflammatory mediators often upregulate the expression of a given chemokine in a synergistic manner. For example, both IP-10 and RANTES are synergistically induced by TNF-α and IFN-γ.[25,26] To analyze cooperation of inflammatory cytokines in the upregulation of chemokine genes in EC, HMEC-1 cells and HUVEC were stimulated for 4 hours with TNF-α, IL-1β, and IFN-γ at 1 U/ml either individually or in all possible combinations. As shown in FIGURE 3 (data are shown for HMEC-1; HUVEC gave similar results), we observed synergism between TNF-α and IFN-γ for RANTES, IP-10, and mig. In addition, TNF-α synergized with IL-1β in the upregulation of RANTES, and IL-1β synergized with IFN-γ in the induction of IP-10. By contrast, no synergism was observed for MCP-1 and IL-8 (data shown for MCP-1 only). Our results suggest that synergistic induction of chemokines is a more general mechanism and reflects the potential of the endothelium to respond to an array of distinct stimuli with different chemokine production.

BORRELIA BURGDORFERI INCREASES CHEMOKINE GENE EXPRESSION IN ENDOTHELIAL CELLS

Upregulation of chemokines in EC results not only from the binding of host-derived soluble mediators but also from interaction with pathogens. The most potent agent is bacterial LPS which induces RANTES, MCP-1, IL-8, gro-α, IP-10, and mig in EC (TABLE 1). Moreover, other bacterial products such as capsular polysaccharide of *Staphylococcus aureus* can induce chemokine expression in EC.[23] We analyzed the potential of the spirochete *B. burgdorferi*, the causative agent of Lyme disease, to induce chemokine expression in EC. Cultured HMEC-1 EC were incubated with either sonicated preparations of *B. burgdorferi* strain ZS7[27] (25 μg/ml, dry weight) or whole organisms (10^8/ml) as described previously.[28] In addition, EC were stimulated with bacterial preparations containing either complete LPS (*Salmonella abortus equi*, 10 μg/ml, dry weight) or only the core polysaccharide of LPS (*E. coli* LE 392, 10 μg/ml, dry weight). *B. burgdorferi* structures, similar to bacteria

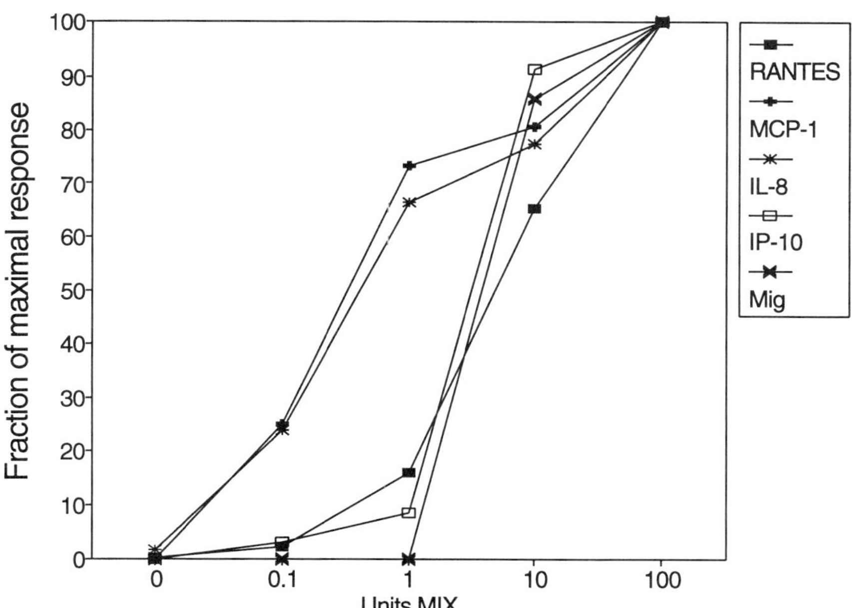

FIGURE 2. Dose response of chemokine genes expressed in cytokine-activated endothelial cells. HMEC-1 cells were stimulated for 4 hours with TNF-α, IL-1β, and IFN-γ (cytokine mix) at the indicated concentrations. Chemokine gene expression was analyzed as described in FIGURE 1. Upregulation of MCP-1 and IL-8 requires only 0.1 U/ml of the cytokine mix; RANTES, IP-10, and mig require between 1 and 10 U/ml.

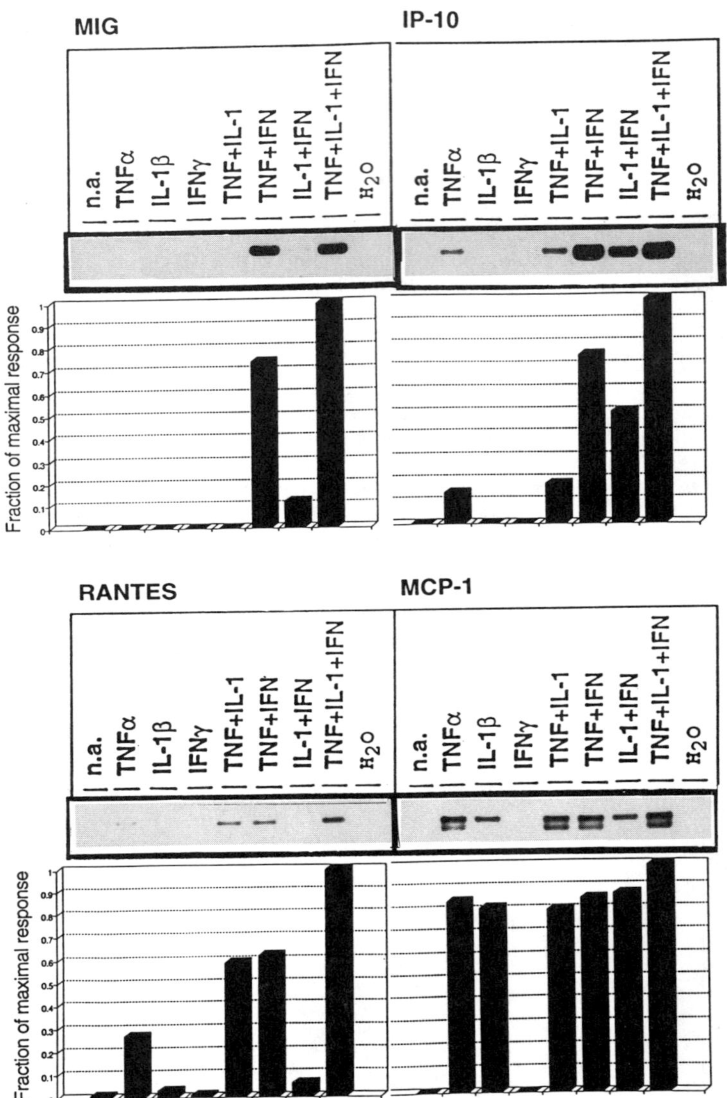

FIGURE 3. Synergistic upregulation of chemokine gene expression in endothelial cells by proinflammatory cytokines. HMEC-1 endothelial cells were stimulated for 4 hours with TNF-α, IL-1β, and IFN-γ either individually or in all possible combinations. Chemokine gene expression was analyzed as described in FIGURE 1. Synergism between proinflammatory cytokines is observed for mig, IP-10, and RANTES.

containing LPS or purified LPS or inflammatory cytokines, upregulated the expression of all six chemokines (FIG. 4). In addition to chemokines, *B. burgdorferi* also induced an increase in the mRNA expression levels of EC surface molecules, that is, E-selectin, ICAM-1, and VCAM-1, which play central roles in the binding of leukocytes to EC. The latter findings are in line with previous observations describing the upregulation of E-selectin, P-selectin, ICAM-1, and VCAM-1 *in vitro* as well as *in vivo*.[28,29]

B. BURGDORFERI UPREGULATES CHEMOKINE GENE EXPRESSION IN FIBROBLASTS

After their deposition in the dermis during the blood meal of ticks and during their dissemination in the body, *B. burgdorferi* organisms encounter different tissues

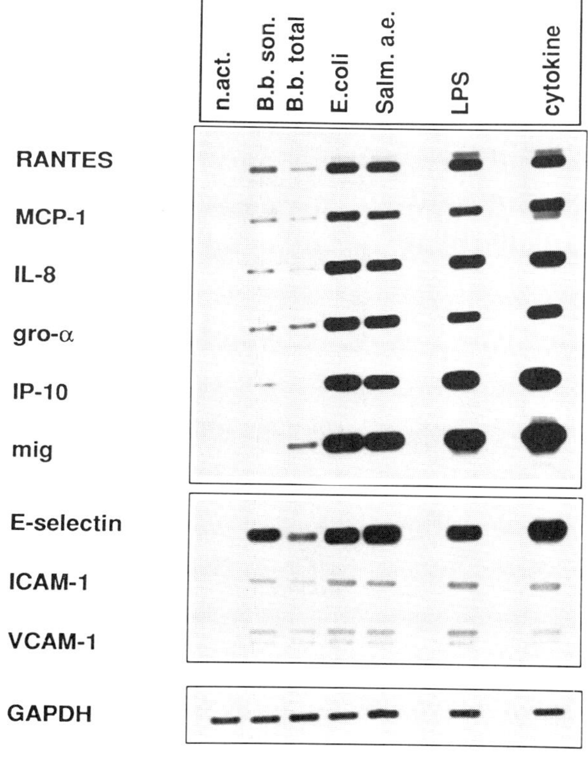

FIGURE 4. Induction of chemokine gene expression in endothelial cells by *B. burgdorferi.* HMEC-1 endothelial cells were incubated with sonicated (B.b. son., 25 μg/ml, dry weight) or intact, (B.b. total, 10^8/ml) preparations of *B. burgdorferi.* Bacterial strains expressing lipopolysaccharide (LPS) (*Escherichia coli* [E. coli] LE392 and *Salmonella abortus equi* [*Salm. a. e.*], each at 10 μg/ml, dry weight), purified LPS (1 μg/ml), and a mix of TNF-α, IL-1β, and IFN-γ (cytokine, 100 U/ml each) were used as controls. Chemokine and adhesion molecule gene expression was analyzed as described in FIGURE 1.

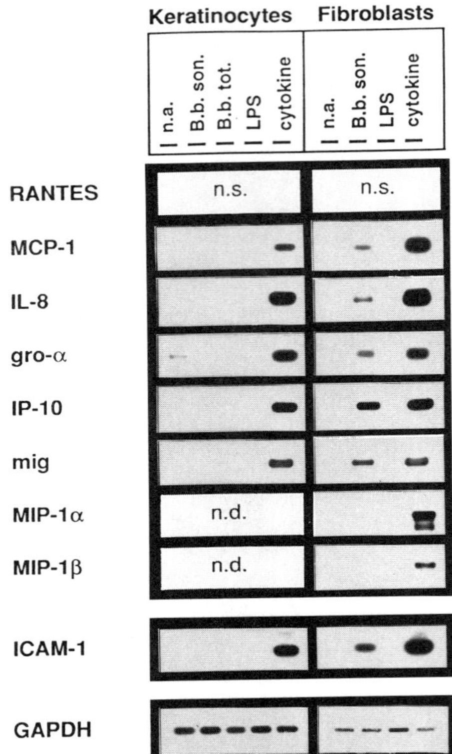

FIGURE 5. Induction of chemokine gene expression in fibroblasts by *B. burgdorferi*. Primary cultures of human keratinocytes and human skin-derived fibroblasts were stimulated in serum-free medium for 4 hours with *B. burgdorferi* sonicate (B.b. son., 25 μg/ml dry weight) or whole *B. burgdorferi* bacteria (B.b. tot., 10^8/ml). A cytokine mix (TNF-α, IL-1β, and IFN-γ, cytokine, 100 u/ml each) was used as positive control. Expression of chemokine and adhesion molecule genes was analyzed as described in FIGURE 1.

and the associated cell types including keratinocytes and fibroblasts in the skin. Because many chemokines can be produced by a variety of cell types,[9] we asked whether *B. burgdorferi* structures could induce chemokine upregulation in human keratinocytes or fibroblasts. Primary cultures of keratinocytes and skin-derived fibroblasts were incubated for 4 hours with *B. burgdorferi* preparations. Cells were harvested and analyzed for the upregulation of chemokine genes. Whereas no upregulation was induced in keratinocytes, genes encoding MCP-1, IL-8, gro-α, IP-10, mig, and ICAM-1 were upregulated in fibroblasts (FIG. 5). MIP-1α and MIP-1β were not induced by *B. burgdorferi* in fibroblasts even though they are inducible by proinflammatory cytokines.

SUMMARY

Chemokines play a central role in the process of leukocyte recruitment to tissues. By their chemotactic activity they guide leukocytes to the site of infection/injury.

Chemokines have been suggested to trigger firm adhesion of leukocytes to activated endothelial cells[12,13] as well as the subsequent diapedesis.[30,31] For these functions, chemokines produced by EC are particularly well suited.

Our experiments with proinflammatory stimuli demonstrate that chemokines are induced in EC by a variety of stimuli including inflammatory cytokines and bacterial structures such as LPS and preparations of *B. burgdorferi.* The induction of chemokines by all of these agents occurs rapidly and does not require new protein synthesis. Two chemokines, MCP-1 and IL-8, respond to very low doses (0.1–1 U/ml) of proinflammatory cytokines which is important at the beginning of an immune response when soluble inflammatory mediators might still be limiting. The chemokines RANTES, IP-10, and mig show synergistic induction by low doses (1 U/ml) of several inflammatory mediators, which again is important when only limiting amounts of inflammatory stimuli are present.

The upregulation of six chemokine genes as well as genes encoding adhesion molecules in two cell types, EC and fibroblasts, by *B. burgdorferi* suggests that chemokines might play a central role in the regulation of spirochete-induced inflammatory responses and the subsequent immune responses. Recent evidence suggests that T cells with pathogenic potential contribute to chronic inflammation at the late stage of Lyme disease.[32] Therefore, the use of therapeutic agents that block chemokine activity might be useful in treating chronic Lyme arthritis.

ACKNOWLEDGMENTS

We thank Dr. E. Ades for providing HMEC-cells, Dr. M. Bartlett for providing HUVECs and helpful comments on the manuscript, and Dr. A. Sarin for helpful comments on the manuscript.

REFERENCES

1. SPRINGER, T. A. 1994. Traffic signals for lymphocyte recirculation and leukocyte emigration: The multistep paradigm. Cell **76:** 301–314.
2. CARLOS, T. M. & J. HARLAN. 1994. Leukocyte endothelial adhesion molecules. Blood **84:** 2068–2101.
3. SHIMIZU, Y., W. NEWMAN, Y. TANAKA & S. SHAW. 1992. Lymphocyte interactions with endothelial cells. Immunol. Today **13:** 106–112.
4. BUTCHER, E. C. 1991. Leukocyte-endothelial cell recognition: Three (or more) steps to specificity and diversity. Cell **67:** 1033–1036.
5. KISHIMOTO, T. K., R. S. LARSON, A. L. CORBI, M. L. DUSTIN, D. E. STAUNTON & T. A. SPRINGER. 1989. The leukocyte integrins. Adv. Immunol. **46:** 149–182.
6. TEDDER, T. F., D. A. STEEBER, A. CHEN & P. ENGEL. 1995. The selectins: Vascular adhesion molecules. FASEB J. **9:** 866–873.
7. BERLIN, C., R. F. BARGATZE, J. J. CAMPBELL, U. H. VON ANDRIAN, M. C. SZABO, S. R. HASSLEN, R. D. NELSON, E. L. BERG, S. L. ERLANDSEN & E. C. BUTCHER. 1995. α4 integrins mediate lymphocyte attachment and rolling under physiologic flow. Cell **80:** 413–422.
8. ALON, R., P. D. KASSNER, M. W. CARR, E. B. FINGER, M. E. HEMLER & T. A. SPRINGER. 1995. The integrin VLA-4 supports tethering and rolling in flow on VCAM-1. J. Cell Biol. **128:** 1243–1253.
9. BAGGIOLINI, M., B. DEWALD & B. MOSER. 1994. Interleukin-8 and related chemotactic cytokines—CXC and CC chemokines. Adv. Immunol. **55:** 97–179.
10. MURPHY, P. M. 1994. The molecular biology of leukocyte chemoattractant receptors. Annu. Rev. Immunol. **12:** 593–633.
11. WITT, D. P. & A. D. LANDER. 1994. Differential binding of chemokines to glycosaminoglycan subpopulations. Curr. Biol. **4:** 394–400.

12. WEBB, L. M. C., M. U. EHRENGRUBER, I. CLARK-LEWIS, M. BAGGIOLINI & A. ROT. 1993. Binding to heparan sulfate or heparin enhances neutrophil responses to interleukin 8. Proc. Natl. Acad. Sci. USA **90:** 7158–7162.

13. TANAKA, Y., D. H. ADAMS, S. HUBSCHER, H. HIRANO, U. SIEBENLIST & S. SHAW. 1993. T-cell adhesion induced by proteoglycan-immobilized cytokine MIP-1β. Nature **361:** 79–82.

14. FURIE, M. B. & G. J. RANDOLPH. 1995. Chemokines and tissue injury. Am. J. Pathol. **146:** 1287–1301.

15. DEVERGNE, O., A. MARFAING-KOKA, T. J. SCHALL, M.-B. LEGER-RAVET, M. SADICK, M. PEUCHMAUR, M.-C. CREVON, T. KIM, P. GALANAUD & D. EMILIE. 1994. Production of the RANTES chemokine in delayed-type hypersensitivity reactions: Involvement of macrophages and endothelial cells. J. Exp. Med. **179:** 1689–1694.

16. NARUMI, S., L. M. WYNER, M. H. STOLER, C. S. TANNENBAUM & T. HAMILTON. 1992. Tissue-specific expression of murine IP-10 mRNA following systemic treatment with interferon γ. J. Leukocyte Biol. **52:** 27–33.

17. WEN, D., A. ROWLAND & R. DERYNCK. 1989. Expression and secretion of gro/MGSA by stimulated human endothelial cells. EMBO J. **8:** 1761–1766.

18. SCHWARTZ, D., A. ANDALIBI, L. CHAVERRI-ALMADA, J. A. BERLINER, T. KIRCHGESSNER, Z.-T. FANG, P. TEKAMP-OLSON, A. J. LUSIS, C. GALLEGOS, A. M. FOGELMAN & M. C. TERRITO. Role of the GRO family of chemokines in monocyte adhesion to MM-LDL-stimulated endothelium. J. Clin. Invest. **94:** 1968–1973.

19. ROLLINS, B. J. & J. S. POBER. 1991. Interleukin-4 induces the synthesis and secretion of MCP-1/JE by human endothelial cells. Am. J. Pathol. **138:** 1315–1319.

20. SIRONI, M., C. MUNOZ, T. POLLICINO, A. SIBONI, F. L. SCIACCA, S. BERNASCONI, A. VECCHI, F. COLOTTA & A. MANTOVANI. 1993. Divergent effects of interleukin-10 on cytokine production by mononuclear phagocytes and endothelial cells. Eur. J. Immunol. **23:** 2692–2695.

21. JEANNIN, P., Y. DELNESTE, P. GOSSET, S. MOLET, P. LASSALLE, Q. HAMID, A. TSICOPOULOS & A. B. TONNEL. 1994. Histamine induces interleukin-8 secretion by human endothelial cells. Blood **84:** 2229–2233.

22. COLOTTA, F., F. L. SCIACCA, M. SIRONI, W. LUINI, M. J. RABIET & A. MANTOVANI. 1994. Expression of monocyte chemotactic protein-1 by monocytes and endothelial cells exposed to thrombin. Am. J. Pathol. **144:** 975–985.

23. SOELL, M., M. DIAB, G. HAAN-ARCHIPOFF, A. BERETZ, C. HERBELIN, B. POUTREL & J.-P. KLEIN. 1995. Capsular polysaccharide types 5 and 8 of Staphylococcus aureus bind specifically to human epithelial (KB) cells, endothelial cells, and monocytes and induce release of cytokines. Infect. Immun. **63:** 1380–1386.

24. ADES, E. A., F. J. CANDAL, R. A. SWERLICK, V. G. GEORGE, S. SUMMERS, D. C. BOSSE & T. J. LAWLEY. 1992. HMEC-1: Establishment of an immortalized human microvascular endothelial cell line. J. Invest. Dermatol. **99:** 683–690.

25. OHMORI, Y. & T. A. HAMILTON. 1995. The interferon-stimulated response element and a κB site mediate synergistic induction of murine IP-10 gene transcription by IFN-γ and TNF-α. J. Immunol. **154:** 5235–5244.

26. MARFAING-KOKA, A., O. DEVERGNE, G. GORGONE, A. PORTIER, T. J. SCHALL, P. GALANAUD & D. EMILIE. 1995. Regulation of the production of the RANTES chemokine by endothelial cells. J. Immunol. **154:** 1870–1878.

27. SCHAIBLE, U. E., M. D. KRAMER, C. MUSETEANU, G. ZIMMER, H. MOSSMAN & M. M. SIMON. 1989. The severe combined immunodeficiency (SCID) mouse: A laboratory model for the analysis of Lyme arthritis and carditis. J. Exp. Med. **170:** 1427–1432.

28. BOEGGEMEYER, E., T. STEHLE, U. E. SCHAIBLE, M. HAHNE, D. VESTWEBER & M. M. SIMON. 1994. Borrelia burgdorferi upregulates the adhesion molecules E-Selectin, P-Selectin, ICAM-1 and VCAM-1 on mouse endothelioma cells in vitro. Cell Adh. Comm. **2:** 145–157.

29. SCHAIBLE, U. E., D. VESTWEBER, E. C. BUTCHER, T. STEHLE & M. M. SIMON. 1994. Expression of endothelial cell adhesion molecules in joints and heart during Borrelia burgdorferi infection in mice. Cell Adh. Comm. **2:** 465–479.

30. HUBER, A. R., S. L. KUNKEL, R. F. TODD III & S. J. WEISS. 1991. Regulation of transendothelial neutrophil migration by endogenous interleukin-8. Science **254:** 99–102.

31. RANDOLPH, G. J. & M. B. FURIE. 1995. A soluble gradient of endogenous monocyte chemoattractant protein-1 promotes the transendothelial migration of monocytes in vitro. J. Immunol. **155:** 3610–3618.

32. LENGL-JANSSEN, B., A. F. STRAUSS, A. C. STEERE & T. KAMRADT. 1994. The T helper cell response in Lyme arthritis: Differential recognition of *Borrelia burgdorferi* outer surface protein A in patients with treatment-resistant or treatment-responsive Lyme arthritis. J. Exp. Med. **180:** 2069–2078.

Systemic and Mucosal Protective Immunity to Pneumococcal Surface Protein A

DAVID E. BRILES,[a–c] REBECCA CREECH TART,[a]
HONG-YIN WU,[a] BETH A. RALPH,[a]
MICHAEL W. RUSSELL,[a,d] AND LARRY S. McDANIEL[a]

*Departments of Microbiology,[a] Comparative Medicine,[b] Pediatrics,[c]
and Oral Biology[d]
University of Alabama at Birmingham
Birmingham, Alabama 35294-2170*

Streptococcus pneumoniae causes more fatal infections worldwide than does almost any other pathogen.[1,2] In the United States, deaths caused by *S. pneumoniae* exceed those caused by AIDS.[2] Most fatal pneumococcal infections in the United States occur in individuals over 65 years of age, in whom *S. pneumoniae* is the most common cause of community-acquired pneumonia. In the developed world, most pneumococcal deaths occur in the elderly or in immunodeficient patients including those with sickle cell disease. In the less developed areas of the world, pneumococcal infection is one of the greatest causes of death among children under 5 years of age.[3–6] The increase in frequency of multiple antibiotic resistance among pneumococci and the prohibitive cost of drug treatment in poor countries make the present prospects for control of pneumococcal disease problematic.[7–9]

Humans acquire pneumococci through aerosols or by direct contact. The organisms first colonize the upper airways and can remain on nasal mucosa for weeks or months. As many as 50% or more of young children and the elderly are colonized with *S. pneumoniae*. In most cases this colonization results in no apparent infection.[10,11] Studies of outbreak strains suggest that even highly virulent strains can colonize without causing disease. In some individuals, however, the organism carried in the nasopharynx can give rise to symptomatic sinusitis or middle ear infections. If pneumococci are aspirated into the lung, especially with food particles or mucus, they can cause pneumonia. Infections in the lung generally shed pneumococci into the blood, which can lead to sepsis especially if organisms continue to enter the blood in large numbers. Blood-borne pneumococci can reach the brain and cause meningitis. Although pneumococcal meningitis is less common than other infections caused by *S. pneumoniae,* it is particularly devastating; 10% of patients die and most survivors have life-long neurologic sequelae.[12,13]

In elderly adults, the present 23-valent capsular polysaccharide (PS) vaccine is about 60% effective against invasive pneumococcal disease with strains of the capsular types included in the vaccine.[14,15] The 23-valent vaccine is not effective in children less than 2 years of age, because of their inability to respond adequately to most polysaccharides.[16,17] Improved vaccines to protect children and adults against invasive infections with pneumococci are needed.

In immunization of young children with *Haemophilus influenzae* group b PS-protein conjugates, carriage was reduced from about 4% to less than 1%,[18] a possible explanation being concomitant herd immunity.[19] If a vaccine could prevent coloniza-

118

tion by pneumococci, it would be expected to prevent virtually all pneumococcal infections in the immunized subjects. Inasmuch as nonimmunized patients must acquire pneumococci from others, a vaccine that reduced carriage should reduce infections in immunocompromised as well as nonimmunized members of the population.

Intramuscular immunization with capsular PS vaccines has been effective in reducing the incidence of pneumococcal sepsis in the elderly,[15] yet it has not been reported to affect pneumococcal carriage rates in children up to 54 months of age.[20,21] Whether the pneumococcal PS-protein conjugate vaccine will reduce carriage in children is not yet known. We recently showed, however, that immunization with pneumococcal surface protein A (PspA) can protect mice against sepsis, intratracheal infections, and carriage of *S. pneumoniae*.

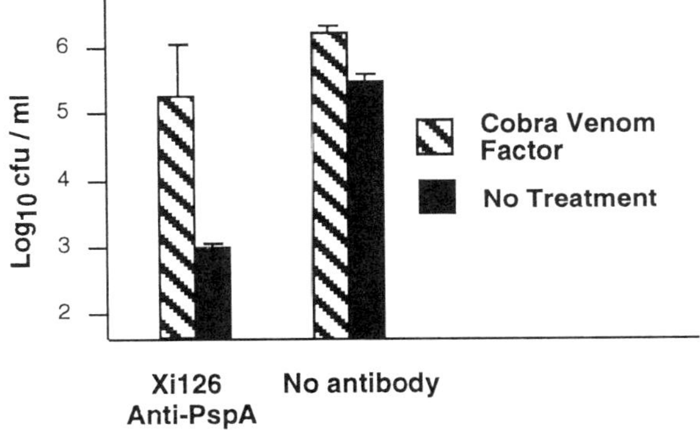

FIGURE 1. Effect of complement depletion with cobra venom factor on anti-PspA–mediated blood clearance of capsular type 3 *Streptococcus pneumoniae* strain WU2 in CBA/N XID mice. A 1/20 dilution of monoclonal anti-PspA antibody Xi126 was injected intraperitoneally 1 hour before intravenous injection of 10^6 cfu strain WU2.

SYSTEMIC IMMUNITY TO PSPA

PspA elicits protection against intravenous (iv) and intraperitoneal (ip) pneumococcal infection in mice.[22–24] PspA is necessary for full virulence, as demonstrated by more efficient clearance of PspA⁻ pneumococci from the blood of nonimmune mice.[25,26] Although the mechanism of action of PspA has not been established, it was shown by van Dijk[27] and colleagues to interfere with complement fixation as detected by the bystander assay for complement fixation. Antibody to PspA results in rapid clearance of pneumococci from the blood,[23] and requires the presence of complement as shown by C3 depletion with cobra venom factor (FIG. 1). PspA is about 70 kD in size,[28] but larger or smaller variants are common.[29] PspA was shown by several criteria to be a surface protein.[30,31] FIGURE 2 depicts a cartoon of what PspA is expected to look like on the pneumococcal cell surface. The COOH-terminal 37% of the molecule is largely composed of ten 20 amino acid repeats,[28] which form a binding site that permits PspA to attach to the phosphocholine residues of pneumococcal lipoteichoic acids.[32] The central region of PspA is rich in prolines and is thought to be the portion of the molecule that passes through the cell wall.[28] The sequence of the NH$_2$-terminal 50% of the molecule is largely α-helical[28] and contains the region of PspA that elicits antibodies that are protective against pneumococcal sepsis in mice.[33]

Although PspAs are almost always at least slightly different from one another, there is sufficient cross-reactivity between them so that antibodies to one PspA detect PspAs of all pneumococci.[34] Moreover, immunization with one PspA can either protect against death or delay death with most challenge strains.[22,35] TABLE 1 shows protection elicited by immunization with three different PspAs. These studies were conducted by ip immunization of CBA/N mice with purified full-length PspA and subsequent iv challenge with 10^4 cfu of each strain. The LD$_{50}$ for each of these strains in CBA/N mice by this route is ≤ 10 cfu. CBA/N mice were used because they

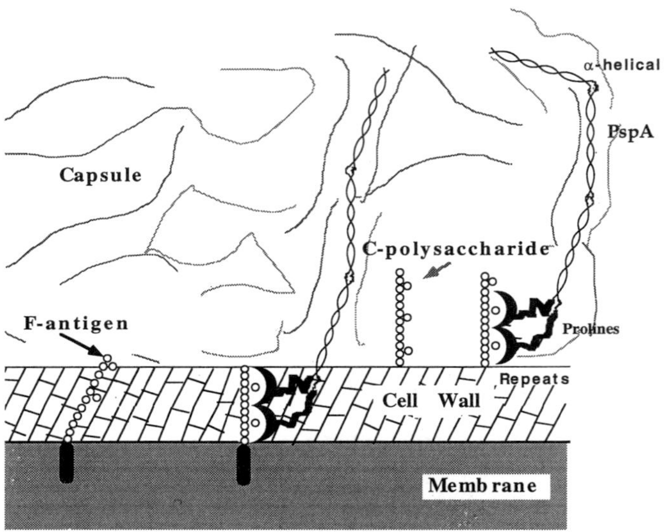

FIGURE 2. Hypothetical conformation of PspA dimers on the surface of pneumococci. Existing evidence indicates that the bulk of PspA is attached to the F-antigen of the pneumococcal membrane,[32] but it is possible that some of the PspA may be attached to similar determinants in the C-polysaccharide of the cell wall.

express the X-linked immunodeficiency (XID) trait and cannot make antibodies to polysaccharide antigens,[36,37] thereby eliminating the possibility that any protection elicited in these animals might be due to anticapsular antibodies.[38] Unlike the sera of immunologically normal mice, the sera of XID mice lack naturally occurring antibodies to the phosphocholine determinant of C-polysaccharide. As a result, they are much more susceptible to infection by encapsulated *S. pneumoniae*.[37]

Pneumococcal strains easiest to protect against following PspA immunization were those of capsular types 3, 6A, and 6B. Those strains for which immunization extended life, but left few survivors were all of capsular types 2, 4, and 5. Although some of the differences in the ability of the immunizations to protect against individual strains are undoubtedly due to serologic differences in the immunizing PspAs, some are apparently due to other factors. For example, even when mice were

TABLE 1. Ability of 3 PspAs to Elicit Protection against 14 *S. pneumoniae* Challenge Strains; Median Days Alive Postchallenge[a]

Challenge Strain	Capsule Type	PspA Type	Vaccine PspA			
			D39	WU2	BG9739	None
D39	2	25	**4.5**	**>21**		2
WU2	3	1	**>21**	**>21**	**>21**	2
A66	3	13	**>21**	**>21**	**>21**	2
EF10197	3	18	**>21**		**>21**	2
ATCC6303	3	7	**>21**			5
BG9739	4	26	**3**	**>21**	**6**	2
EF3296	4	20	5	5	5	2
EF5668	4	12	**6**	2	**>21**	3
L81905	4	23	5	5	**8**	2
DBL5	5	33	**4**		3	2
EF6796	6A	1	**>21**			1
DBL6A	6A	19	**>21**	9	13	6
BG9163	6B	21	**>21**		**>21**	9
BG7322	6B	24	**>21**	**>21**	15	7

[a]Boldface = statistically different times of death from none at $p < 0.05$, Wilcoxon two-sample rank test.

immunized ip with D39 or BG9739 PspA, it was difficult to protect against iv challenge with D39 or BG9739 pneumococci. The difficulty in eliciting protection against capsular type 2, 4, and 5 strains is likely related to their increased virulence in immunodeficient CBA/N mice. Evidence to support this hypothesis comes from a single study in which BALB/cJ mice were immunized with D39 PspA and challenged with strain D39. PspA immunization protected against death due to *S. pneumoniae* D39 challenge in immunologically normal BALB/cJ mice.

The protection-eliciting residues of PspA were detected in the NH_2-terminal half of the molecule. This was indicated initially by the demonstration that immunization with a fragment containing the NH_2-terminal 245 amino acids of PspA could protect mice from infection.[39] Subsequent studies demonstrated that the epitopes detected by a panel of five protective monoclonal antibodies to PspA were all present in the NH_2-terminal 260 amino acids. The epitopes detected by four of the five protective antibodies were mapped between amino acids 192 and 260. Recent studies have shown that fragments of PspA comprising amino acids 192–299 and 192–588 can elicit cross-protection against a diverse panel of pneumococci. TABLE 2 depicts the results obtained by immunization with the 192–299 PspA fragment (BAR416).

TABLE 2. Protection of Mice by Immunization with BAR416[a] from Rx1 PspA

Challenge Strain	BAR416-Immunized			Sham-Immunized			P Value[b]
	Alive (n)/ Dead (n)	% Survival	Median Days Alive	Alive (n)/ Dead (n)	% Survival	Median Days Alive	
WU2	4/1	80%	>21	0/3	0%	1	0.002
ATCC6303	2/3	40%	13	1/4	20%	4	0.048
A66	5/0	100%	>21	0/5	0%	2	0.004
BG7322	3/2	60%	>21	0/4	0%	7	0.02
EF6796	3/2	60%	>21	0/5	0%	5	0.004
DBL6A	0/5	0%	7	0/5	0%	2	0.008

[a]BAR416; Rx1 PspA fragment containing amino acids 192–299.
[b]p values calculated using a one-tailed Wilcoxon two-sample rank test.

MUCOSAL IMMUNITY TO PspA

To determine if PspA could elicit protection against pneumococcal carriage, we developed a mouse carriage model.[40] *S. pneumoniae* strains exhibiting a range of virulence, when injected parenterally, were tested for their ability to exhibit carriage in CBA/N mice following intranasal (in) infection. Some of the strains used, those of capsular types 14, 19, and 23, were so poorly virulent that they did not cause sepsis even when injected iv at doses as great as 10^7 cfu. Others were highly virulent; no more than 10 cfu given iv were sufficient to cause fatal sepsis.

Seven days after in inoculation with these strains, the mice were sacrificed, and saline solution injected into their cut tracheas was used to wash out the nasal tissues. The area washed represents the pharynx and nasal tissues. Bacteria recovered from nasal washes were identified as pneumococci based on their colony morphology, gentamicin resistance,[41] and optochin sensitivity. Unchallenged control mice yielded no gentamicin-resistant, optochin-sensitive bacteria in their nasal washes.[40]

The results obtained by the in inoculation of CBA/N mice with *S. pneumoniae* strains are depicted in TABLE 3. A66, a highly virulent capsular type 3 pneumococcus,

TABLE 3. Carriage of *S. pneumoniae* in CBA/N (XID) Mice (10^7 cfu in)

Strain/ Capsular Type	Log_{10} LD_{50} iv	Alive:Dead	% with Carriage	Median cfu in Nose	Maximum cfu/ml Blood
A66/3	<2	0:4	—	—	—
BG9739/4	<2	3:1	67	1,000	<3
L82106/6B	≥7	6:0	100	2,000	<3
BG9163/6B	3.5	2:0	100	2,000	<3
TJ0893/14	~4	4:0	100	4,000	<3
L82013/19	≥7	4:0	100	200	<3
BG8826/23F	≥7	2:0	100	20,000	<3

NOTE: Carriage and blood colony-forming units determined after 7 days. Greater than 10 cfu of pneumococci were recovered from the nares of all mice judged as carriers.

killed all four of the mice within 3 days.[40] The observation that A66 was able to kill all XID mice inoculated in was not surprising, because it is known that injection of 10 or more of these pneumococci into the blood of CBA/N mice results in death from sepsis in just a few days. What was surprising was that carriage of type 4 strain BG9739, which is as virulent in XID mice as is strain A66 based on LD_{50}, did not also produce fatal sepsis in all mice. This finding suggests that the two strains may differ significantly in their ability to invade nasal tissue and reach the blood. The fact that capsular type 14, 19, and 23 strains established carriage indicates that the virulence properties required for carriage must be different from those required to cause sepsis.

Carriage was rapidly established and remained stable for at least 6 days. By 14 days, over 80% of mice still carried pneumococci, but the numbers of organisms were greatly reduced (TABLE 4). Despite transient bacteremia and pulmonary infection at day 1, pulmonary infection or bacteremia was not detectable after this time point. Thus, it seemed clear that the presence of pneumococci in the nose was the result of carriage in the nasopharynx rather than generalized sepsis or bacteremia.[40] However, as the dose of pneumococci was decreased, the median numbers of pneumococci in

TABLE 4. Log_{10} cfu Recovered from the Nasopharynx of Mice Infected in with 10^7 cfu L82106 *S. pneumoniae*

Source	Day 1	Day 3	Day 6	Day 14	Day 19
Nasal	4.2 ± .5	4.1 ± .3	4.3 ± .3	1.7 ± .6	2.5 ± .2
Blood	2.9 ± 1.6	<1.3	<1.3	<1.3	<1.3
Lungs	3.9 ± 1.6	<2.3	<2.3	nd	nd

NOTE: nd = not done. Data expressed as total colony-forming units in the 50 µl nasal wash, 10 ml lung homogenate, or 1 ml blood. Different mice were assayed at each timepoint. Values preceded by a < sign are cases in which no pneumococci were observed. The number given is the log of the highest number of colony-forming units that could have been present without detection.

mice exhibiting carriage remained about the same. This finding and the studies of the duration of carriage make it clear that carriage is a steady-state phenomenon, in which the numbers of *S. pneumoniae* appear to be locally regulated.[40]

Protection against pneumococcal carriage can be elicited by in immunization with purified PspA. PspA was purified by choline-Sepharose chromatography and was demonstrated to be at least 90% homogeneous by silver-stained polyacrylamide gel.[24,32] CBA/N mice received 150 ng of PspA isolated from strain L82016 in three in immunizations at 10-day intervals. Commercially obtained cholera toxin B subunit (CTB; List Biological Laboratories, Inc., Campbell, California) was given with the first two injections as an adjuvant. Two weeks following the last immunization mice were inoculated with 10^8 cfu *S. pneumoniae* L82016. Seven days later the mice were sacrificed, bled, and assayed for carriage in the nasopharynx. Control mice were immunized with a similarly isolated fraction from a PspA⁻ pneumococcus, CTB alone, or they received no immunization. TABLE 5 shows that neither PspA-immunized nor control mice exhibited detectable pneumococci in the blood. Carriage was seen in all mice except the group immunized in with PspA and CTB. This study was repeated with larger numbers of mice and identical results were obtained. Subcutaneous immunization with PspA did not protect against carriage even though it elicited high levels of serum IgG antibody to PspA.[42]

Intranasal immunization elicited detectable salivary IgG and IgA antibody responses to PspA. Saliva from mice immunized with PspA and CTB contained PspA-specific IgA. Immunizations with CTB only or with CTB plus mock-isolated material from a PspA⁻ strain did not elicit detectable antibody to PspA in the saliva of these control mice.[42]

To extend these studies to lung infection, BALB/cJ mice were challenged intratracheally (it) with *S. pneumoniae* strain A66 following in immunization with R36A PspA. The challenge strain A66 has a different PspA from that of R36A; R36A is an unencapsulated strain expressing the PspA from capsular type 2 strain

TABLE 5. Elicitation of Protection against Carriage: L82016 PspA Immunization; Challenge with 10^8 cfu L82016 *S. pneumoniae*

Immunogen	Geometric Mean cfu from the Nasal Wash	cfu/ml Blood
L82016 PspA + CTB	<0.4 ×/÷ 1.0	<20
PspA⁻ (WG44.1) + CTB	5,000 ×/÷ 6.3	<20
CTB	13,000 ×/÷ 3.1	<20
None	2,900 ×/÷ 7.9	<20

D39. Mice immunized in with PspA plus CTB were protected against death following challenge by the it and iv route with at least 100 times the LD_{50} of *S. pneumoniae*. When mice were challenged 5 months after the last of three PspA in immunizations, they were protected against fatal infection.[42] Therefore, immunity to PspA elicited by in immunization appears to be of long duration.

SUMMARY AND CONCLUSIONS

To date our studies demonstrate that PspA is a highly immunogenic molecule in mice and that it can elicit immunity to otherwise fatal infections following iv, ip, in, and it challenge. Although the molecule is serologically variable, it is sufficiently cross-reactive so that immunization with a single PspA can protect against strains of highly diverse serotypes. It is anticipated that a vaccine composed of a mixture of carefully chosen PspA molecules will be able to elicit protective immunity to virtually all pneumococci.

If this vaccine proved efficacious in man, it would provide a more simple and less costly means of immunizing against pneumococcal infection than using recombinant vaccines. This could be especially important in the developing world where the cost of successful vaccines must be no more than pennies per dose. If PspA is found to be less efficacious than capsular polysaccharides, it may be valuable as a protein component of a PS-protein conjugate vaccine. In this capacity, PspA might expand the breath of protection elicited by a vaccine composed of only a few polysaccharide-protein conjugates representing capsule types most commonly associated with infectious pneumococci.

REFERENCES

1. FRASER, D. W. 1982. What are our bacterial disease problems? *In* Bacterial Vaccines. J. B. Robbins, J. C. Hill & J. C. Sadoff, Eds. Thieme-Stratton. New York.
2. ANONYMOUS. 1991. Centers for Disease Control HIV/AIDS Surveillance Report.
3. GREENWOOD, B. M., A. M. GREENWOOD, A. K. BRADLEY, S. TULLOCH, R. HAYES & F. S. J. OLDFIELD. 1987. Deaths in infancy and early childhood in a well vaccinated, rural, West African population. Ann. Trop. Pediatr. **7:** 91.
4. SPIKA, J. S., M. H. MUNSHI, B. WOJTYANIAK, D. A. SACK, A. HOSSAIN, M. RAHMAN & S. K. SAHA. 1989. Acute lower respiratory infections: A major cause of death in children in Bangladesh. Ann. Trop. Pediatr. **9:** 33.
5. BALE, J. R. 1990. Etiology and epidemiology of acute respiratory tract infections in children in developing countries. Rev. Infect. Dis. **12** (Suppl 8): S861.
6. BERMAN, S. & K. MCINTOSH. 1985. Selective primary health care: Strategies for control of disease in the developing world. XXI acute respiratory infections. Rev. Infect. Dis. **7:** 647.
7. KLUGMAN, K. P. 1990. Pneumococcal resistance to antibiotics. Clin. Microbiol. Rev. **3:** 171.
8. MARTON, A., M. GULYAS, R. MUNOZ & A. TOMASZ. 1991. Extremely high incidence of antibiotic resistance in clinical isolates of *Streptococcus pneumoniae* in Hungary. J. Infect. Dis. **163:** 542.
9. MUNOZ, R., J. M. MUSSER, M. CRAIN, D. E. BRILES, A. MARTON, A. J. PARKINSON, U. SORENSEN & A. TOMASZ. 1992. Geographic distribution of penicillin-resistant clones of *Streptococcus pneumoniae*: Characterization by penicillin-binding protein profile, surface protein A typing, and multilocus enzyme analysis. Clin. Infect. Dis. **15:** 112.
10. HENDLEY, J. O., M. A. SANDE, P. M. STEWART & J. GWALTNEY, JR. 1975. Spread of *Streptococcus pneumoniae* in families. I. Carriage rates and distribution of types. J. Infect. Dis. **132:** 55.

11. GRAY, B. M., G. M. CONVERSE, III & H. C. DILLON. 1980. Epidemiologic studies of *Streptococcus pneumoniae* in infants: Acquisition, carriage, and infection during the first 24 months of life. J. Infect. Dis. **142:** 923.

12. KLEIN, J. O. 1981. The epidemiology of pneumococcal diseases in infants and children. Rev. Infect. Dis. **3:** 246.

13. BOHR, V., N. RASMUSSEN, B. HANSEN, A. GADE, H. KJERSEM, N. JOHSEN & O. PAULSON. 1985. Pneumococcal meningitis: An evaluation of prognostic factors in 164 cases based on mortality and on a study of lasting sequelae. J. Infect. Dis. **10:** 143.

14. BOLAN, G., C. V. BROOME, R. R. FACKLAM, B. D. PLIKAYTIS, W. D. FRASER & W. F. I. SCHLECH. 1986. Pneumococcal vaccine efficacy in selected populations in the United States. Ann. Intern. Med. **104:** 1.

15. SHAPIRO, E. D., A. T. BERG, R. AUSTRIAN, D. SCHROEDER, V. PARCELLS, A. MARGOLIS, R. K. ADAIR & J. D. CLEMMENS. 1991. Protective efficacy of polyvalent pneumococcal polysaccharide vaccine. N. Engl. J. Med. **325:** 1453.

16. GOTSCHLICH, E. C., I. GOLDSCHNEIDER, M. L. LEPOW & R. GOLD. 1977. The immune response to bacterial polysaccharides in man. *In* Antibodies in Human Diagnosis and Therapy. E. Haber & R. M. Krause, Eds. :391. Raven Press. New York.

17. COWAN, M. J., A. J. AMMANN, D. W. WARA, V. M. HOWIE, L. SCHULTZ, N. DOYLE & M. KAPLAN. 1978. Pneumococcal polysaccharide immunization in infants and children. Pediatrics **62:** 721.

18. BARBOUR, M. L., R. T. MAYON-WHITE, D. W. CROOK, C. COLES & E. R. MOXON. 1993. The influence of *Haemophilus influenzae* type b (Hib) conjugate vaccine (PRP-T) on oropharyngeal carriage of Hib in infants under 12 months of age. ICAAC Abstr. **33:** 175.

19. CHIU, S. S., P. D. GREENBERG, S. M. MARCY, V. K. WONG, S. J. CHANG, C. Y. CHIU & J. I. WARD. 1994. Mucosal antibody responses in infants following immunization with *Haemophilus influenzae.* Pediatr. Res. Abstr. **35:** 10.

20. DOUGLAS, R. M., H. D. H. B. MILES & J. C. PATON. 1986. Pneumococcal carriage and type-specific antibody: Failure of a 14-valent vaccine to reduce carriage in healthy children. Am. J. Dis. Child. **140:** 1183.

21. DOUGLAS, R. M. & H. B. MILES. 1984. Vaccination against *Streptococcus pneumoniae* in childhood: Lack of demonstrable benefit in young Australian children. J. Infect. Dis. **149:** 861.

22. McDANIEL, L. S., J. S. SHEFFIELD, P. DELUCCHI & D. E. BRILES. 1991. PspA, a surface protein of *Streptococcus pneumoniae,* is capable of eliciting protection against pneumococci of more than one capsular type. Infect. Immun. **59:** 222.

23. BRILES, D. E., C. FORMAN, J. C. HOROWITZ, J. E. VOLANAKIS, W. H. BENJAMIN, JR., L. S. McDANIEL, J. ELDRIDGE & J. BROOKS. 1989. Antipneumococcal effects of C-reactive protein and monoclonal antibodies to pneumococcal cell wall and capsular antigens. Infect. Immun. **57:** 1457.

24. BRILES, D. E., J. D. KING, M. A. GRAY, L. S. McDANIEL, E. SWIATLO & K. A. BENTON. 1996. PspA, a protection-eliciting pneumococcal protein: immunogenicity of isolated native PspA in mice. Vaccine **14:** 858–867.

25. McDANIEL, L. S., J. YOTHER, M. VIJAYAKUMAR, L. McGARRY, W. R. GUILD & D. E. BRILES. 1987. Use of insertional inactivation to facilitate studies of biological properties of pneumococcal surface protein A (PspA). J. Exp. Med. **165:** 381.

26. BRILES, D. E., J. YOTHER & L. S. McDANIEL. 1988. Role of pneumococcal surface protein A in the virulence of *Streptococcus pneumoniae.* Rev. Infect. Dis. **10:** S372.

27. VAN DIJK, H. Unpublished observations.

28. YOTHER, J. & D. E. BRILES. 1992. Structural properties and evolutionary relationships of PspA, a surface protein of *Streptococcus pneumoniae,* as revealed by sequence analysis. J. Bacteriol. **174:** 601.

29. WALTMAN, W. D., II, L. S. McDANIEL, B. M. GRAY & D. E. BRILES. 1990. Variation in the molecular weight of PspA (pneumococcal surface protein A) among *Streptococcus pneumoniae.* Microb. Pathog. **8:** 61.

30. McDANIEL, L. S., G. SCOTT, K. WIDENHOFER, J. M. CARROLL & D. E. BRILES. 1986. Analysis of a surface protein of *Streptococcus pneumoniae* recognized by protective monoclonal antibodies. Microb. Pathog. **1:** 5.

31. GRAY, B. M. 1995. Pneumococcal infections in an era of multiple antibiotic resistance. Adv. Pediatr. Infect. Dis. **11:** 55.

32. YOTHER, J. & J. M. WHITE. 1994. Novel surface attachment mechanism for the *Streptococcus pneumoniae* protein PspA. J. Bacteriol. **176:** 2976.

33. McDANIEL, L. S., B. A. RALPH, D. O. McDANIEL & D. E. BRILES. 1994. Localization of protection-eliciting epitopes on PspA of *Streptococcus pneumoniae* between amino acid residues 192 and 260. Microb. Pathog. **17:** 323.

34. CRAIN, M. J., W. D. WALTMAN, II, J. S. TURNER, J. YOTHER, D. E. TALKINGTON, L. M. McDANIEL, B. M. GRAY & D. E. BRILES. 1990. Pneumococcal surface protein A (PspA) is serologically highly variable and is expressed by all clinically important capsular serotypes of *Streptococcus pneumoniae*. Infect. Immun. **58:** 3293.

35. RALPH, B. A., D. E. BRILES & L. S. McDANIEL. 1996. A cross-reactive, protection-eliciting, region is present between amino acids 192 and 299 of PspA of *Streptococcus pneumoniae*. Manuscript in preparation.

36. AMSBAUGH, D. F., C. T. HANSEN, B. PRESCOTT, P. W. STASHAK, D. R. BARTHOLD & P. J. BAKER. 1972. Genetic control of the antibody response to type III pneumococcal polysaccharide in mice. I. Evidence that an X-linked gene plays a decisive role in determining responsiveness. J. Exp. Med. **136:** 931.

37. BRILES, D. E., M. NAHM, K. SCHROER, J. DAVIE, P. BAKER, J. KEARNEY & R. BARLETTA. 1981. Antiphosphocholine antibodies found in normal mouse serum are protective against intravenous infection with type 3 *Streptococcus pneumoniae*. J. Exp. Med. **153:** 694.

38. McDANIEL, L. S., G. SCOTT, J. F. KEARNEY & D. E. BRILES. 1984. Monoclonal antibodies against protease sensitive pneumococcal antigens can protect mice from fatal infection with *Streptococcus pneumoniae*. J. Exp. Med. **160:** 386.

39. TALKINGTON, D. F., D. L. CRIMMINS, D. C. VOELLINGER, J. YOTHER & D. E. BRILES. 1991. A 43-kilodalton pneumococcal surface protein, PspA isolation, protective abilities, and structural analysis of the amino-terminal sequence. Infect. Immun. **59:** 1285.

40. WU, H.-Y., A. VIROLAINEN, J. KING, M. RUSSELL & D. E. BRILES. 1996. A model of pneumococcal carriage in adult mice. Manuscript in preparation.

41. CONVERSE, G. M., III & H. C. DILLON, JR. 1977. Epidemiological studies of *Streptococcus pneumoniae* in infants: Methods of isolating pneumococci. J. Clin. Microbiol. **5:** 293.

42. WU, H.-Y., M. NAHM, Y. GUO, M. W. RUSSELL & D. E. BRILES. 1996. Intranasal immunization can prevent carriage and infection with *Streptococcus pneumoniae*. J. Infect. Dis. Submitted.

Heparan Sulfate in Immune Responses[a]

RATHINAM S. SELVAN,[b] NATHAN S. IHRCKE,[b]
AND JEFFREY L. PLATT[b,e]

Departments of Surgery,[b] Pediatrics,[c] and Immunology[d]
Duke University Medical Center
Durham, North Carolina 27710

Heparan sulfate proteoglycans are acidic polysaccharide-protein conjugates associated with cell membranes and extracellular matrices. They bind avidly to a variety of biologic effector molecules, including extracellular matrix components, growth factors, growth factor binding proteins, cytokines, cell adhesion molecules, proteins of lipid metabolism, degradative enzymes, and protease inhibitors (TABLE 1). Owing to these interactions, heparan sulfate proteoglycans play a dynamic role in biology, contributing to cell-cell interactions and cell growth and differentiation in a number of systems. In this review, we focus on the role of heparan sulfate proteoglycans in diverse processes involving the immune system and immune reactions.

STRUCTURE AND TYPES OF HEPARAN SULFATE PROTEOGLYCAN

Heparan sulfate is a linear copolymer consisting of repeating disaccharides of glucosamine and hexuronic acid. The saccharides are extensively modified by N- and O-sulfation and by epimerization of the glucuronic acid, resulting in extraordinary structural heterogeneity.[1] This structural heterogeneity translates into functional variability; the heparan sulfate chain possesses discrete functional domains and distinct binding sites for proteins such as type I collagen, antithrombin III, lipoprotein lipase, fibroblast growth factors, and hepatocyte growth factor which may vary by cell type and by state of differentiation.[2–11] Heparan sulfate chains are covalently linked to a variety of core proteins including integral membrane proteins (the syndecans and betaglycan), glycosylphosphatidylinositol-linked proteins (glypican, OCI-5, and cerebroglycan), and the large basement membrane proteoglycan perlecan.[10,12–15] Most functions of the proteoglycans are attributable to the heparan sulfate chains.

HEPARAN SULFATE PROTEOGLYCANS IN IMMUNE CELL DEVELOPMENT AND DIFFERENTIATION

Role in Hematopoietic Cell Development

Hematopoiesis is regulated by two sets of signals, those generated by cytokines and those generated when precursor cells interact with bone marrow stroma.

[a]This work was supported by grants from the National Institutes of Health (HL 46810, HL50985, and DK38108).
[e]Address for correspondence: Jeffrey L. Platt, MD, Department of Surgery, Duke University Medical Center, Box 2605, Durham, NC 27710. Tel: 919/681–3857; fax: 919/681–7263.

Heparan sulfate proteoglycans may play a role in both types of signals.[16–18] The close contact between precursors and bone marrow stroma appears to be mediated by a variety of receptor-ligand binding events.[17,19–26] The model system of A4 progenitor cells in coculture with 3T3 fibroblasts provides clues to molecules involved in the interaction of myeloid progenitors with stromal fibroblasts and hematopoiesis.[27] A4 progenitor cells survive, proliferate, and differentiate by adhering to 3T3 fibroblasts through adhesion molecules MAC-1 (CD11b/CD18) and CD45 which mediate adhesion through heparan sulfate in the absence of exogenous interleukin-3 (IL-3).[28] In this system, however, endogenous cytokines could have promoted adhesion of A4 progenitor cells to 3T3 stromal cells. For instance, heparan sulfate binds and presents cytokines such as IL-3 and granulocyte/macrophage colony-stimulating factor (GM-CSF) to hematopoietic cells.[16] Thus, heparan sulfate proteoglycans play an important role in cell adhesion and cytokine function during hematopoiesis.

TABLE 1. Heparan Sulfate Proteoglycans Bind and Modulate the Functions of a Variety of Biologic Effector Molecules

ECM components	Fibronectin, vitronectin, laminin, and collagens
Growth factors	Hepatocyte, fibroblast, epithelial and endothelial growth factors
Growth factor binding proteins	Follistatin
Cytokines	IL-3, TNFα, TGFβ, GM-CSF, and IFNγ
Chemokines	α-Chemokines (PF-4, IL-8, MGSA, IP-10, and NAP-2) and β-chemokines (MCP-1, MIP-1α, MIP-1β, and RANTES)
Adhesion molecules	CD45 and Mac-1 (CD11b/CD18)
Proteins of lipid metabolism	Apolipoproteins
Degradative enzymes	Thrombin, lipoprotein lipase, cathepsin G, and elastase
Protease inhibitors	Antithrombin III, heparin cofactor II, nexin-1, and plasminogen activator inhibitor type I

Role in B-cell Differentiation

B-cell precursor differentiation into plasma cells is a multistep process involving localization of precursor cells within a series of distinct microenvironments. B cells detach from one location, migrate, and attach to cells at another location in a process of precise coordination of both cell-cell and cell-matrix interactions.[29] Such interactions may be mediated in part by syndecan which is expressed by B cells at distinct stages of differentiation only when and where B cells associate with matrix.[30] B-cell syndecan is structurally and functionally distinct from other syndecans. It has a lower molecular mass than does syndecan from epithelial cells and binds to type I collagen but not type IV collagen, laminin, or fibronectin.[31] Thus, changes in heparan sulfate proteoglycan, particularly syndecan expression, during B cell differentiation may control B-cell localization within specific microenvironments.

Role in T-Cell Differentiation

T-cell precursors colonize the murine fetal thymus and shortly thereafter express T-cell antigen receptor (TCR) complex, CD4 and CD8. The events controlling the initial expression of these molecules on T-cell precursors are not well understood;

however, interactions of T-cell precursors with cortical epithelial cells and the production of cytokines such as IL-1α and IL-7 may play a role.[32,33] Recently, Wrenshall *et al.*[34] found that inhibition of the synthesis of heparan sulfate results in a decrease in the production of IL-1. The lack of IL-1, in turn, prevents the synthesis of CD4, CD8, and the T-cell receptor molecules. These studies indicate that heparan sulfate proteoglycans produced by cortical epithelial cells along with other components of the thymic microenvironment contribute to T-cell differentiation.

Role in Macrophage Function

Heparan sulfate proteoglycans interact directly with receptors on antigen presenting cells (APC), leading to modulation of cell function. Wrenshall *et al.*[35–37] demonstrated that heparan sulfate activates murine macrophages and as a result modulates T-cell–mediated cytotoxicity and splenocyte proliferation. T-cell–mediated cytotoxicity increases 3- to 10-fold due in part to cytokines produced by heparan sulfate-stimulated APC and in part to direct interaction between T cells and heparan sulfate-stimulated APC. Cytotoxicity is downregulated when heparan sulfate is present during the later days in mixed lymphocyte culture due to the production of prostaglandin (PGE$_2$) by heparan sulfate-stimulated macrophages.[36] Heparan sulfate also modulates splenocyte proliferation.[35] During the initial 1–2 days of a mixed lymphocyte culture, heparan sulfate amplifies the proliferative response by stimulating elaboration of IL-1 and IL-6.

Heparan sulfate stimulates macrophages through at least two signaling pathways.[37] First, heparan sulfate stimulates the synthesis of IL-1α by activating macrophages via a pathway involving NF-kB and a tyrosine kinase. Later (> 72 hours) in mixed lymphocyte culture, heparan sulfate stimulates production of PGE$_2$ by macrophages through a pathway involving protein kinase C and elevation of intracellular calcium. This later process may provide an important brake on T-cell proliferation which might otherwise be driven continuously. Administering nonanticoagulant heparin, which is essentially a more modified form of heparan sulfate, to mice following trauma and hemorrhage improves splenocyte and macrophage function as determined by measuring the secretion of IL-2, IL-3, and IL-6.[38]

HEPARAN SULFATE PROTEOGLYCAN IN LEUKOCYTE ADHESION AND TRAFFICKING

Heparan Sulfate Proteoglycans Localize and Present Chemokines to Leukocytes

Migration to and local accumulation of leukocytes at sites of inflammation are important steps in the reaction cascade during infectious or inflammatory responses. Cell migration from circulation into tissue involves a coordinated sequence of events involving molecules on the leukocytes and molecules on the endothelium such as adhesion molecules, heparan sulfate proteoglycans, and cytokines.[39–43] Major steps involved in this process are shown in FIGURE 1. The first step is the "loose binding" of leukocytes to endothelium via one of the selectin family. The second step involves "triggering," in which signals transduced to the leukocyte convert the functionally inactive integrin molecules to an active adhesive configuration. The third step is "strong adhesion" mediated by leukocyte integrins binding to endothelial cell receptors. The fourth step is "extravasation" of leukocytes through activated endo-

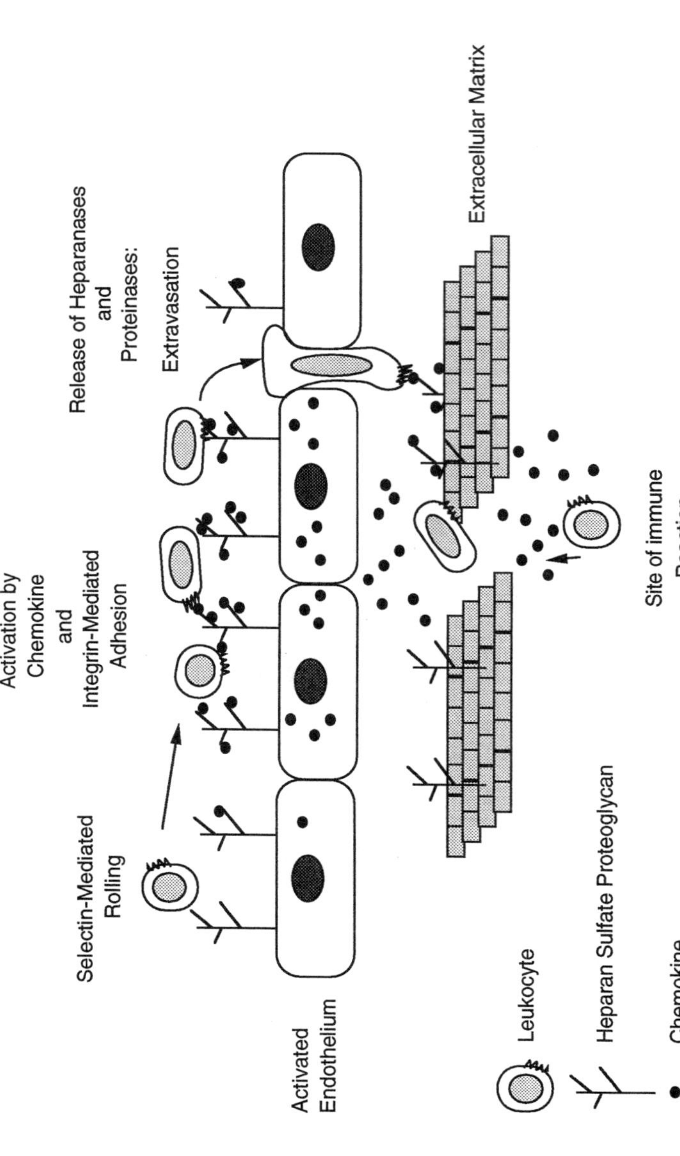

FIGURE 1. Schematic diagram of the role of heparan sulfate-bound chemokine in leukocyte attraction, adhesion, and extravasation: (a) Chemokines bind on the surface of endothelial cells via heparan sulfate proteoglycans, attracting passing leukocytes; (b) heparan sulfate-bound chemokines activate leukocytes, leading to adhesion; and (c) activated leukocytes release heparanases and proteinases which facilitate transmigration across endothelial cells and extracellular matrices.

thelial cells and extracellular matrices to the site of inflammation or tissue injury. Chemokines, a large family of structurally and functionally related heparin-binding cytokines, are active players in these processes and are secreted by a variety of cell types including leukocytes and tissue cells such as endothelial cells, fibroblasts, mesangial cells, and smooth muscle cells in response to inflammatory stimuli.[44–47] Chemokines attract passing leukocytes and upregulate integrin avidity, and this contributes to the "triggering step" in cell migration.[48] Additionally, chemokines, by way of their chemoattractive and haptotactic properties, may also direct transmigration of cells toward extravascular tissue in physiologic or pathologic situations.

Chemokines are anchored to heparan sulfate on the surface of the endothelium and extracellular matrices. Heparan sulfate proteoglycans in the extracellular matrices pool, protect, and present growth factors and cytokines to passing leukocytes and to tissue cells in the microenvironment.[49,50] Rot[51] demonstrated that interleukin-8 (IL-8), an α-chemokine, binds selectively to the luminal surface of small vessel endothelium, the site of transmigration of recruited cells. Macrophage inflammatory protein (MIP-1β), a β-chemokine, localizes at the high endothelial venules of reactive lymph nodes which are the sites of lymphocyte migration into lymph nodes.[52] T-cell adhesion to purified vascular cell adhesion molecule-1 (VCAM-1) is induced by MIP-1β tethered to heparan sulfate proteoglycans.[52] Recent studies demonstrate that chemokines such as MIP-1β and RANTES (regulated upon activation of normal T-cell expressed and secreted) interact with extracellular matrices via heparan sulfate proteoglycans, and this interaction facilitates the binding of resting CD4+ human T cells. The adhesive effect of heparan sulfate-bound chemokines can be abrogated by exposing the extracellular matrices to heparanase before or after the addition of chemokines.[53]

Heparan Sulfate Proteoglycan Binding Influences Chemokine Function

Heparan sulfate proteoglycans not only bind and present chemokines to passing leukocytes but also influence the function of chemokines. Using *in vitro* vessel wall construct, Huber and colleagues[48] demonstrated that IL-8 bound to endothelial cells, but not soluble IL-8, activates neutrophil β₂-integrins, promoting transendothelial cell migration. Other *in vitro* studies have shown that IL-8 specifically binds to endothelial cells via heparan sulfate proteoglycans, and such binding enhances the chemotactic response of neutrophils to IL-8.[54] Heparan sulfate proteoglycan may act as an accessory binding site on cells, facilitating the binding of chemokines to their receptors and thereby enhancing the function of chemokines, as was shown for basic fibroblast growth factor (bFGF).[55,56]

Differential Binding of Chemokines to Heparan Sulfate Proteoglycans

The specificity of chemokine-heparan sulfate proteoglycan interactions may play a role in regulating the recruitment and the homing of specific leukocytes to sites of inflammation. Using affinity coelectrophoresis, Witt and Lander[57] demonstrated that IL-8 preferentially bound to a subfraction of heparin chains that also had heightened affinity for another chemokine, melanocyte growth-stimulating activity (MGSA; also known as GRO or GROα). The same subfraction of heparin did not bind significantly to some other chemokines in the same subfamily, such as platelet factor-4 (PF-4) or neutrophil-activating peptide-2 (NAP-2). The ability to discriminate between heparin chains may be associated with the presence of paired glutamic acid residues within the putative glycosaminoglycan binding site of the chemokine. Other studies demonstrate that IL-8 binds to endothelial cells and fibroblasts but not to smooth muscle cells; however, all three cell types express heparan sulfate proteoglycans and IL-8.[58] Because the binding of IL-8 is mediated by heparan sulfate, these results suggest the existence of differential expression of heparan sulfate proteoglycan which binds to IL-8. The variable capacity of endothelial cells and smooth muscle cells to produce and express IL-8 binding sites indicates that vascular cell-derived IL-8 may contribute to differential regulation of infectious and inflammatory responses in the vessel wall. Thus, the affinity of heparan sulfate proteoglycans for specific subsets of chemokines might determine which chemokines are presented to leukocytes and therefore may direct leukocyte trafficking.

Competition for binding to specific heparan sulfate chains influences the function of chemokines. PF-4 bound to cell surface heparan sulfate proteoglycans inhibits angiogenesis and megakaryocytopoesis.[59-61] Recent studies demonstrate that PF-4 specifically inhibits bFGF-induced fibroblast proliferation.[62] Excess bFGF or heparin overcome the inhibition by PF-4, suggesting competition for cell surface heparan sulfate proteoglycans by these proteins. Gamma interferon (IFNγ) inducible protein-10 (IP-10), another α-chemokine, shares the angiostatic property of PF-4 by sharing the binding sites on heparan sulfate proteoglycans.[63] IP-10 binding to cells is inhibited by heparin and heparan sulfate, is eliminated by treatment with heparanase, and IP-10 does not bind to mutant chinese hamster ovary cells that do not express cell surface heparan sulfate proteoglycans. PF-4 but not IL-8, monocyte chemotactic protein (MCP-1), RANTES, MIP-1α, or MIP-1β can compete effectively with IP-10 for binding to the cell surface.[63] These studies suggest that specific heparan sulfate chains or sequences or domains within heparan sulfate chains regulate the function of a subset of chemokines or cytokines having similar or opposite function.

HEPARAN SULFATE PROTEOGLYCANS BIND AND MODIFY THE FUNCTION OF OTHER INFLAMMATORY MEDIATORS

Heparan sulfate may also modify immune reactions by regulating the function of inflammatory enzymes. Heparan sulfate regulates vasotension and protects tissues from superoxide radicals by tethering superoxide dismutase to the endothelium and extracellular matrices.[64-66] Heparan sulfate directly inhibits enzymes such as elastase and cathepsin.[54,67] It also inhibits by activating proteinase inhibitors such as antithrombin III, heparin co-factor II, plasminogen activator inhibitor type I, and protease nexin-1, thereby protecting the surrounding tissues from the inflammatory reactions.[4,68-71]

HEPARAN SULFATE METABOLISM IN IMMUNE REACTIONS

Heparan Sulfate Metabolism

Changes in the metabolism of heparan sulfate appear to be a common event during immune reactions and are one mechanism by which immune cells control the development and progression of immune reactions.[72,73a] The metabolism of heparan sulfate is altered by enzymes secreted by immune cells and cells within tissues in response to stimulation by immune complexes, antigens, growth factors, and inflammatory molecules such as thrombin and C5a.[73b] Glycosylphosphatidylinositol (GPI)-linked heparan sulfate proteoglycans are released from bone marrow stromal cells by GPI-specific phospholipase D.[74a] Activated neutrophils, T cells, and endothelial cells elaborate proteinases that cleave heparan sulfate proteoglycan core proteins.[74b,c] The action of the proteinases is selective: proteinases from neutrophils degrade the core protein of proteoglycans preferentially over other cell-surface proteins, and proteinases from endothelial cells may selectively cleave proteoglycans either on the surface of cells or in the basement membrane.[74c–78] Activated platelets, macrophages, neutrophils, T cells, and B cells secrete heparanases whose activity appears to be tightly regulated.[73,78–82] Connective tissue activating peptide III, an α-chemokine, can act as a heparanase, and some heparanases act as adhesion molecules or as degradative enzymes depending on the pH of the microenvironment.[83,84]

The synthesis of heparan sulfate is influenced by inflammatory mediators such as endotoxin, thrombin, and cytokines. Thrombin, IL-1β, and TNFα inhibit synthesis of heparan sulfate by endothelial and smooth muscle cells.[85–89] Heparin, endotoxin and transforming growth factor (TGFβ) stimulate synthesis of heparan sulfate, and TGFβ suppresses the inhibitory effect of IL-1β and TNFα.[87,90–93] Heparan sulfate expression changes as a result of injury to cells and during cell migration.[10] During cell migration and after hypoxic shock injury, the synthesis of heparan sulfate decreases.[94] Furthermore, during cell migration, cells express more cell-membrane heparan sulfate proteoglycans associated with adhesion plaques and heparan sulfate chains that appear to be free of core protein.[95–97]

Impact of Heparan Sulfate Metabolism on Immune Reactions

Changes in the metabolism of heparan sulfate have profound effects on immune reactions. Changes in the synthesis of heparan sulfate may modify its ability to bind to chemokines such as PF-4 and IL-8 and to matrix proteins such as type I collagen and tenascin.[9,10,31,57,58,63] The loss of heparan sulfate facilitates the extravasation of blood cells by depriving the endothelium of barrier function.[73,81,82,98–101] The release of heparan sulfate-chemokine complexes stimulates leukocyte chemotaxis mediated by IL-8, and as immune reactions progress, the lack of heparan sulfate might inhibit transmigration due to the loss of heparan sulfate-chemokine complexes associated with endothelium and extracellular matrix.[42,54] The loss of heparan sulfate may make tissues more susceptible to complement-mediated injury and may promote coagulation due to the loss of antithrombin III and to the cleavage of the antithrombin III binding domain within heparan sulfate.[4,102,103] The release of heparan sulfate-bound superoxide dismutase C might increase vasoconstriction and might aggravate tissue injury mediated by superoxide radicals generated by activated neutrophils and endothelial cells.[64,104–106] The release of heparan sulfate deprives tissues of protection from enzymes such as elastase and cathepsin G.[54,67,70]

CONCLUSIONS

Heparan sulfate plays a variety of roles in immune reactions. It contributes to immune cell development and differentiation. Heparan sulfate proteoglycan maintains tissue integrity and endothelial cell function. It serves as an adhesion molecule and presents adhesion-inducing cytokines (especially chemokines), facilitating localization and activation of leukocytes. It modulates the activation and the action of enzymes secreted by inflammatory cells. The function of heparan sulfate changes during the course of the immune response due to changes in the metabolism of heparan sulfate and to the differential expression of and competition between heparan sulfate-binding molecules.

REFERENCES

1. LINDAHL, U. & L. KJELLEN. 1991. Heparin or heparan sulfate: What is the difference? Thromb. Haemostasis **66:** 44–48.
2. KATO, M., H. WANG, M. BERNFIELD, J. T. GALLAGHER & J. E. TURNBULL. 1994. Cell surface syndecan-1 on distinct cell types differs in fine structure and ligand binding of its heparan sulfate chains. J. Biol. Chem. **269:** 18881–18890.
3. PARTHASARATHY, N., I. J. GOLDBERG, P. SIVARAM, B. MULLOY, D. M. FLORY & W. D. WAGNER. 1994. Oligosaccharide sequences of endothelial cell surface heparan sulfate proteoglycan with affinity for lipoprotein lipase. J. Biol. Chem. **269:** 22391–22396.
4. MARCUM, J. A. & R. D. ROSENBERG. 1987. Anticoagulantly active heparan sulfate proteoglycan and the vascular endothelium. Semin. Thromb. Hemostasis. **13:** 464–474.
5. MACH, H., D. B. VOLKIN, C. J. BURKE, C. R. MIDDAUGH, R. J. LINDHARDT, J. R. FROMM & D. LOGANATHAN. 1993. Nature of interaction of heparin with acidic fibroblast growth factor. Biochemistry **32:** 5480–5489.
6. TURNBULL, J. E., D. G. FERNIG, Y. KE, M. C. WILKINSON & J. T. GALLAGHER. 1992. Identification of the basic fibroblast growth factor binding sequence in fibroblast heparan sulfate. J. Biol. Chem. **267:** 10337–10341.
7. LYON, M., J. A. DEAKIN, K. MIZUNO, T. NAKAMURA & J. T. GALLAGHER. 1994. Interaction of hepatocyte growth factor with heparan sulfate. J. Biol. Chem. **269:** 11216–11223.
8. LINDBLOM, A., G. BENGTSSON-OLIVECRONA & L. FRANSSON. 1991. Domain structure of endothelial cell heparan sulfate. Biochem. J. **279:** 821–829.
9. SALMIVIRTA, M., K. ELENIUS, S. VAINIO, U. HOFER, R. CHIQUET-EHRISMANN, I. THESLEFF & M. JALKANEN. 1991. Syndecan from embryonic tooth mesenchyme binds tenascin. J. Biol. Chem. **266:** 7733–7739.
10. BERNFIELD, M., M. T. HINKES & R. L. GALLO. 1993. Developmental expression of the syndecans: Possible function and regulation. Development (Suppl.): 205–212.
11. BAI, X. M., B. VAN DER SCHUEREN, J. CASSIMAN, H. VAN DEN BERGHE & G. DAVID. 1994. Differential expression of multiple cell-surface heparan sulfate proteoglycans during embryonic tooth development. J. Histochem. Cytochem. **42:** 1043–1056.
12. BERNFIELD, M., R. KOKENYESI, M. KATO, M. T. HINKES, J. SPRING, R. L. GALLO & E. J. LOSE. 1992. Biology of the syndecans: A family of transmembrane heparan sulfate proteoglycans. Annu. Rev. Cell Biol. **8:** 365–393.
13. DAVID, G., V. LORIES, B. DECOCK, P. MARYNEN, J. CASSIMAN & H. VAN DEN BERGHE. 1990. Molecular cloning of phosphatidylinositol-anchored membrane heparan sulfate proteoglycan from human lung fibroblast. J. Cell Biol. **111:** 3165–3176.
14. STIPP, C. S., E. D. LITWACK & A. D. LANDER. 1994. Cerebroglycan: An integral membrane heparan sulfate proteoglycan that is unique to the developing nervous system and expressed specifically during neuronal differentiation. J. Cell Biol. **124:** 149–160.
15. MURDOCH, A. D., G. R. DODGE, I. COHEN, R. S. TUAN & R. V. IOZZO. 1992. Primary structure of the human heparan sulfate proteoglycan from basement membrane (HSPG-2/perlecan). J. Biol. Chem. **267:** 8544–8557.
16. ROBERTS, R., J. GALLAGHER, E. SPOONCER, T. D. ALLEN, F. BLOOMFIELD & T. M. DEXTER. 1988. Heparan sulphate bound growth factors: A mechanism for stromal cell mediated haematopoiesis. Nature **332:** 376–378.
17. GORDON, M. Y., G. P. RILEY & D. CLARKE. 1988. Heparan sulfate is necessary for

adhesive interactions between human early hematopoietic progenitor cells and the extracellular matrix of the microenvironment. Leukemia **2:** 804–809.

18. KOLSET, S. O. & J. T. GALLAGHER. 1990. Proteoglycans in haemopoietic cells. Biochem. Biophys. Acta **1032:** 191–211.

19. MIYAKE, K., K. L. MEDINA, S. HAYASHI, S. ONO, T. HAMAOKA & P. W. KINCADE. 1990. Monoclonal antibodies to pgp-1/CD44 block lympho-hemopoiesis in long-term bone marrow cultures. J. Exp. Med. **171:** 477–488.

20. MIYAKE, K., C. B. UNDERHILL, J. LESLEY & P. W. KINCADE. 1990. Hyaluronate can function as a cell adhesion molecule and CD44 participates in hyaluronate recognition. J. Exp. Med. **172:** 69–75.

21. RYAN, D. H., B. L. NUCCIE, C. N. ABBOUD & J. M. WINSLOW. 1991. Vascular cell adhesion molecule-1 and the integrin VLA-4 mediate adhesion of human B cell precursors to cultured bone marrow adherent cells. J. Clin. Invest. **88:** 995–1004.

22. BALLARD, L. L., E. J. BROWN & V. M. HOLERS. 1991. Expression of the fibronectin receptor VLA-5 is regulated during human B cell differentiation and activation. Clin. Exp. Immunol. **84:** 336–346.

23. MIYAKE, K., I. L. WEISSMAN, J. S. GREENBERGER & P. W. KINCADE. 1991. Evidence for a role of the integrin VLA-4 in lympho-hemopoiesis. J. Exp. Med. **173:** 599–607.

24. MIYAKE, K., K. MEDINA, K. ISHIHARA, M. KIMOTO, R. AUERBACH & P. W. KINCADE. 1991. A VCAM-like adhesion molecule on murine bone marrow stromal cells mediates binding of lymphocyte precursors in culture. J. Cell Biol. **114:** 557–565.

25. SICZKOWSKI, M., D. CLARKE & M. Y. GORDON. 1992. Binding of primitive hematopoietic progenitor cells to marrow stromal cells involves heparan sulfate. Blood **80:** 912–919.

26. WATT, S. M., J. WILLIAMSON, H. GENEVIER, J. FAWCETT, D. L. SIMMONS, A. HATZFELD, S. A. NESBITT & D. R. COOMBE. 1993. The heparin binding PECAM-1 adhesion molecule is expressed by CD34$^+$ hematopoietic precursor cells with early myeloid and B-lymphoid cell phenotypes. Blood **82:** 2649–2663.

27. ROBERTS, R. A., E. SPOONCER, E. K. PARKINSON, B. I. LORD, T. D. ALLEN & T. M. DEXTER. 1987. Metabolically inactive 3T3 cells can substitute for marrow stromal cells to promote the proliferation and development of multipotent haemopoietic stem cells. J. Cell. Physiol. **132:** 203–214.

28. COOMBE, D. R., S. M. WATT & C. R. PARISH. 1994. Mac-1 (CD11b/CD18) and CD45 mediate the adhesion of hematopoietic progenitor cells to stromal cell elements via recognition of stromal heparan sulfate. Blood **3:** 739–752.

29. KINCADE, P. W., G. LEE, C. E. PIETRANGELI, S. HAYASHI & J. M. GIMBLE. 1989. Cells and molecules that regulate B-lymphopoiesis in bone marrow. Ann. Rev. Immunol. **7:** 111–143.

30. SANDERSON, R. D., P. LALOR & M. BERNFIELD. 1989. B-lymphocytes express and lose syndecan at specific stages of differentiation. Cell Reg. **1:** 27–35.

31. SANDERSON, R. D., T. B. SNEED, L. A. YOUNG, G. L. SULLIVAN & A. D. LANDER. 1992. Adhesions of B-lymphoid (MPC-11) cells to type 1 collagen is mediated by the integral membrane proteoglycan, syndecan. J. Immunol. **148:** 3902–3911.

32. PALACIOS, R., S. STUDER, J. SAMARIDIS & J. PELKONEN. 1989. Thymic epithelial cells induce in vitro differentiation of pro-T lymphocyte clones into TCRα,β/T3$^+$ and TCRγ,δ/T3$^+$ cells. EMBO J. **8:** 4053–4063.

33. GUTIERREZ, J. C. & R. PALACIOS. 1991. Heterogeneity of thymic epithelial cells in promoting T-lymphocyte differentiation in vivo. Proc. Natl. Acad. Sci. USA **88:** 642–646.

34. WRENSHALL, L. E., F. B. CERRA, P. RUBINSTEIN & J. L. PLATT. 1993. Regulation by heparan sulfate and interleukin-1α of the ontogenic expression of T-cell receptor, CD4, and CD8 in developing thymus. Hum. Immunol. **38:** 165–171.

35. WRENSHALL, L. E., F. B. CERRA, A. CARLSON, F. H. BACH & J. L. PLATT. 1991. Regulation of murine splenocyte responses by heparan sulfate. J. Immunol. **147:** 455–459.

36. WRENSHALL, L. E., A. CARLSON, F. B. CERRA & J. L. PLATT. 1994. Modulation of cytolytic T-cell responses by heparan sulfate. Transplantation **57:** 1087–1094.

37. WRENSHALL, L. E., F. B. CERRA, R. K. SINGH & J. L. PLATT. 1995. Heparan sulfate

initiates signals in murine macrophages leading to divergent biological outcomes. J. Immunol. **154:** 871–880.

38. ZELLWEGER, R., A. AYALA, X. ZHU, K. R. HOLME, C. M. DEMASO & I. H. CHAUDRY. 1995. A novel nonanticoagulant heparin improves splenocyte and peritoneal macrophage immune function after trauma-hemorrhage and resuscitation. J. Surg. Res. **59:** 211–218.

39. BUTCHER, E. C. 1991. Leukocyte-endothelial cell recognition: Three (or more) steps to specificity and diversity. Cell **67:** 1033–1036.

40. SHIMIZU, Y., W. NEWMAN, Y. TANAKA & S. SHAW. 1992. Lymphocyte interactions with endothelial cells. Immunol. Today **13:** 106–112.

41. PARDI, R., L. INVERARDI & J. R. BENDER. 1992. Regulatory mechanisms in leukocyte adhesion: Flexible receptors for sophisticated travelers. Immunol. Today **13:** 224–230.

42. TANAKA, Y., D. ADAMS & S. SHAW. 1993. Proteoglycans on endothelial cells present adhesion-inducing cytokines to leukocytes. Immunol. Today **14:** 111–115.

43. SPRINGER, T. A. 1994. Traffic signals for lymphocyte recirculation and leukocyte emigration: The multistep paradigm. Cell **76:** 301–314.

44. SCHALL, T. J. 1991. Biology of the RANTES/SIS cytokine family. Cytokine **3:** 165–183.

45. MILLER, M. D. & M. S. KRANGEL. 1992. Biology and biochemistry of the chemokines: A family of chemotactic and inflammatory cytokines. Crit. Rev. Immunol. **12:** 17–46.

46. BAGGIOLINI, M., B. DEWALD & B. MOSER. 1994. Interleukin-8 and related chemotactic cytokines-CXC and CC chemokines. Adv. Immunol. **55:** 97–179.

47. KELNER, G. S., J. KENNEDY, K. B. BACON, S. KLEYENSTEUBER, D. A. LARGAESPADA, N. A. JENKINS, N. G. COPELAND, J. F. BAZAN, K. W. MOORE, T. J. SCHALL & A. ZLOTNIK. 1994. Lymphotactin: A cytokine that represents a new class of chemokine. Science **266:** 1395–1399.

48. HUBER, A. R., S. L. KUNKEL, R. F. TODD & S. J. WEISS. 1991. Regulation of transendothelial neutrophil migration by endogenous interleukin-8. Science **254:** 99–102.

49. NATHAN, C. & M. SPORN. 1991. Cytokines in context. J. Cell Biol. **113:** 981–986.

50. LORTAT-JACOB, H. & J. A. GRIMAUD. 1991. Interferon-gamma C-terminal function: new working hypothesis. Heparan sulfate and heparin, new targets for IFN-gamma, protect, relax the cytokine and regulate its activity. Cell. Mol. Biol. **37:** 253–260.

51. ROT, A. 1992. Endothelial cell binding of NAP-1/IL-8: role in neutrophil emigration. Immunol. Today **13:** 291–294.

52. TANAKA, Y., D. H. ADAMS, S. HUBSCHER, H. HIRANO, U. SIEBENLIST & S. SHAW. 1993. T-cell adhesion induced by proteoglycan-immobilized cytokine MIP-1b. Nature **361:** 79–82.

53. GILAT, D., R. HERSHKOVIZ, Y. A. MEKORI, I. VLODAVSKY & O. LIDER. 1994. Regulation of adhesion of CD4$^+$ T lymphocytes to interact or heparinase-treated subendothelial extracellular matrix by diffusible or anchored RANTES and MIP-1β. J. Immunol. **153:** 4899–4906.

54. WEBB, L. M. C., M. U. EHRENGRUBER, I. CLARK-LEWIS, M. BAGGIOLINI & A. ROT. 1993. Binding to heparan sulfate or heparin enhances neutrophil responses to interleukin-8. Proc. Natl. Acad. Sci. USA **90:** 7158–7162.

55. YAYON, A., M. KLAGSBRUN, J. D. ESKO, P. LEDER & D. M. ORNITZ. 1991. Cell surface, heparin-like molecules are required for binding of basic fibroblast growth factor to its high affinity receptor. Cell **64:** 841–848.

56. AVIEZER, D., D. HECHT, M. SAFRAN, M. EISINGER, G. DAVID & A. YAYON. 1994. Perlecan, basal lamina proteoglycan, promotes basic fibroblast growth factor-receptor binding, mitogenesis, and angiogenesis. Cell **79:** 1005–1013.

57. WITT, D. P. & A. D. LANDER. 1994. Differential binding of chemokines to glycosaminoglycan subpopulations. Curr. Biol. **4:** 394–400.

58. SCHONBECK, U., E. BRANDT, F. PETERSEN, H. D. FLAD & H. LOPPNOW. 1995. IL-8 specifically binds to endothelial but not to smooth muscle cells. J. Immunol. **154:** 2375–2383.

59. HANDIN, R. I. & H. J. COHEN. 1976. Purification and binding properties of human platelet factor-4. J. Biol. Chem. **251:** 4273–4282.

60. MAIONE, T. E., G. S. GRAY, J. PETRO, A. J. HUNT, A. L. DONNER, S. I. BAUER, H. F.

CARSON & R. J. SHARPE. 1990. Inhibition of angiogenesis by recombinant human platelet factor-4 and related peptides. Science **247:** 77–79.

61. HAN, Z. C., L. SENSEBE, J. F. ABRGALL & J. BRIERE. 1990. Platelet factor-4 inhibits human megakaryocytopoiesis in vitro. Blood **75:** 1234–1239.

62. WATSON, J. B., S. B. GETZIER & D. F. MOSHER. 1994. Platelet factor-4 modulates the mitogenic activity of basic fibroblast growth factor. J. Clin. Invest. **94:** 261–268.

63. LUSTER, A. D., S. M. GREENBERG & P. LEDER. 1995. The IP-10 chemokine binds to a specific cell surface heparan sulfate site shared with platelet factor-4 and inhibits endothelial cell proliferation. J. Exp. Med. **182:** 219–231.

64. NAKAZONO, K., N. WATANABE, K. MATSUNO, J. SASAKI, T. SATO & M. INOUE. 1991. Does superoxide underlie the pathogenesis of hypertension? Proc. Natl. Acad. Sci. USA **88:** 10045–10048.

65. ABRAHAMSSON, T., U. BRANDT, S. L. MARKLUND & P. SJOQUIST. 1992. Vascular bound recombinant extracellular superoxide dismutase type C protects against the detrimental effects of superoxide radicals on endothelium-dependent arterial relaxation. Circ. Res. **70:** 264–271.

66. KARLSSON, K. & S. L. MARKLUND. 1988. Plasma clearance of human extracellular-superoxide dismutase C in rabbits. J. Clin. Invest. **82:** 726–766.

67. REDINI, F., J. TIXIER, M. PETITOU, J. CHOAY, L. ROBERT & W. HORNEBECK. 1988. Inhibition of leucocyte elastase by heparin and its derivatives. Biochem. J. **252:** 515–519.

68. PETZELBAUER, E., D. SEIFFERT, R. BECKMANN, B. PUSCH, M. GEIGER & B. R. BINDER. 1992. Modulation of heparin cofactor II activity by glycosaminoglycans and adhesive glycoproteins. Thromb. Res. **66:** 559–567.

69. EHRLICH, H. J., J. KEIJER, K. T. PREISSNER, R. K. GEBBINK & H. PANNEKOEK. 1991. Functional interactions of plasminogen activator inhibitor type 1 (PAI-1) and heparin. Biochemistry **30:** 1021–1028.

70. FARRELL, D. H. & D. D. CUNNINGHAM. 1986. Human fibroblasts accelerate the inhibition of thrombin by protease nexin-1. Proc. Natl. Acad. Sci. USA **83:** 6858–6862.

71. FARRELL, D. H. & D. D. CUNNINGHAM. 1987. Glycosaminoglycans on fibroblasts accelerate thrombin inhibition by protease nexin-1. Biochem. J. **245:** 543–550.

72. IHRCKE, N. S., L. E. WRENSHALL, B. J. LINDMAN & J. L. PLATT. 1993. Role of heparan sulfate in immune system-blood vessel interactions. Immunol. Today **14:** 500–505.

73. (a) VLODAVSKY, I., A. ELDOR, A. HAIMOVITZ-FRIEDMAN, R. ISHAI-MICHAELI, O. LIDER, Y. NAPARSTEK, I. R. COHEN & Z. FUKS. 1992. Expression of heparanase by platelets and circulating cells of the immune system: Possible involvement in diapedesis and extravasation. Invasion & Metastasis **12:** 112–127.

    (b) PLATT, J. L., A. P. DALMASSO, B. J. LINDMAN, N. S. IHRCKE & F. H. BACH. 1991. The role of C5a and antibody in the release of heparan sulfate from endothelial cells. Eur. J. Immunol. **21:** 2887–2890.

74. (a) METZ, C. N., G. BRUNNER, N. H. CHOI-MUIRA, H. NGUYEN, J. GABRILOVE, I. W. CARAS, N. ALTSZULER, D. B. RIFKIN, E. L. WILSON & M. A. DAVITZ. 1994. Release of GPI-anchored membrane proteins by a cell-associated GPI-specific phospholipase D. EMBO J. **13:** 1741–1751.

    (b) PLATT, J. L., G. M. VERCELLOTTI, B. J. LINDMAN, T. R. OEGEMA, JR., F. H. BACH & A. P. DALMASSO. 1990. Release of heparan sulfate from endothelial cells: Implications for pathogenesis of hyperacute rejection. J. Exp. Med. **171:** 1363–1368.

    (c) IHRCKE, N. S. & J. L. PLATT. 1996. Shedding of heparan sulfate proteolgycan by stimulated endothelial cells: Evidence for proteolysis of cell surface molecules. J. Cell. Physiol. In press.

75. KEY, N. S., J. L. PLATT & G. M. VERCELLOTTI. 1992. Vascular endothelial cell proteoglycans are susceptible to cleavage by neutrophils. Arterioscler. Thromb. **12:** 836–842.

76. SAKSELA, O. & D. RIFKIN. 1990. Release of basic fibroblast growth factor-heparan sulfate complexes from endothelial cells by plasminogen activator-mediated proteolytic activity. J. Cell Biol. **110:** 767–775.

77. RIFKIN, D. 1992. Plasminogen activator expression and matrix degradation. Matrix **1:** 20–22.

78. GELLER, R. L., N. S. IHRCKE & J. L. PLATT. 1994. Release of endothelial cell-associated heparan sulfate proteoglycan by activated T cells. Transplantation **57:** 770–774.

79. HAIMOVITZ-FRIEDMAN, A., D. J. FALCONE, A. ELDOR, V. SCHMIRRMACHER, I. VLODAVSKY & Z. FUKS. 1991. Activation of platelet heparitinase by tumor cell-derived factors. Blood **78:** 789–796.

80. WASTESON, A., B. GLIMELIUS, C. BUSCH, B. WESTERMARK, C. HELDIN & B. NORLING. 1977. Effect of platelet endoglycosidase on cell surface associated heparan sulphate of human cultured endothelial and glial cells. Thromb. Res. **11:** 309–321.

81. NAPARSTEK, Y., I. R. COHEN, Z. FUKS & I. VLODAVSKY. 1984. Activated T-lymphocytes produce a matrix-degrading heparan sulfate endoglycosidase. Nature **310:** 241–244.

82. LASKOV, R., R. I. MICHAELI, H. SHARIR, E. YEFENOF & I. VLODAVSKY. 1991. Production of heparanse by normal and neoplastic murine B-lymphocytes. Int. J. Cancer **47:** 92–98.

83. HOOGEWERF, A. J., J. W. LEONE, I. M. REARDON, W. J. HOWE, D. ASA, R. L. HEINRIKSON & S. R. LEDBETTER. 1995. CXC chemokines connective tissue activating peptide-III and neutrophil activating peptide-2 are heparin/heparan sulfate-degrading enzymes. J. Biol. Chem. **270:** 3268–3277.

84. GILAT, D., R. HERSHKOVIZ, I. GOLDKORN, L. CAHALON, G. KORNER, I. VLODAVSKY & O. LIDER. 1995. Molecular behavior adapts to context: Heparanase functions as an extracellular matrix-degrading enzyme or as a T-cell adhesion molecule, depending on the local pH. J. Exp. Med. **181:** 1929–1934.

85. COLBURN, P., E. KOBAYASHI & V. BUONASSISI. 1994. Depleted level of heparan sulfate proteoglycan in the extracellular matrix of endothelial cell cultures exposed to endotoxin. J. Cell. Physiol. **159:** 121–130.

86. RAMASAMY, S., D. W. LIPKE, C. J. MCCLAIN & B. HENNIG. 1995. Tumor necrosis factor reduces proteoglycan synthesis in cultured endothelial cells. J. Cell. Physiol. **162:** 119–126.

87. KOBAYASHI, M., K. SHIMADA & T. OZAWA. 1992. Human platelet-derived transforming growth factor-β stimulates synthesis of glycosaminoglycans in cultured porcine aortic endothelial cells. Gerontology **38**(Suppl. 1): 36–42.

88. AKAI, T., T. KAJI, Y. HAYAKAWA, T. HAYASHI & N. SAKURAGAWA. 1991. Antithrombin III modulates the effect of thrombin on the metabolism of glycosaminoglycans in cultured endothelial cells. Thromb. Res. **62:** 707–716.

89. KAJI, T., S. HIRAGA, C. YAMAMOTO, M. SAKAMOTO, Y. NAKASHIMA, K. SUEISHI & F. KOIZUMI. 1993. Tumor necrosis factor alpha-induced alteration of glycosaminoglycans in cultured vascular smooth-muscle cells. Biochim. Biophys. Acta **1176:** 20–26.

90. SHIMADA, K., M. KOBAYASHI & T. OZAWA. 1989. The modulation of heparin-like activity of endothelial cells in experimental systems. Acta Haematol. Jpn. **52:** 1337–1342.

91. NADER, H. B., L. TOMA, M. A. S. PINHAL, V. BUONASSISI, P. COLBURN & C. P. DIETRICH. 1991. Effect of heparin and dextran sulfate on the synthesis and structure of heparan sulfate from cultured endothelial cells. Semin. Thromb. Hemostasis **17**(Suppl. 1): 47–56.

92. NADER, H. B., V. BUONASSISI, P. COLBURN & C. P. DIETRICH. 1989. Heparin stimulates the synthesis and modifies the sulfation pattern of heparan sulfate proteoglycan from endothelial cells. J. Cell. Physiol. **140:** 305–310.

93. BOUDREAU, N., N. CLAUSELL, J. BOYLE & M. RABINOVITCH. 1992. Transforming growth factor-β regulates increased ductus arteriosus endothelial glycosaminoglycan synthesis and a post-transcriptional mechanism controls increased smooth muscle fibronectin, features associated with intimal proliferation. Lab. Invest. **67:** 350–359.

94. HUMPHERIES, D. E., S. LEE, B. L. FANBURG & J. E. SILBERT. 1986. Effects of hypoxia and hyperoxia on proteoglycan production by bovine pulmonary artery endothelial cells. J. Cell. Physiol. **126:** 249–253.

95. LARK, M. W. & L. A. CULP. 1984. Turnover of heparan sulfate proteoglycans from substratum adhesion sites of murine fibroblasts. J. Biol. Chem. **259:** 212–217.

96. KINSELLA, M. G. & T. N. WIGHT. 1986. Modulation of sulfated proteoglycan synthesis by bovine aortic endothelial cells during migration. J. Cell Biol. **102:** 679–687.

97. LARK, M. W. & L. A. CULP. 1984. Multiple classes of heparan sulfate proteoglycans from fibroblast substratum adhesion sites. J. Biol. Chem. **259:** 6773–6782.

98. NAKAJIMA, M., A. DeCHAVIGNY, C. E. JOHNSON, J. HAMADA, C. A. STEIN & G. L.

NICOLSON. 1991. Suramin: A potent inhibitor of melanoma heparanase and invasion. J. Biol. Chem. **266:** 9661–9666.

99. BAR-NER, M., M. D. KRAMER, V. SCHIRRMACHERR, R. ISHAI-MICHAELI, Z. FUKS & I. VLODAVSKY. 1985. Sequential degradation of heparan sulfate in the subendothelial extracellular matrix by highly metastatic lymphoma cells. Int. J. Cancer **35:** 483–491.

100. MATZNER, Y., M. BAR-NER, J. YAHALOM, R. ISHAI-MICHAELI, Z. FUKS & I. VLODAVSKY. 1985. Degradation of heparan sulfate in the subendothelial extracellular matrix by a readily released heparanase from human neutrophils: Possible role in invasion through basement membranes. J. Clin. Invest. **76:** 1306–1313.

101. KANWAR, Y. S., A. LINKER & M. G. FARQUHAR. 1980. Increased permeability of the glomerular basement membrane to ferritin after removal of glycosaminoglycans (heparan sulfate) by enzyme digestion. J. Cell Biol. **86:** 688–693.

102. WEILER, J. M. & R. J. LINHARDT. 1991. Antithrombin III regulates complement activity in vitro. J. Immunol. **146:** 3889–3894.

103. THUNDBERG, L., G. BACKSTROM, A. WASTESON, H. C. ROBINSON, S. OGREN & U. LINDAHL. 1982. Enzymatic depolymerization of heparin-related polysaccharides. J. Biol. Chem. **257:** 10278–10282.

104. PLATT, J. L. 1995. Xenotransplantation: The need, the immunologic hurdles and the prospects for success. ILAR J. **37:** 22–31.

105. RADI, R., P. C. PANUS, J. A. ROYALL, A. PALER-MARTINEZ & B. A. FREEMAN. 1992. Generation of Reactive Species by Vascular Endothelium. Biological Oxidants: Generation and Injurious Consequences. C. G. Cochrane & M. A. Gimbrone, Jr., Eds.: 83–118. Academic Press, Inc. New York.

106. ZWEIER, J. L., P. KUPPUSAMY & G. A. LUTTY. 1988. Measurement of endothelial cell free radical generation: Evidence for a central mechanism of free radical injury in post-ischemic tissue. Proc. Natl. Acad. Sci. USA **85:** 4046–4050.

Antibody Responses of Rats and Humans to Flagella-less Cells and OspA Protein of *Borrelia burgdorferi*[a]

ARIADNA SADZIENE,[b] PATRICIA A. THOMPSON,[b]
AND ALAN G. BARBOUR[b-d]

Departments of [b]Microbiology and [c]Medicine
University of Texas Health Science Center at San Antonio
San Antonio, Texas 78284

Lyme disease is now the most frequently reported arthropod-borne disease in the United States and Europe (reviewed in ref. 1). It is caused by the spirochete *Borrelia burgdorferi sensu lato,* and its distribution correlates closely with the occurrence of *Ixodes* species hard ticks that are infected with this microorganism. In the United States the annual risk of Lyme disease varies from highs of 0.1–1% in some communities, particularly those along the northeastern coast, to practically nil in other regions, such as the northern Rocky Mountains. In suburban areas that are highly endemic for Lyme disease, persons are exposed to the infection around their homes. In this situation personal protection measures, such as repellents and special clothing, are not practical or safe on a daily basis. For persons at high risk of the disease because of their residence or occupation, a safe vaccine would be an alternative for protection.

The focus to date for a human vaccine has been on single recombinant protein products. The first candidate is OspA, a surface-exposed outer membrane lipoprotein of *B. burgdorferi.*[2-6] Mice have been protected against syringe and tick challenge by *B. burgdorferi* by immunizations with recombinant OspA. Human trials of recombinant OspA are now under way.[7]

Although experimental animals, including dogs, have been protected by killed whole cell vaccines,[8-10] there is concern about the possible induction of autoimmune reactions in humans from whole cell vaccines.[1] One antigen that is present in a whole cell preparation and that possibly may lead to untoward reactions is flagellin, the major structural protein of the periplasmic flagella of these spirochetes. The monoclonal antibody H9724,[11] which was raised in mice immunized with borrelias, binds to both the *Borrelia* flagellin and to at least one component of human nerve cells.[12-14] Because of these concerns about safety of a whole cell vaccine as well as other concerns about the efficacy of an antibacterial vaccine based on a single protein, we have been investigating the potential of an attenuated live vaccine based on a flagella-less mutant of *B. burgdorferi.*[15] Immunization with isolated flagellin did not confer immunity to challenge with *B. burgdorferi* in one study.[16] Here we report on the immunogenicity of the flagella-less mutant in rats. In this study we found that *in vitro* exposure of *B. burgdorferi* to the sera of some humans immunized with

[a]This work was supported by National Institutes of Health grant AI37248 from the United States Public Health Service.

[d]Address for correspondence: Department of Microbiology & Molecular Genetics, University of California Irvine College of Medicine, Irvine, CA 92697-4025; e-mail: abarbour@uci.edu.

recombinant OspA leads to the appearance of flagella-less cells in the spirochete population.

MATERIALS AND METHODS

Strains and Culture Conditions

B. burgdorferi sensu stricto isolates were high-passage (HP) strain B31 (ATCC 35210), low-passage (LP) and HP isolates of strain HB19, a human blood isolate,[17] and a flagella-less mutant of strain HB19,[15] which was designated HB19Fla⁻ in this study. Populations that were passed in medium for no more than 30 generations were considered low passage. HB19HP had been passed continuously since 1983 and had been cloned four times by limiting dilution or colony plating. HB19Fla⁻ had been cloned twice by colony plating and stored in small aliquots at −135°C until use. The *B. hermsii* isolate was strain HS1 serotype C (ATCC 35209) and was abbreviated BhC. Borrelias were grown in BSK I or BSK II broth medium and harvested by methods previously described.[15,17] Cells were counted in a Petroff-Hauser chamber by phase-contrast microscopy.

Rat Immunizations

Six- to eight-week-old female Lewis (LEW/N) rats were obtained from Harlan Sprague-Dawley (Indianapolis, Indiana) and housed under pathogen-free conditions; food and water were provided ad libitum. Harvested borrelias were washed three times in phosphate-buffered saline solution (PBS), pH 7.2, with 5 mM MgCl (PBS/Mg) and resuspended in PBS. The total cellular protein in the suspension was estimated with Bradford reagent (Bio-Rad Laboratories, Richmond, California). The cell suspension was adjusted with PBS for a total cellular protein concentration of 200 μg/ml; 0.5 ml was mixed and emulsified with an equal volume of complete Freund's adjuvant (CFA; Gibco Laboratories, Grand Island, New York) and administered as six subcutaneous injections. Control rats received CFA and PBS alone. After 4 weeks the rats were boosted subcutaneously at six sites with 100 μg of total borrelia protein in 1 ml of PBS without adjuvant. Rats were bled under ether anesthesia by eye sinus puncture before immunization and at 2, 3, 4, 5, 6, 7, 8, 10, and 12 weeks after first vaccination. If enzyme-linked immunosorbent assay (ELISA; see below) values of a given bleeding were within 5% of each other, sera of rats immunized with the same isolate were pooled. Pooled sera were heat treated (56°C for 30 minutes) and stored in small aliquots at −70°C until use.

ELISA

For the ELISA 50 μl of borrelial suspension in PBS at a protein concentration of 1.4 μg/ml were dried onto polystyrene 96-well microtiter plates at 37°C for 18 hours. After overnight incubation of the plates at 37°C, 200 ml of 1% (w/v) dried nonfat milk in PBS (milk/PBS) were added to each well. The plates were incubated for an additional 2 hours at 37°C, the wells were washed eight times with PBS, and 60-ml volumes of sera serially diluted twofold in milk/PBS were added to each empty well. After incubation for 2 hours at 37°C, the wells were washed eight times with PBS.

Bound antibody was measured using rabbit alkaline phosphatase-conjugated anti-rat IgG (heavy and light chains) sera (Sigma Chemical Co., St. Louis, Missouri) in milk/PBS buffer and p-nitrophenyl phosphate as the substrate. Absorbance values were recorded at 490 nm on an ELISA reader (model 580; Dynatech Laboratories, Inc., Alexandria, Virginia). Wells having absorbance values equal to or greater than 0.300 were considered positive.

Growth Agglutination and Inhibition Assays

The agglutination assay was performed as described.[18] The growth inhibition assay (GIA) *in vitro* was performed essentially as described before.[18] Borrelias in late log-phase growth in BSK II medium were counted, and the cell concentration was adjusted to 5×10^6/ml by the addition of fresh medium. In each well of polystyrene, flat-bottomed, 96-well microtiter plates were placed 100-μl volumes of the adjusted cell culture. To the wells were added equal volumes of sterile immune sera serially diluted twofold in BSK II medium. Plates were covered with adhesive clear plastic seals (Sensititre Microbiologic Systems, Westlake, Ohio) and incubated for 72 hours at 34°C in a 1% CO_2 atmosphere without additional humidity. Growth was evaluated by observing changes in the phenol red indicator and by phase-contrast microscopy. In some experiments 2 hemolytic units (CH_{50}) of guinea pig complement (Diamedix, Miami, Florida) was added to wells after the addition of antibody. The end titer was the dilution of immune serum at which BSK II medium remained the pink color and there were at least 20-fold fewer cells than in the well with the next dilution. Growth inhibition titers were expressed in log2 values of the arithmetical mean ($\pm$ standard error of the mean) of the individual sera.

Polyacrylamide Gel Electrophoresis (PAGE) and Western Blot

Whole cell lysates were subjected to PAGE and Western blot analysis as previously described[19]; the acrylamide concentration was 12.5%. After blotting the nitrocellulose membranes were blocked with 3% (w/v) dried nonfat milk in 10 mM Tris-HCl, pH 7.4–150 mM NaCl (milk/TS) for 2 hours. After the membranes were washed in milk/TS, they were incubated with immune rat sera diluted 1:500 in the same buffer. Blots were then washed and incubated for 1 hour with alkaline phosphatase-conjugated ImmunoPure Protein A/G (Pierce, Rockford, Illinois) diluted in milk/TS. Immunoblots were developed using the ImmunoPure nitroblue tetrazolium-5-bromo-4-chloro-indolylphosphate Substrate Kit (Pierce, Rockford, Illinois). The locations of flagellin, OspA, OspB, and OspD protein were identified with monoclonal antibodies H9724,[11] H5332,[20] H614,[17] and 1C8[21] (C. Luke and A.G.B., unpublished findings), respectively. Protein P39 was identified in the blots by antibody kindly provided by Dr. Tom Schwan.[22]

Mutant Selection

Borrelias in late log-phase growth in BSK II medium were counted, and the cell concentration was adjusted to values of between 2×10^2 and 2×10^7/ml by the addition of fresh medium. In each well of polystyrene, flat-bottomed, 96-well microtiter plates were placed 100-μl volumes of the adjusted cell culture and 2 hemolytic units (CH_{50}) of guinea pig complement (Diamedix, Miami, Florida). To the wells were then added equal volumes of sera that had been serially diluted twofold in BSK II medium and filtered through the 0.22-mm filter. Human sera were provided by Dr. Frederick Koster of the University of New Mexico and Dr. Lorne Erdile of Connaught Laboratories (Swiftwater, Pennsylvania). Human volunteers had been immunized with recombinant OspA (vaccinees 6 and 12) or placebo as described by Keller *et al.*[7]; OspA was that of strain B31. The plates were covered with adhesive clear plastic seals and incubated for 72 hours at 34°C in a 1% CO_2 atmosphere without additional humidity. Growth in the wells was evaluated by observing changes in the phenol red indicator by eye as well as with the ELISA reader and a 405-nm filter. Color discrimination was best after the plates had been at 4°C for 2–3 hours. An absorbance value of 0.15 or higher on the instrument was the cut-off point for growth in a well. Spirochete motility, aggregation, and morphology were evaluated by examination of wet mounts by phase-contrast microscopy.

Scanning Electron Microscopy

Cell suspensions in broth medium were incubated over nitrocellulose membrane filters (Millipore, Bedford, Massachusetts) in a petri dish. Filters were then gently washed in PBS to remove excess cells and medium. The filters were fixed in 2% (v/v) glutaraldehyde in 0.1 M cacodylate buffer (pH 7.2) for approximately 12 hours at 4°C. The specimen was dehydrated in Polaron E3100 critical point dryer and then coated with platinum-gold to a thickness of approximately 1,000 nm. The specimens were examined on a model 840A JEOL scanning electron microscope as described.[23]

Immunofluorescence Assay

Indirect immunofluorescence assay of fixed, dried cells was performed as described.[11,20] Harvested, fresh borrelias were washed with RPMI 1640 medium, mixed with a suspension of washed rat erythrocytes in 50% RPMI 1640–50% fetal calf serum, and a thin smear of the suspension was coated on the slides. Slides were fixed in methanol, air dried, and kept in a desiccator at −20°C until use. Murine monoclonal antibodies H9724, H6831, and H5332, which are specific for flagellin,[11] OspB,[24] and OspA,[19] respectively, were used.

RESULTS

Antibody Responses of Rats Immunized with Whole Cells

Antibody responses of rats to killed cells of HB19 and HB19Fla⁻ were characterized. To enhance detection of antibodies to a wide variety of antigens the immunizing cells were administered with an adjuvant. To identify antigens unique to LP *B. burgdorferi* and antigens common to more than one *Borrelia* spp., HB19LP and *B. hermsii* were included as immunogens. Sera were collected before immunization and then at 2, 3, 4, 5, 6, 7, 8, 10, and 12 weeks after the first immunization.

The results of ELISA, agglutination, and GIA with rat antisera are presented in FIGURE 1. The antigens in these assays were *B. burgdorferi* HB19 HP (left panel) or *B. hermsii* (BhC) (right panel). Reciprocal antibody titers for homologous reactions, for example, anti-HB19 HP against HB19 HP antigen, reached peak values by or after the fifth week of 131,072 for ELISA, 2,048 for growth inhibition, and 1,024 for agglutination. Beginning week 8–10 after the first immunization and week 4–6 after the booster, antibody titers declined in each assay. The immune responses of rats immunized with HB19LP, HB19HP, and HB19Fla⁻ were essentially the same. The mutant lacking flagella elicited the same high and longlasting titers by ELISA, GIA, and agglutination assays as its wild-type parents, a finding that suggests that antibodies against flagella were irrelevant for protective immunity.

When heterologous reactions were examined, ELISA indicated substantial cross-reactivity of the anti-BhC antibodies against the two flagella-bearing *B. burgdorferi* isolates. By contrast, the titers of anti-BhC sera against the flagella-less isolate of *B. burgdorferi* were several-fold lower than those of its flagella-bearing counterparts, a finding that indicated that anti-flagellar antibodies contributed to ELISA cross-reactions.

Pooled serum samples obtained at 6 weeks were also analyzed by Western blots with HB19LP and HB19HP as antigens (FIG. 2). The major distinction between blots with sera from rats immunized with HB19HP and HB19Fla⁻ was the lack of

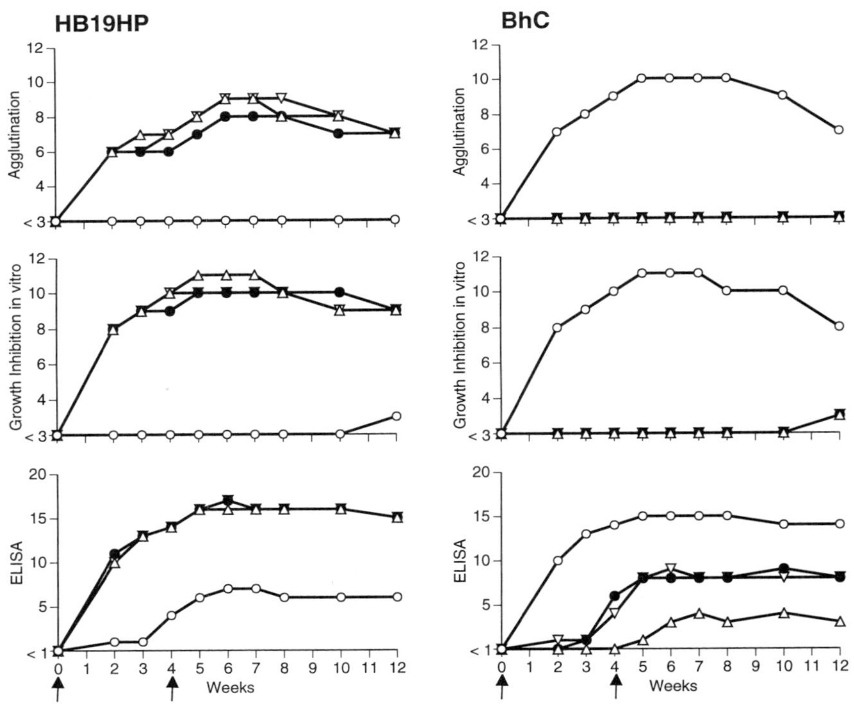

FIGURE 1. Reciprocal titers (log₂) of pooled rat antisera by growth inhibition *in vitro*, agglutination, and ELISA to either *Borrelia burgdorferi* HP19HP or *Borrelia hermsii* (BhC). Rats were immunized the start of weeks 0 and 4 (*arrows*) with whole cells of one of the following isolates: *B. burgdorferi* HB19HP (●), HB19 LP (△), HB19Fla⁻ (▽), or *B. hermsii* (BhC) (○).

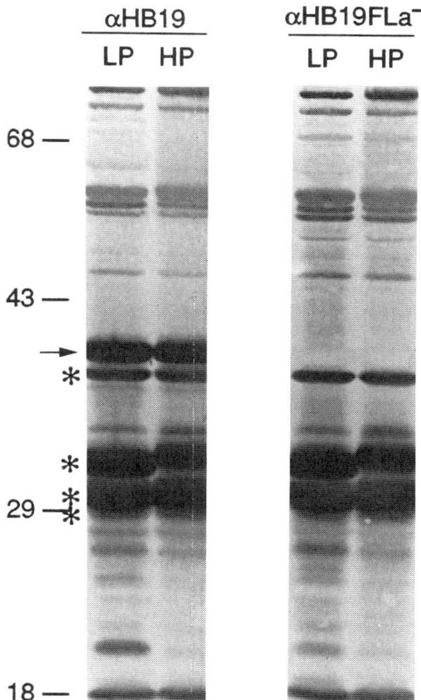

FIGURE 2. Western blot analysis of *B. burgdor-feri* strain HB19HP and HB19LP. As an antibody served pooled rat serum samples obtained at 6 weeks after immunization with whole cell lysates of HB19HP (αHB19) and HB19Fla⁻ (αHB19Fla⁻) emulsified in complete Freund's adjuvant. *Arrow-head* indicates the binding of antibodies in the HB19HP antisera to flagellin. *Asterisks* identify the P39, OspA, OspB, and OspD proteins in descending order of apparent size. Molecular size standards (in kilodaltons) were bovine serum albumin,[68] ovalbumin,[43] and carbonic anhydrase[29] and are shown on the *left*.

antibodies towards flagellin in the latter antisera. Both antisera gave similar reactions to OspA, OspB, OspD, and P39 as well as to other proteinaceous antigens detected by Western blot.

Selection of Populations of B. burgdorferi with Human Sera

Sera from two human volunteers (vaccinees 6 and 12) immunized with recombinant OspA were examined for their ability to inhibit the growth of strain B31 of *B. burgdorferi*. The reciprocal GIA titer in the presence of complement for a human volunteer who received placebo was 4. The reciprocal GIA titers for vaccinees 6 and 12 were 1024 and 512, respectively, in the presence or absence of complement. The morphologic effects of these sera and a placebo serum on *B. burgdorferi* cells are shown in FIGURE 3. Borrelias exposed to sera 6 and 12 have multiple large and small outer membrane blebs. These sera were then used to select for isolates that were resistant to growth-inhibiting antibodies.

To determine the approximate frequency of such mutants, strain B31 cells were exposed to human serum 6 at a dilution of 1:100 with complement in 96-well microtiter plates. With a control plate of complement alone, 35 of 96 wells inoculated with an estimated 0.3 cell per well had growth. In the presence of #6 sera, plates inoculated with 0.3×10^2, 10^3, 10^4, and 10^5 cells per well showed no growth after 1 week of incubation. When an estimated 0.3×10^6 were used as the inocula, 5 of the 96 wells containing serum 6 had growth. The frequency of antibody-resistant cells in the original inoculum was between 10^{-5} and 10^{-6}. Cells from five wells that had growth in the presence of human serum 6 were then exposed to immune serum 12; all of them were susceptible to immune serum 12 by GIA.

In the second experiment both sera from vaccinees 6 and 12 were used at a dilution of 1:60 in the absence of complement to select from strain B31 population cells resistant to the antibodies in broth medium. Wells were inoculated with an estimated 0.1 cells per well. The results are shown in TABLE 1. Correcting for the efficiency of growth in the control wells, we calculated the frequency of cells that were resistant to the growth-inhibiting activity of the vaccinee sera to be 2–5×10^{-6}.

Antibody-resistant cells that were recovered from the wells after exposure to antisera were passed in 1:10 dilutions to the microtiter wells containing medium with the antiserum or broth medium alone for a total of six passages. In most of the surviving populations, 80–90% of cells in the wells were straight and nonmotile. In this appearance the cells were identical to the flagella-less mutant HB19Fla⁻.[15] The remainder of the cells in the population were wavy and motile. When IFA was performed on these populations, the straight, nonmotile cells were bound by anti-OspA and anti-OspB monoclonal antibodies but not by the anti-flagellin antibody. B31 cells unexposed to the antisera were bound by all three antibodies (not shown).

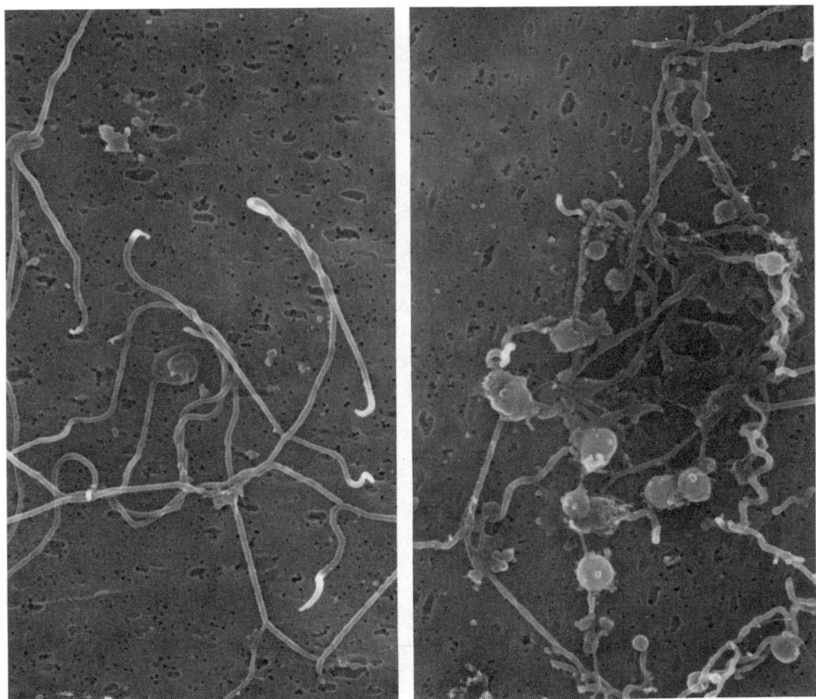

FIGURE 3. Scanning electron microscopy of *B. burgdorferi* strain B31 exposed for 2 hours to control serum (*left*) and serum from a human immunized with recombinant OspA protein (*right*). Magnification 6,000×.

TABLE 1. Frequency of Mutants Resistant to Human anti-OspA Sera among *Borrelia burgdorferi* Strain B31 in Broth Medium

Estimated Cells	Human Serum		
per Well at t_0	Vaccinee 6	Vaccinee 12	Placebo
10^{-1}	—[a]	—	$4/96^b$
			$(4.0 \times 10^{-2})^c$
10^3	0/96	0/96	—
10^4	1/96	1/96	—
	(1.0×10^{-6})	(1.0×10^{-6})	
10^5	31/96	19/96	—
	(3.0×10^{-6})	(2.0×10^{-6})	

[a]Not done.

[b]Wells with growth/total wells inoculated per microtiter plate.

[c]Frequency of cells with growth potential at t_0.

DISCUSSION

The study of rats immunized with flagella-bearing and flagella cells of *B. burgdorferi* showed that the immunogenicity of the flagella-less cells was equivalent to that of the wild type as assessed by ELISA as well as the functional assays of agglutination and growth inhibition. The only discernible difference between the antisera obtained from the rats was in reactivity with the flagellin protein by Western blot. These findings indicate that antibodies to flagellin do not detectably contribute to agglutinating and growth-inhibiting activities of antisera to whole cells of *B. burgdorferi*. From this we conclude that flagellin or flagella may not be needed for an effective vaccine against infection by *B. burgdorferi*.

With regard to the diagnosis of Lyme disease or *B. burgdorferi* infection, a vaccine based on a flagella-less mutant offers a way to assess whether an immunized animal or person became infected with a Lyme disease *Borrelia* spp. before or after vaccination. Assuming no prior infection with *Borrelia* spp., we would expect that an individual immunized with HB19Fla⁻, or similar mutant, would not have antibody to species-specific epitopes of flagellin of *B. burgdorferi*. The absence of anti-flagellin antibodies was found in rats and mice immunized with the flagella-less mutant in the present study. If that is generally the case, then a diagnostic assay based on the flagella of Lyme disease *Borrelia* spp. could be used to diagnose intercurrent Lyme disease in an immunized person or animal. The flagella-less mutant might also be useful in reducing antibody cross-reactions in matrix-based assays, such as ELISA, for distinguishing between Lyme disease and relapsing fever *Borrelia* spp.

We began our studies of human sera with the aim to determine the frequency of antibody-resistant mutants in populations of *B. burgdorferi* exposed to antibodies from persons immunized with recombinant OspA. From our previous studies of polyclonal and monoclonal antibodies from rats and mice we expected to find mutants lacking OspA entirely or possessing OspA with mutations in the gene itself.[21,25,26] These may occur, but the surprising finding was that among the cells that survived exposure to the vaccinees' sera and further passage in medium with or without the selecting antiserum, the majority of cells present possessed OspA but not flagellin. Some or most of these cells may have OspA proteins that differ in their reactivity from the OspA of wild-type cells in their reactivities with some antibodies to OspA; this remains to be determined. Of relevance here is the occurrence of cells with the flagella-less phenotype by the criteria of morphology and antibody reactivity after exposure to antisera to another antigen *in vitro*. The flagella-less cells selected in this way from a population of strain B31 were similar to the original flagella-less cells selected from strain HB19 in the apparent high frequency of reversion to the flagella-bearing, motile phenotype. We do not know the genetic or epigenetic basis for the flagella-less cells of either B31 or HB19. The flagellin gene operon of HB19Fla⁻ is identical to that of HB19 (A.S. and A.G.B., unpublished findings).

Why would antisera to OspA lead to the appearance in the surviving cells of a high proportion of flagella-less cells? One possible clue is the effect of the human sera on the borrelias (FIG. 3). In the absence of complement the sera from the vaccinees substantially perturbed the membrane of the cells. This was similar to the effect observed with Fab fragments of a monoclonal antibody to the OspB protein of *B. burgdorferi*.[25] It is possible that the apparent lower metabolic state of the nonmotile, flagella-less cells[15] provides the cell with escape not from the binding of the antibodies to OspA (or other surface component) but from the subsequent cell autolysis that follows binding of an antibody to the outer membrane.[25] In an earlier study one of the authors (A.G.B.) and colleagues showed that any of a number of mutations that might lead to a slower growth rate in *Escherichia coli* could also produce a phenotype of resistance to the beta-lactam antibiotic mecillinam.[27] The antibiotic had its intended direct effect on cell wall synthesis, but the slower growing cells could continue to divide.

Whether the flagella-less phenotype observed here *in vitro* with human antisera to OspA could occur *in vivo* during the course of infection is unknown. If the antibody resistance provided by the flagella-less phenotype is not limited to anti-OspA antibodies, then it is possible that flagella-less cells occur during chronic infections with *B. burgdorferi*. This would explain the paradox of the presence of neutralizing antibodies[28,29] and the persistence of microorganisms in the body that are thought to have extracellular ecologic niches.[30]

ACKNOWLEDGMENTS

We thank Drs. Frederick Koster and Lorne Erdile for providing human sera and Dan Guerro for electron microscopy.

REFERENCES

1. BARBOUR, A. G. & D. FISH. 1993. The biological and social phenomenon of Lyme disease. Science **260:** 1610–1616.
2. FIKRIG, E., S. W. BARTHOLD, F. S. KANTOR & R. A. FLAVELL. 1990. Protection of mice against the Lyme disease agent by immunizing with recombinant OspA. Science **250:** 553–556.
3. SCHAIBLE, U. E., M. D. KRAMER, K. EICHMANN, M. MODOLELL, C. MUSETEANU & M. M. SIMON. 1990. Monoclonal antibodies specific for the outer surface protein A (OspA) of *Borrelia burgdorferi* prevent Lyme borreliosis in severe combined immunodeficiency (scid) mice. Proc. Natl. Acad. Sci. USA **87:** 3768–3772.
4. SIMON, M. M., U. E. SCHAIBLE, M. D. KRAMER, C. ECKERSKORN, C. MUSETEANU, H. MULLER-HERMELINK & R. WALLICH. 1991. Recombinant outer surface protein A from *Borrelia burgdorferi* induces antibodies protective against spirochetal infection in mice. J. Infect. Dis. **164:** 123–132.
5. ERDILE, L. F., M.-A. BRANDT, D. J. WARAKOMSKI, G. J. WESTRACK, A. SADZIENE, A. G. BARBOUR & J. P. MAYS. 1993. The role of attached lipid in the immunogenicity of *Borrelia burgdorferi* OspA. Infect. Immun. **61:** 81–90.

6. STOVER, C. K., G. P. BANSAL, M. S. HANSON, J. E. BURLEIN, S. R. PALASZYNSKI, J. F. YOUNG, S. KOENIG, D. B. YOUNG, A. SADZIENE & A. G. BARBOUR. 1993. Protective immunity elicited by recombinant bacille Calmette-Guerin (BCG) expressing outer surface protein A (OspA) lipoprotein: A candidate Lyme disease vaccine. J. Exp. Med. **178:** 197–209.

7. KELLER, D., F. T. KOSTER, D. H. MARKS, P. HOSBASCH, L. F. ERDILE & J. P. MAYS. 1994. Safety and immunogenicity of a recombinant outer surface protein A Lyme vaccine. JAMA **271:** 1764–1768.

8. JOHNSON, R. C., C. KODNER & M. RUSSEL. 1986. Active immunization of hamsters against experimental infection with *Borrelia burgdorferi.* Infect. Immun. **54:** 897–898.

9. CHU, H. J., L. G. CHAVEZ, B. M. BLUMER, R. W. SEBRING, T. L. WASMOEN & W. M. ACREE. 1992. Immunogenicity and efficacy study of a commercial *Borrelia burgdorferi* bacterin. J. Am. Vet. Med. Assoc. **201:** 403–411.

10. HUGHES, C. A., S. M. ENGSTROM, L. A. COLEMAN, C. B. KODNER & R. C. JOHNSON. 1993. Protective immunity is induced by a *Borrelia burgdorferi* mutant that lacks OspA and OspB. Infect. Immun. **61:** 5115–5122.

11. BARBOUR, A. G., S. F. HAYES, R. A. HEILAND, M. E. SCHRUMPF & S. L. TESSIER. 1986. A *Borrelia* genus-specific monoclonal antibody binds to a flagellar epitope. Infect. Immun. **52:** 549–554.

12. ABERER, E., C. BRUNNER, G. SUCHANEK, H. KLADE, A. BARBOUR, G. STANEK & H. LASSMANN. 1989. Molecular mimicry and Lyme borreliosis: A shared antigenic determinant between *Borrelia burgdorferi* and human tissue. Ann. Neurol. **26:** 732–737.

13. FIKRIG, E., R. BERLAND, M. CHEN, S. WILLIAMS, L. H. SIGAL & R. A. FLAVELL. 1993. Serologic response to the *Borrelia burgdorferi* flagellin demonstrates an epitope common to a neurablastoma cell line. Proc. Natl. Acad. Sci. USA **90:** 183–187.

14. SIGAL, L. H. 1990. Molecular mimicry and Lyme borreliosis. Ann. Neurol. **28:** 195–196.

15. SADZIENE, A., D. D. THOMAS, V. G. BUNDOC, S. H. HOLT & A. G. BARBOUR. 1991. A flagella-less mutant of *Borrelia burgdorferi.* J. Clin. Invest. **88:** 82–92.

16. FIKRIG, E., S. W. BARTHOLD, N. MARCANTONIO, K. DEPONTE, F. S. KANTOR & R. A. FLAVELL. 1992. Roles of OspA, OspB, and flagellin in protective immunity to Lyme borreliosis in laboratory mice. Infect. Immun. **60:** 657–661.

17. BUNDOC, V. G. & A. G. BARBOUR. 1989. Clonal polymorphisms of outer membrane protein OspB of *Borrelia burgdorferi.* Infect. Immun. **57:** 2733–2741.

18. SADZIENE, A., P. A. THOMPSON & A. G. BARBOUR. 1993. In vitro inhibition of *Borrelia burgdorferi* growth by antibodies. J. Infect. Dis. **167:** 165–172.

19. BARBOUR, A. G., W. BURGDORFER, E. GRUNWALDT & A. C. STEERE. 1983. Antibodies of patients with Lyme disease to components of the *Ixodes dammini* spirochete. J. Clin. Invest. **72:** 504–515.

20. BARBOUR, A. G., S. L. TESSIER & W. J. TODD. 1983. Lyme disease spirochetes and Ixodes tick spirochetes share a common surface antigen determinant defined by a monoclonal antibody. Infect. Immun. **41:** 795–804.

21. SADZIENE, A., P. A. ROSA, P. A. THOMPSON, D. M. HOGAN & A. G. BARBOUR. 1992. Antibody-resistant mutants of *Borrelia burgdorferi: In vitro* selection and characterization. J. Exp. Med. **176:** 799–809.

22. SIMPSON, W. J., M. E. SCHRUMPF & T. G. SCHWAN. 1990. Reactivity of human Lyme borreliosis sera with 39-kilodalton antigen specific to *Borrelia burgdorferi.* J. Clin. Microbiol. **28:** 1329–1337.

23. KINDER, S. A. & S. C. HOLT. 1989. Characterization of coaggregation between *Bacteroides gingivalis* T22 and *Fusobacterium nucieatum* T18. Infect. Immun. **57:** 3425–3433.

24. SADZIENE, A., M. JONSSON, S. BERGSTRÖM, R. K. BRIGHT, R. C. KENNEDY & A. G. BARBOUR. 1994. A bactericidal antibody is directed against a variable region of the OspB protein. Infect. Immun. **62:** 2037–2045.

25. SADZIENE, A., A. G. BARBOUR, P. A. ROSA & D. D. THOMAS. 1993. An OspB mutant of *Borrelia burgdorferi* has reduced invasiveness *in vitro* and reduced infectivity *in vivo.* Infect. Immun. **61:** 3590–3596.

26. SADZIENE, A., D. D. THOMAS & A. G. BARBOUR. 1995. *Borrelia burgdorferi* mutant lacking Osp: Biological and immunological characterization. Infect. Immun. **63:** 1573–1580.

27. BARBOUR, A. G., L. W. MAYER & B. G. SPRATT. 1981. Mecillinam resistance in *Escherichia coli:* Dissociation of growth inhibition and morphologic change. J. Infect. Dis. **143:** 114–121.
28. BARTHOLD, S. W. & L. K. BOCKENSTEDT. 1993. Passive immunizing activity of sera from mice infected with *Borrelia burgdorferi.* Infect. Immun. **61:** 4696–4702.
29. FIKRIG, E., L. K. BOCKENSTEDT, S. W. BARTHOLD, M. CHEN, H. TAO, P. ALI-SALAAM, S. R. TELFORD & R. A. FLAVELL. 1994. Sera from patients with chronic Lyme disease protect mice from Lyme borreliosis. J. Infect. Dis. **169:** 568–574.
30. BARBOUR, A. G. & S. F. HAYES. 1986. Biology of *Borrelia* species. Microbiol. Rev. **50:** 381–400.

Immunopathogenesis and Immunoregulation in Schistosomiasis

Distinct Chronic Pathologic Syndromes in CBA/J Mice

G. L. FREEMAN, JR.,[a] M. A. MONTESANO,[a] W. E. SECOR,[a]
D. G. COLLEY,[a,b] M. J. HOWARD,[c] AND
S. C. BOSSHARDT[c]

[a]*Division of Parasitic Diseases*
National Center for Infectious Diseases
Centers for Disease Control and Prevention
Public Health Service
U.S. Department of Health and Human Services
4770 Buford Hwy. NE, MS-F22
Atlanta, Georgia 30341

[c]*Vanderbilt University*
Nashville, Tennessee 37232

Human schistosomiasis is a helminthic infection of over 200 million people.[1] The pathogenesis of infection is largely determined by host T-cell–mediated responses, such as the granulomatous response to tissue-deposited eggs[2] and subsequent fibrogenesis.[3–6] The severity of human disease is spectral, with more than 90% of those with chronic infections presenting with the less severe "intestinal" form, whereas 5–10% develop severe, hepatosplenic disease. Hepatosplenic disease is characterized by hepatosplenomegaly, Symmers' or "clay pipestem" fibrosis, portal hypertension, and esophageal varices, which may lead to hematemesis and death.[5] We reported on a chronic (20-week) mouse model that appears to parallel chronic human infections in that two different "clinical" forms occur.[7] In inbred, male CBA/J mice infected with low-to-moderate worm burdens, there is a repeatable, characteristic set of observable differences in a small (±20%) subset that develop a spleen of >550 mg (or a spleen-to-body ratio >1.2%). We refer to this subgroup as having the hypersplenomegaly syndrome (HSS). The other ±80% of mice have splenomegaly, but with spleens <550 mg and spleen-to-body ratios of <1.2%. This latter group displays what we term the moderate splenomegaly syndrome (MSS).[7] There are obvious histopathologic differences between MSS and HSS mice. Hepatic lesions in MSS mice are largely granulomatous, whereas HSS mice have more extensive hepatic fibrosis, which is not limited to the area surrounding deposited eggs but is periportal. HSS mice are also anemic, exhibit frank splenic congestion, and have extensive lymph node plasmacytosis. The two syndromes also differ immunologically, in that anti-*schistosome* soluble egg antigens (SEA) antibodies from MSS mice and those from HSS mice express different sets of idiotypes.[7]

To characterize other possible pathophysiologic and immunologic differences between these two distinct forms of chronic, experimental schistosomiasis, we examined pulmonary histopathology, spleen cell phenotypes by flow cytometry, the isotypic patterns of anti-SEA antibody responses, and the cytokine responsiveness of

[b]Tel: 770/488-7750; fax: 770/488-7794; e-mail: DXC@CIDDPD2.EM.CDC.GOV

spleen cell cultures of uninfected mice, mice with acute (8-week) infections, and either MSS or HSS chronic infections.

MATERIALS AND METHODS

Male CBA/J mice (Jackson Laboratories, Bar Harbor, Maine) were maintained in the AAALAC-approved animal care facilities of either the Veterans Administration Medical Center (Nashville, Tennessee) or the Centers for Disease Control and Prevention. Monoclonal antibodies were purchased commercially and are listed in TABLE 1. Uninfected mice or those infected by subcutaneous injection of ±45 cercariae of *Schistosoma mansoni* were killed by an overdose of methoxyflurane (Pitman-Moore, Mundelein, Illinois) and exsanguinated from the retroorbital plexus. Spleens were removed and weighed, and single cell suspensions were prepared.[8] Erythrocytes were eliminated from the cell suspensions prior to flow cytometry using red blood cell lysing buffer (Sigma Chemical Co., St. Louis, Missouri).

TABLE 1. Monoclonal Antibodies Used in Flow Cytometry Assay

Description	Clone	Source
Anti-mouse CD4	RM-4-5	Pharmingen (San Diego, California)
Anti-mouse CD8a	53-6.7	Pharmingen (San Diego, California)
Anti-mouse CD45RB	YCD45R-1	GIBCO BRL (Grand Island, New York)
Anti-mouse CD44	IM7	Pharmingen (San Diego, California)
Anti-mouse CD62L (LECAM1)	MEL-14	Pharmingen (San Diego, California)
Anti-mouse Ia	OX-6	GIBCO BRL (Grand Island, New York)
Anti-mouse CD25	AMT-13	GIBCO BRL (Grand Island, New York)
Anti-mouse CD3ϵ	145-2C11	Pharmingen (San Diego, California)
Anti-mouse B7-2 (CD86)	GL1	Pharmingen (San Diego, California)
Anti-mouse CD45R (B220)	RA3-6B2	Pharmingen (San Diego, California)

Spleen cells (1×10^6) were stained for flow cytometry after centrifugation in a chilled 13×75 mm polystyrene tube (Falcon #2058; Becton-Dickinson Labware, San Jose, California), and 0.1 ml of appropriately labeled antibodies were diluted in FACS buffer (0.01 M Dulbecco's phosphate buffered saline solution [GIBCO-BRL, Grand Island, New York] and 2% bovine serum albumin [Sigma], with 0.02% sodium azide [Sigma]) and added at 10 μg/ml. After 30 minutes on ice in the dark, 1 ml of FACS buffer was added and then underlayered with 1 ml of heat-inactivated (56°C/30 minutes) fetal bovine serum. Cells were centrifuged at $130 \times g$ for 8 minutes at 4°C, the supernatant fluid was removed, and cells were resuspended and stored overnight in 0.01 M phosphate-buffered saline (PBS) solution containing 1% paraformaldehyde. Flow cytometric data were acquired and analyzed on a FACScan flow cytometer using Lysis II software (Becton-Dickinson).

Statistical comparisons were made using analysis of variance, contrasting the data from the acute infection group to the other three groups. This was done because the acute time point (8 weeks postinfection) is a commonly studied time in experimental schistosomiasis. Livers and lungs were fixed in buffered formalin, sectioned and stained, and examined microscopically as previously described.

Sera from mice at 20 weeks of infection (segregated into MSS and HSS by spleen weight) were collected and stored at −20°C. Antibody isotype analyses were performed by specific ELISAs used to detect anti-SEA activity. SEA was adsorbed on flat-bottom Immunolon II microtiter plates (Dynatech Laboratories, Inc., Chantilly, Virginia). Following a blocking step of PBS with 0.3% Tween 20 (Sigma), plates were incubated with optimized dilutions of infected mouse sera. Optimal sera dilutions for each isotype were determined by testing serial serum dilutions and plotting absorbance against dilution. A dilution that fell on the linear portion of this curve was chosen for each isotype and used for all further determinations. Anti-SEA antibodies bound to the SEA-plate were detected using peroxidase-conjugated IgG fractions of isotype-specific goat anti-mouse IgM (Boehringer Mannheim, Indianapolis, Indiana), anti-mouse IgG1, anti-mouse IgG2a or anti-mouse IgG2b (Fisher Scientific, Pittsburgh, Pennsylvania), the addition of TMB peroxidase substrate solution (Kirkegaard & Perry Laboratories, Gaithersburg, Maryland), development, and reading of the subsequent color reaction at 450 nm on a microplate reader (Molecular Devices Corp., Menlo Park, California). Results from the sera of MSS and HSS mice were analyzed by a two-tailed t test. P values < 0.05 were considered significant.

For cytokine production systems, spleen cell suspensions were cultured in triplicate in 96-well U-bottomed microtiter plates (Costar, Cambridge, Massachusetts) at 2×10^6 cells/well in 0.2 ml/well RPMI 1640 supplemented with 2% fetal bovine serum and 2% penicillin/streptomycin (GIBCO, Grand Island, New York) at 37°C in a humidified atmosphere of 5% CO_2 in medium alone, medium with 0.5 μg/ml hamster anti-mouse CD3, or 50 ng/ml PMA + 6 μg/ml Ionomycin (Sigma). Cultures were also exposed to anti-CD3 plus 0.5 μg/ml of either rat anti-mouse B7-2, hamster anti-mouse CD28, rat IgG2a, or hamster IgG. All antibodies were purchased from Pharmingen (San Diego, California).

Cytokines levels were measured by capture ELISAs in culture fluids after 24 hours (interleukin-2 [IL-2], IL-4) or 48 hours (IL-10, gamma interferon [IFN-γ]). Culture fluids were harvested from cells and directly transferred to anti-cytokine ELISA plates previously coated with 2–2.5 μg/ml anti-mouse cytokine monoclonal antibody (Pharmingen) in 0.1 M $NaHCO_3$, pH 9.6. Plates were sealed and incubated with shaking overnight at room temperature. Bound cytokines were detected by the sequential incubation of 1 μg/ml in 0.01 M PBS–0.05% Tween (PBS-T) biotinylated anti-cytokine monoclonal antibody (Pharmingen) specific for each cytokine, 1:4000 dilution in PBS-T of horseradish peroxidase-conjugated streptavidin (Sigma), and TMB peroxidase substrate solution. Plates were washed three times with PBS-T between each incubation period. Change in optical density of each well was measured at 650 nm with a V_{max} kinetic microplate reader (Molecular Devices) and kinetic ELISA protocol.[9] Levels of supernatant cytokines were calculated from $\log_2$ dilution curves of homologous recombinant cytokine standards (BioSource International, La Jolla, California) that were included with each assay.

RESULTS

Evidence of Portal Hypertension. We previously observed periportal fibrosis, ascites fluid, and esophageal varices in HSS mice. Histopathologic evaluation of the lungs of MSS and HSS animals indicated that lungs from MSS mice contained only a few egg-focused granulomas, whereas HSS mouse lungs contained numerous granulomas. Similarly, approximately 80% of the HSS animals, but none of the MSS mice, had adult schistosome worms in the vasculature of their lungs (FIG. 1). The presence of numerous eggs and even adult schistosomes in the lung further establishes that portal shunting is occurring in HSS animals, resulting in collateral circulation by which blood, eggs, and worms can reach the lung.

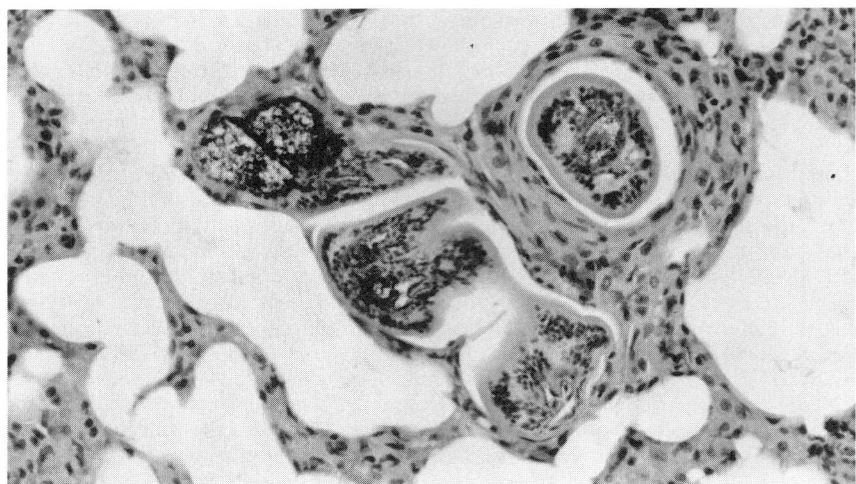

FIGURE 1. Section of paraffin-fixed and hematoxylin and eosin stained lung from HSS mouse showing adult *Schistosoma mansoni* worm cut in multiple cross-sections.

Spleen Cell Phenotyping. As seen in FIGURE 2, mice infected with *S. mansoni* exhibit lower mean percentages of CD3$^+$ cells (T lymphocytes) in the spleen than do uninfected mice, but remain relatively constant in the percentage of B220$^+$ cells (B lymphocytes), except for the HSS mice. The T- to B-cell ratios are essentially the same in mice with acute or either form of chronic infection (FIG. 2). The total of T- and B-cell percentages stays relatively the same in uninfected, acute, and MSS animals (93.6%, 86.6%, and 87.8%, respectively). However, in the HSS group the total is only 70%. Thus, within the spleen cell lymphocyte gate of HSS animals, ±30% of the cells are neither CD3$^+$ nor B220$^+$. As shown in FIGURE 3, in acute infection the ratio of splenic CD4$^+$ cells to CD8$^+$ cells is slightly higher than that in age-matched controls (1.96 vs 1.79). However, by the time chronic infections have been established, this ratio decreases to 1.47 in MSS mice and 1.20 in HSS mice. As the overall numbers of total nucleated spleen cells in infected mice (especially HSS mice) are higher, this decreased CD4:CD8 ratio is most likely due to a disproportional relative increase in the number of CD8$^+$ cells and a less marked increase in CD4$^+$ cells.

FIGURE 4 presents the mean percentages of CD4$^+$ cells that coexpress either of two cell adhesion molecules, CD44^{hi} (PgP-1)[10-12] or CD62L^{lo}(L-selectin),[13,14] that are characteristic of memory CD4$^+$ cells. The mean group expression patterns of CD44^{hi} and CD62L^{lo} are very similar. Low expression of CD45RB[15] by CD4$^+$ spleen cells is more common on cells from all infected groups of mice than on cells from age-matched control (uninfected) mice (FIG. 4). The mean percentages of small CD4$^+$ cells that express activation markers (Ia; CD25)[16-18] on their surface are presented in FIGURE 5. Acutely infected and HSS small CD4$^+$ spleen cell populations each have higher proportions of cells expressing these markers of activation. Small CD4$^+$ spleen cells from uninfected and MSS mice show significantly less expression of these indicators of an activated state.

The expression of the B7-2 costimulatory molecule[19] is a marker for activated B220$^+$ cells.[20] A higher percentage of B220$^+$ spleen cells from 8-week infected mice express B7-2 than do B220$^+$ spleen cells from normal or chronically infected mice (FIG. 6). Also, the mean channel fluorescence (MCF) of B7-2 on B220$^+$ cells from acutely infected animals is higher than that in the other groups. B220$^+$ cells from HSS mice did not express as much B7-2 as did 8-week mice, but they do have a higher percentage of B7-2$^+$ B220 cells that also have a higher MCF for B7-2 than do MSS animals.

Isotypic Profiles of Anti-SEA Antibodies. Previously observed differences in idiotypic expression[7] suggested that there may be variations in the extent of isotype switching observed in MSS and HSS mice. To evaluate this, sera from 15 individual mice were screened on an SEA ELISA (FIG. 7). Sera from MSS mice and HSS mice contained comparable mean levels of IgM and IgG1 anti-SEA antibody. However, mean levels of IgG2a and IgG2b anti-SEA were higher in sera from MSS mice than in sera from HSS mice ($p < 0.05$).

Cytokine Production. When spleen cells from schistosome-infected animals are stimulated with a combination of PMA and ionomycin, they produce levels of IL-2 comparable to those produced by spleen cells from normal animals (FIG. 8). However, on exposure to anti-CD3, spleen cells of 8-week infected MSS and (to an even greater extent) HSS mice exhibit severe deficits in their ability to make IL-2 compared to spleen cells from age-matched controls. Exogenous, direct costimulation by anti-CD28 partially overcomes this deficit by spleen cells from acutely infected or MSS mice (yielding a return to 50%–65% of normal mouse spleen cell production capacity). By contrast, the addition of anti-CD28 only restores HSS IL-2

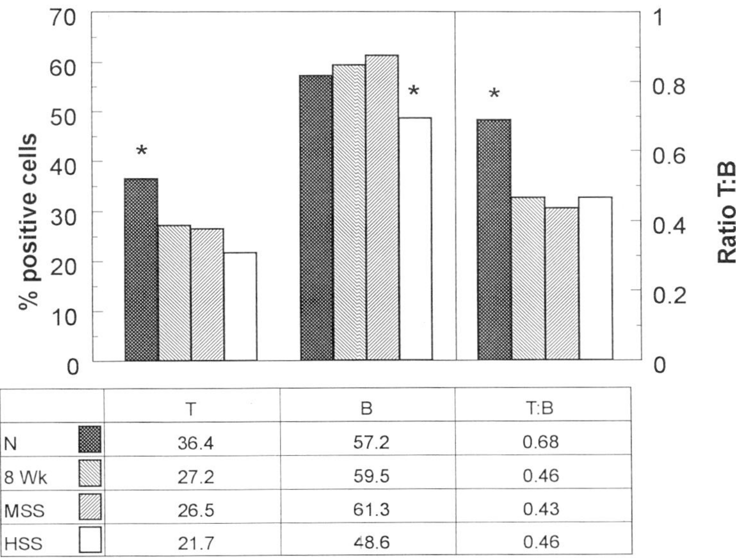

		T	B	T:B
N		36.4	57.2	0.68
8 Wk		27.2	59.5	0.46
MSS		26.5	61.3	0.43
HSS		21.7	48.6	0.46

FIGURE 2. T-cell and B-cell profiles on small, splenic cells from normal ($n = 13$), 8-week infected ($n = 6$), MSS ($n = 6$), and HSS ($n = 6$) mice. *Asterisk* denotes significance ($p < 0.05$) using analysis of variance contrasting the 8-week infected group with the other groups.

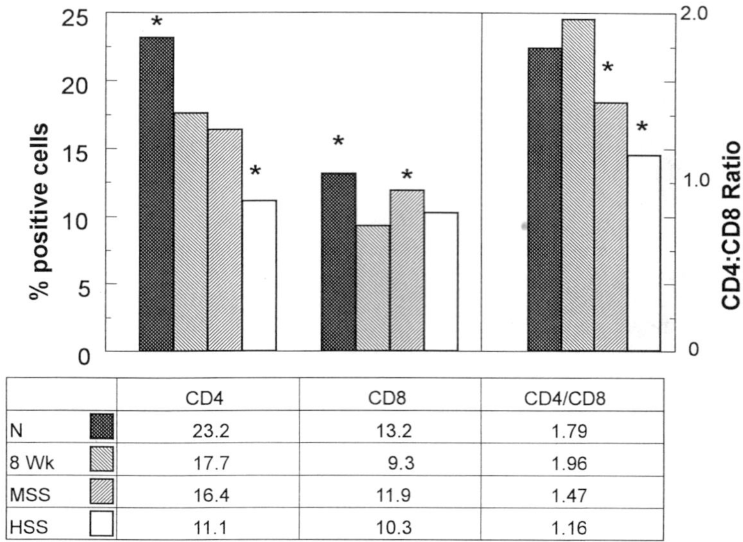

		CD4	CD8	CD4/CD8
N		23.2	13.2	1.79
8 Wk		17.7	9.3	1.96
MSS		16.4	11.9	1.47
HSS		11.1	10.3	1.16

FIGURE 3. CD4[+] and CD8[+] profiles on small, splenic cells from normal (n = 25), 8-week infected (n = 20), MSS (n = 18), and HSS (n = 19) mice. *Asterisk* denotes significance (p <0.05) using analysis of variance contrasting the 8-week infected group with the other groups.

production to 25% of the capacity of normal mouse cells. Anti-CD3 stimulation of spleen cells from normal and all infected mice is essentially eliminated (>90% reduced from full production capacity) in the presence of anti-B7-2 (FIG. 8).

Levels of IFN-γ production in response to anti-CD3 are moderately decreased by acute *S. mansoni* infection (FIG. 9), but this minimal deficit is effectively reversed by exogenous costimulation with anti-CD28 monoclonal antibodies. Cells from neither chronic infection group exhibit this moderate decrease in IFN-γ production, but IFN-γ yield by these cells is also somewhat elevated in the presence of anti-CD28. Coexposure of cells to anti-CD3 and anti-B7-2 reduces IFN-γ production by approximately threefold for spleen cells from all mice (FIG. 9).

Spleen cells from unifected mice make very little IL-4 upon exposure to anti-CD3 (FIG. 10) as compared to spleen cells from mice with acute *S. mansoni* infections. Anti-CD3–stimulated cells from MSS and HSS mice make higher levels of IL-4 than do cells from normal mice but less than cells from mice with 8-week infections. None of these IL-4 production capabilities is appreciably altered by the presence of either anti-CD28 or anti-B7-2 (FIG. 10).

Spleen cells from mice with acute infections respond with more than twofold greater IL-10 production on exposure to anti-CD3 than do those from uninfected mice (FIG. 11). Splenocytes of MSS and HSS mice produce IL-10 similarly (±20% less than mice with infections) on exposure to anti-CD3. Like IL-4 production, these responses are not appreciably altered in the presence of anti-CD28 and are reduced only about 25% by the addition of anti-B7-2 (FIG. 11). These results with anti-CD3 exposure differ from data on specific antigen (SEA) stimulation of spleen cells, where cells from HSS mice produce much less IL-10 than do cells from MSS mice.[21]

DISCUSSION

Analysis of the immunologic parameters of animals displaying MSS or HSS phenotypes has revealed some possibly important immunologic characteristics associated with, and potentially responsible for, these distinct syndromes. Most HSS animals generally display a more activated phenotype, whereas MSS animals appear to express characteristics more associated with immunoregulation. A similar pattern exists in human schistosomiasis in which individuals who are developing hepatosplenic disease have vigorous immune responses and persons with the less severe intestinal disease form exhibit immune responses that appear to be regulated.[22] Thus, the MSS and HSS model resembles human disease forms not only clinically,[7] but also immunologically.

Spleen cells from MSS and HSS mice have a variety of differences in the proportions of various cell phenotypes observed. In particular, there are two differences of potential immunologic import. The first is seen when examining the coexpression patterns of CD4[+] cells in regard to surface markers associated with memory[10–15] (CD44, CD62L, and CD45RB; FIG. 4) and activation[16–18] (Ia and CD25; FIG. 5) functions. Not surprisingly, these markers are much more highly expressed on CD4[+] cells from animals with acute infection than on CD4[+] cells from normal animals. After the acute hyperresponsive phase, however, the characteristic phenotypes decrease as most animals progress to the MSS phase. By contrast, a higher proportion of cells retain these characteristics of immunologic memory and CD4[+] cell activation in HSS mice. The second observation is similar to the first in that the

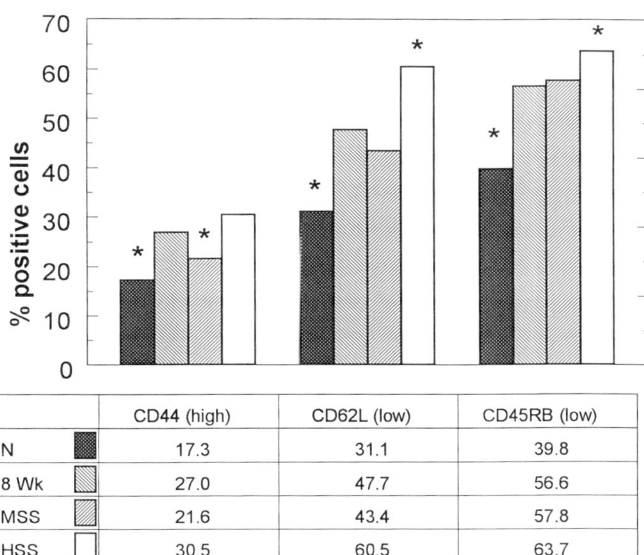

		CD44 (high)	CD62L (low)	CD45RB (low)
N		17.3	31.1	39.8
8 Wk		27.0	47.7	56.6
MSS		21.6	43.4	57.8
HSS		30.5	60.5	63.7

FIGURE 4. Memory markers on small, splenic CD4[+] cells from normal (CD44, $n = 26$; CD62L, $n = 7$; CD45RB, $n = 25$), 8-week infected (CD44, $n = 20$; CD62L, $n = 7$; CD45RB, $n = 18$), MSS (CD44, $n = 17$; CD62L, $n = 7$; CD45RB, $n = 18$), and HSS (CD44, $n = 18$; CD62L, $n = 7$; CD45RB, $n = 19$) mice. *Asterisk* denotes significance ($p < 0.05$) using analysis of variance contrasting the 8-week infected group with the other groups.

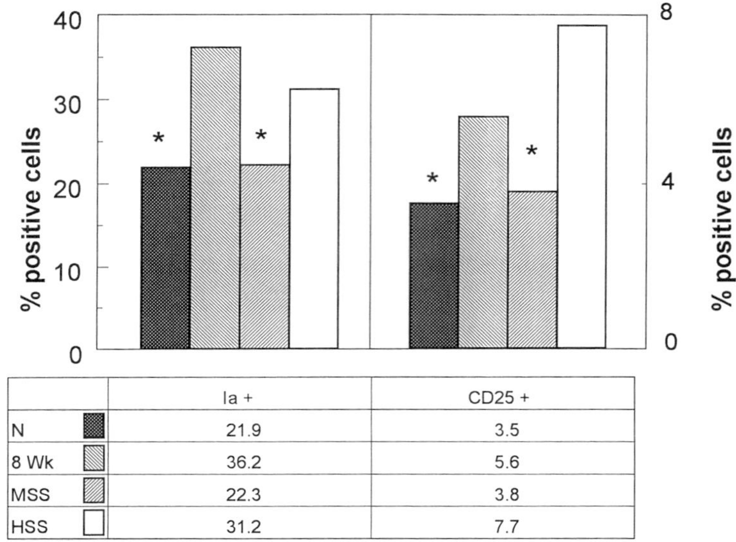

		Ia +	CD25 +
N		21.9	3.5
8 Wk		36.2	5.6
MSS		22.3	3.8
HSS		31.2	7.7

FIGURE 5. T-cell activation markers on small, splenic CD4$^+$ cells from normal (Ia$^+$, $n = 21$; CD25, $n = 19$), 8-week infected (Ia$^+$, $n = 18$; CD25$^+$, $n = 18$), MSS (Ia$^+$, $n = 13$; CD25$^+$, $n = 13$), and HSS (Ia$^+$, $n = 15$; CD25$^+$, $n = 15$) mice. *Asterisk* denotes significance ($p < 0.05$) using analysis of variance contrasting the 8-week infected group with the other groups.

B-cell activation marker B7-2 is more highly expressed on small B220$^+$ cells from acute and HSS animals than they are on such cells from normal or MSS animals. Downmodulation of B7-2 has been associated with regulatory events in schistosomiasis, as loss of B7-2 results in a decreased costimulatory potential.[23] The fact that both the percentage of small B220$^+$, B7-2$^+$ cells and the level of expression of B7-2 on positive cells (as reflected by MCF; FIG. 6) is greater in acute and HSS animals suggests that B220$^+$ cells from these mice may be more able to optimally stimulate T cells in antigen-specific responses than are small B220$^+$ cells from MSS mice.

When these memory and activation patterns are used as markers for immune status, cells from acutely infected mice are similar to those of HSS mice. Cells from MSS mice appear to have returned to a more quiescent state and are more similar to cells from uninfected mice. This pattern suggests that HSS mice may not adequately regulate an earlier, activated (acute) state of disease.

We also investigated whether proposed differences in activation and regulation between MSS and HSS animals could be observed in regard to the humoral response (FIG. 7). Antibody isotype profiles are often considered indicators of the type of Th lymphocyte dominance in a given setting, because of the influence of cytokines on immunoglobulin isotypic switching in B cells. In mice with acute schistosomiasis, the dominance of Th2 responses becomes apparent at the onset of egg deposition.[24,25] We now report that different anti-SEA isotypic profiles exist in the sera of MSS and HSS mice with chronic infection. In the mouse, IgG2a/b production is promoted by IFN-γ,[26] and IFN-γ is often associated with Th1 subset activity.[27] Therefore, the dichotomous pattern of responses in these chronically infected mice implies that MSS mice (higher levels of SEA-specific IgG2a and IgG2b) express a more Th1-like dominance. Interestingly, IFN-γ has also been associated with downregulation of the anti-egg granulomatous response in schistosomiasis. Treatment of animals with recombinant IFN-γ results in formation of smaller granulomas, and treatment with antibodies specific for IFN-γ results in the formation of larger granulomas.[28] Furthermore, the dramatic granuloma-regulating effect of IL-12 is likely mediated through an IFN-γ pathway.[29] Thus, the pattern of class switching that we now report for antibodies specific for those antigens that drive the granulomatous response may be either a marker correlated with or participating in the regulatory development of MSS.

Our comparisons of cytokine production by spleen cells from uninfected mice or mice with acute (8-week) or chronic (20-week) MSS or HSS *S. mansoni* have revealed some interesting differences in the production of various cytokines. The first observation, that cells from infected mice appear severely impaired in their abililty to produce IL-2, was surprising (FIG. 8). Although consistent with observations that little IL-2 is produced in the liver of mice with either acute or chronic schistosome infections,[30] we expected that this was an antigen-specific phenomenon and that cells from infected animals stimulated with anti-CD3 would not differ from cells of normal animals. However, although the PMA/ionomycin stimulations proved that cells from all the mouse groups had the capacity to produce IL-2, these data indicate that cells from all infected animals were impaired in their ability to produce IL-2 in response to a very strong T-cell stimulant, anti-CD3. By contrast, cells from mice with acute infections produced higher levels of IL-4 and IL-10 on exposure to anti-CD3 than did cells from uninfected animals (FIGS. 10 and 11). These findings are consistent with previous reports of a shift in T-cell responses towards a Th2-type environment in mice with patent *S. mansoni* infections.[24,31] Furthermore, our data indicate that a

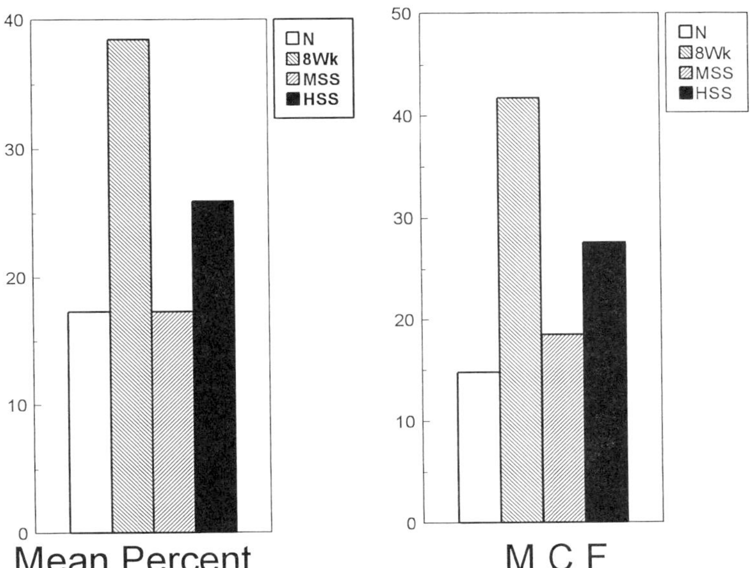

FIGURE 6. B7-2 marker on small, splenic B220[+] cells from normal (*n* = 4), 8-week infected (*n* = 10), MSS (*n* = 12), and HSS (*n* = 12) mice. **(Left)** Percentage of positive cells obtained by subtracting out an isotypic (Rat IgG2a) control. **(Right)** Mean channel fluorescence after subtracting out the isotypic control

modest decrease in *in vitro* spleen cell production of IL-4 and IL-10 in response to anti-CD3 occurs in mice with chronic infections compared with cells from mice with acute infections, potentially signifying a partial downregulation of this Th2 response. Flow cytometry data indicating reduced numbers of total $CD3^+$ T cells in spleen cell preparations from mice with chronic *S. mansoni* infections might only partially account for these observed decreases in *in vitro* production of anti-CD3–induced IL-4 and IL-10. A third pattern was observed in that cells from uninfected, acutely infected, or chronically infected mice produced comparable levels of IFN-γ (FIG. 9). Unfortunately, although cells from uninfected and infected mice produced different patterns of cytokines, no striking distinctions have yet been observed in the cytokine production profile between MSS and HSS mice. However, all of these experiments were performed with nonspecific stimuli. We have data that IL-10 production by HSS

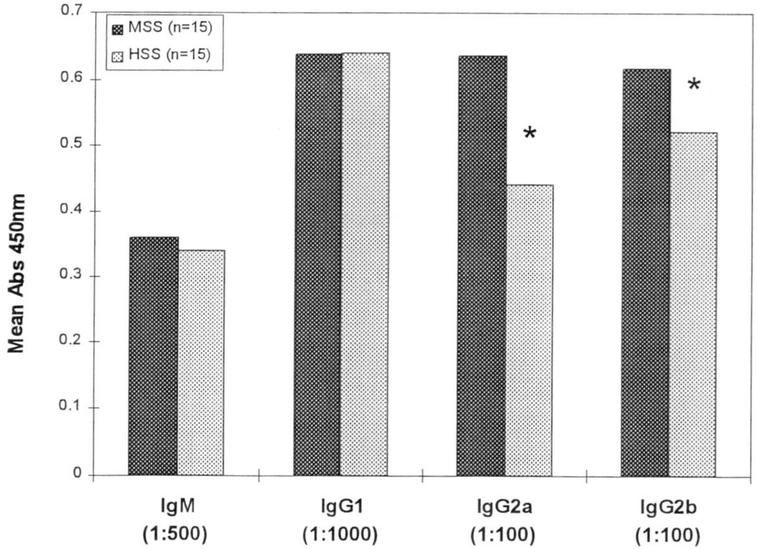

FIGURE 7. Mean anti-SEA isotype profiles in sera from MSS or HSS mice. *Asterisk* denotes significance ($p < 0.05$) using a two-tailed *t* test (n of each group = 15).

spleen cells is low upon SEA exposure, whereas it is higher in MSS animals.[21] Thus, it remains possible that differential regulation of cytokine responses may exist for a specific antigen.

Although nonspecific T-cell stimulation did not reveal distinct cytokine production patterns in MSS and HSS mice, these experiments revealed some interesting differences in the ways in which costimulation for different cytokines may occur in animals with schistosome infections. Production of Th1-type cytokines IL-2 and IFN-γ in response to anti-CD3 appeared to utilize the B7-2/CD28 costimulation pathway as CD28 cross-linking enhanced production of these cytokines and blockage of B7-2 severely inhibited it. Conversely, production of the Th2-type cytokines was not enhanced by CD28 cross-linking or inhibited by B7-2 blockage. These results, as implied by others,[32] indicate that regulation of different sets of cytokines may occur via different costimulatory pathways.

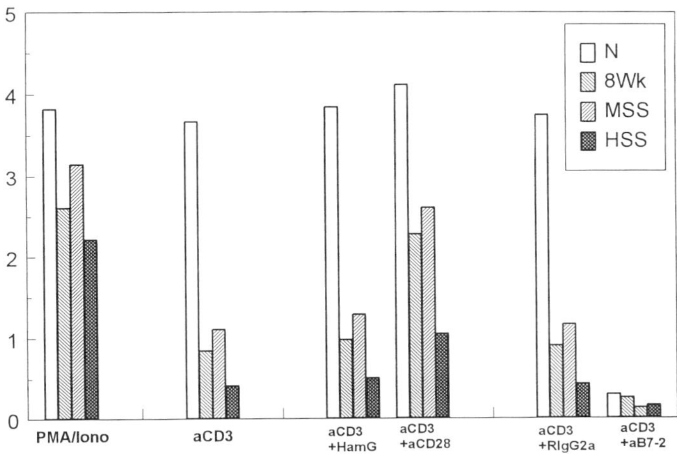

FIGURE 8. Spleen cell IL-2 levels: normal, 8-week infected, MSS, and HSS spleen cell responses to PMA/Iono; anti-CD3 ± anti-CD28 or ± anti-B7-2. HamG (hamster IgG) and RIgG2a (rat IgG2a) are the isotypic controls to anti-CD28 and anti-B7-2, respectively.

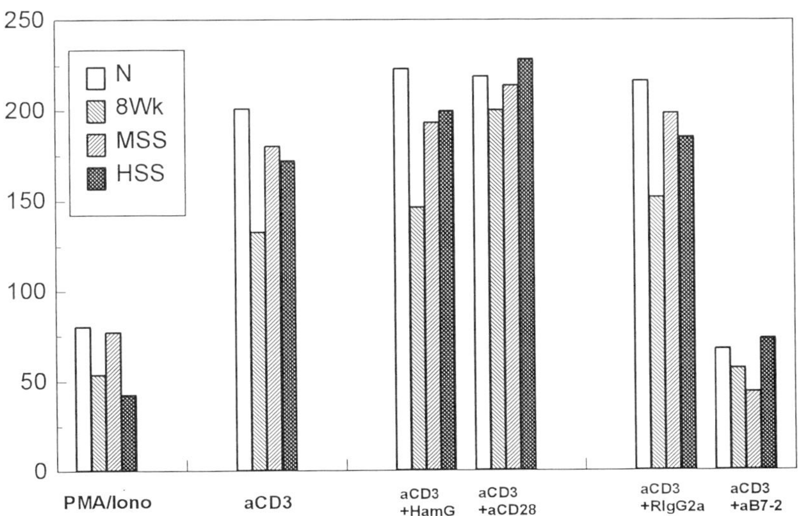

FIGURE 9. Spleen cell IFN-γ levels: normal, 8-week infected, MSS, and HSS spleen cell responses to PMA/Iono; anti-CD3 ± anti-CD28 or ± anti-B7-2. HamG (hamster IgG) and RIgG2a (rat IgG2a) are the isotypic controls to anti-CD28 and anti-B7-2, respectively.

Mean IL-4 (ng/ml)

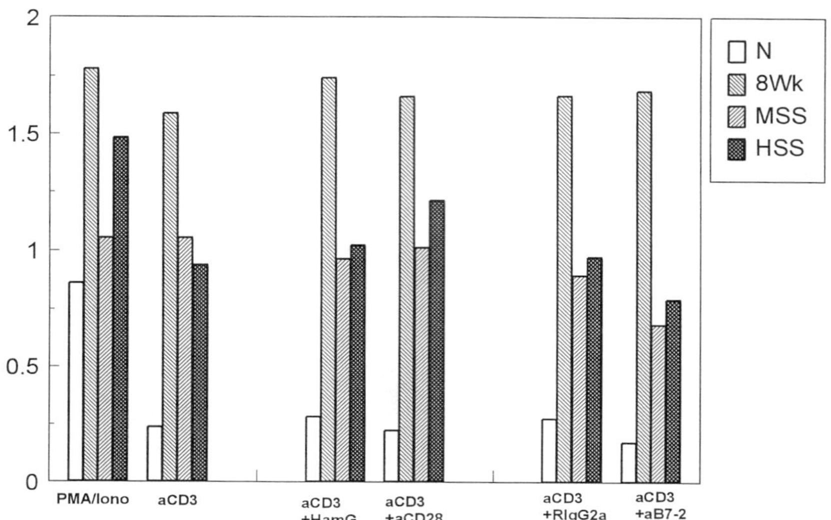

FIGURE 10. Spleen cell IL-4 levels: normal, 8-week infected, MSS, and HSS spleen cell responses to PMA/Iono: anti-CD3 ± anti-CD28 or ± anti-B7-2. HamG (hamster IgG) and RIgG2a (rat IgG2a) are the isotypic controls to anti-CD28 and anti-B7-2, respectively.

Mean IL-10 (U/ml)

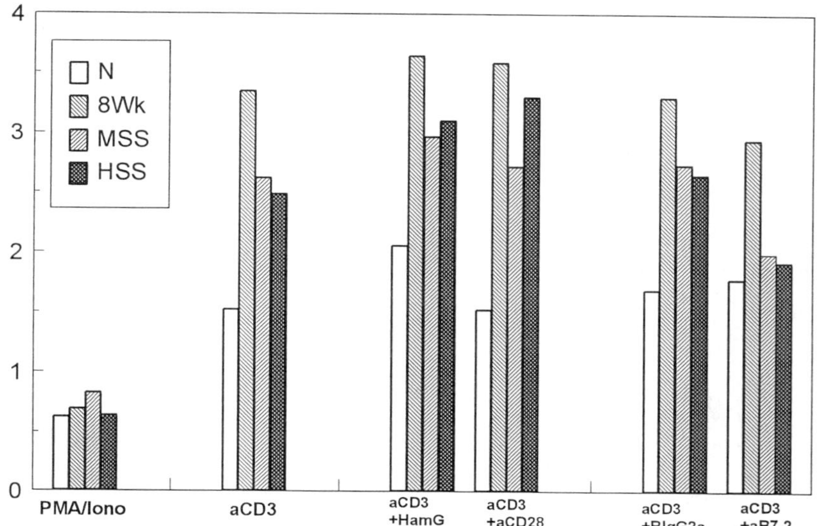

FIGURE 11. Spleen cell IL-10 levels: normal, 8-week infected, MSS, and HSS spleen cell responses to PMA/Iono: anti-CD3 ± anti-CD28 or ± anti-B7-2. HamG (hamster IgG) and RigG2a (rat IgG2a) are the isotypic controls to anti-CD28 and anti-B7-2, respectively.

FIGURE 12 summarizes the currently known characteristics of MSS and HSS mice as well as those of mice with acute infections. Many questions, such as how there could be such a drastic dichotomy in inbred mice and what event(s) drives chronic infection to one syndrome or the other, remain unanswered. However, it is hoped that further investigation of this model will reveal important insights into the severe pathology of schistosomiasis and eventually aid in the prevention of severe disease in humans.

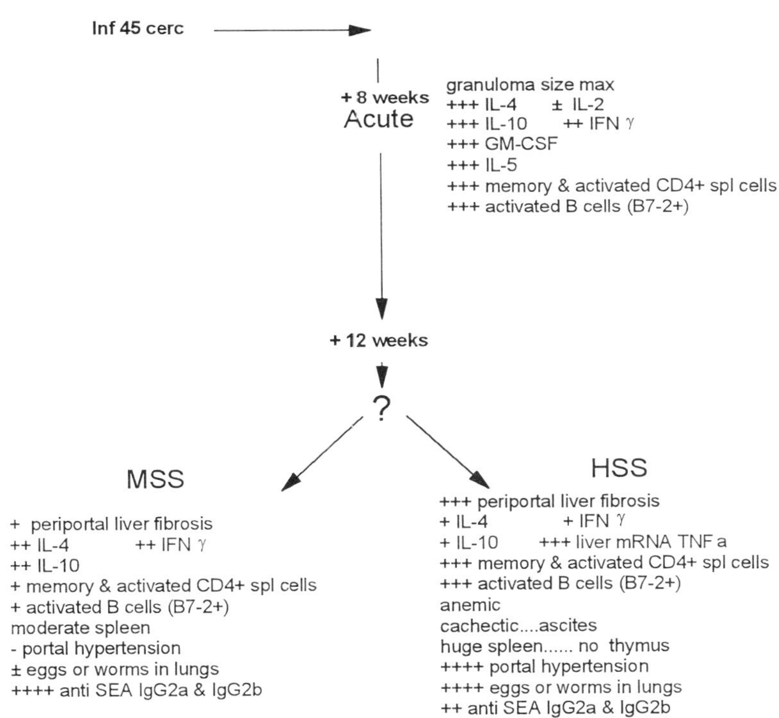

FIGURE 12. Summary of the MSS/HSS model of murine schistosomiasis.

SUMMARY

Inbred CBA/J mice with chronic (20-week) *Schistosoma mansoni* infections demonstrate two distinct syndromes. Hypersplenomegaly syndrome (HSS), characterized by a massive spleen, liver fibrosis, ascites, and anemia, resembles hepatosplenic human schistosomiasis, complete with portal hypertension and shunting. Moderate splenomegaly (MSS) syndrome, with less severe pathology, parallels most chronic human infections. Phenotypic analyses of spleen cells for CD44, CD62L, CD45RB, Ia, and CD25 indicate that HSS mice have more activated and memory CD4$^+$ T cells than do MSS mice. HSS animals also have more B cells that highly express B7-2. Anti-CD3 stimulated spleen cells from 8-week or chronically infected mice produce IL-4 and IL-10 in a manner that appears not to involve the CD28/B7-2 costimulation pathway. By contrast, IFN-γ production is augmented in the presence of anti-CD28 and decreased in the presence of anti-B7-2. Infected mice make very little IL-2 to anti-CD3, even with added anti-CD28. As cytokines affect resultant B-cell responses and HSS and MSS mice display distinctive isotypes, differential regulatory or anergy hypotheses may best explain MSS/HSS differences.

REFERENCES

1. THE CONTROL OF SCHISTOSOMIASIS. SECOND REPORT OF THE WHO EXPERT COMMITTEE. 1993. Technical Report Series No. 830, World Health Organization.
2. BOROS, D. L. 1989. Clin. Microbiol. Rev. **2:** 250–269.
3. GRIMAUD, J. A., D. L. BOROS, C. TAKIYA, R. C. MATHEW & H. EMONARD. 1987. Am. J. Trop. Med. Hyg. **37:** 335–344.
4. WYLER, D. J., H. P. ERLICH, A. E. POSTLETHWAITE, R. RAGHOW & M. M. MURPHY. 138. J. Immunol. **138:** 1581–1586.
5. CHEEVER, A. W. 1972. Trans. R. Soc. Trop. Med. Hyg. **66:** 947–948.
6. ANDRADE, Z. A. 1987. Mem. Inst. Oswaldo Cruz **82:** 325–334.
7. HENDERSON, G. S., N. A. NIX, M. A. MONTESANO, D. GOLD, G. L. FREEMAN, T. L. MCCURLY & D. G. COLLEY. 1993. J. Pathol. **142:** 703–714.
8. POWELL, M. R. & D. G. COLLEY. 1985. J. Immunol. **134:** 4140–4145.
9. TSANG, V. C. W., B. C. WILSON & S. E. MADDISON. 1980. Clin. Chem. **26:** 1255.
10. MACDONALD, H. R., R. C. BUDD & J. C. CEROTTINI. 1990. Curr. Top. Microbiol. Immunol. **159:** 97–109.
11. SWAIN, S. L., A. D. WEINBERG & M. ENGLISH. 1990. J. Immunol. **144:** 1788–1799.
12. SWAIN, S. L., L. M. BRADLEY, M. CROFT, S. TONKONOGY, G. ATKINS, A. D. WEINBERG, D. D. DUNCAN, S. M. HEDRICK, R. W. DUTTON & G. HUSTON. 1991. Immunol. Rev. **123:** 115–144.
13. LEE, W. T. & E. S. VITETTA. 1991. Cell. Immunol. **132:** 215–222.
14. BRADLEY, L. M., G. G. ATKINS & S. L. SWAIN. 1992. J. Immunol. **148:** 324–331.
15. LEE, W. T. & E. S. VITETTA. 1990. Cell. Immunol. **130:** 459–471.
16. SCHWARTZ, B. D. 1984. J. Mol. Cell. Immunol. **1:** 155–156.
17. PARISH, C. R. & I. F. C. MCKENZIE. 1977. Cell. Immunol. **33:** 134–144.
18. HENRY, C., B. DOE, J. KIMURA, J. NORTH & L. WOFSY. 1980. Cell. Immunol. **53:** 125–137.
19. LENSCHOW, D. J., A. I. SPERLING, M. P. COOKE, G. FREEMAN, L. RHEE, D. C. DECKER, G. GRAY, L. M. NADLER, C. C. GOODNOW & J. A. BLUESTONE. 1994. J. Immunol. **153:** 1990–1997.
20. HATHCOCK, K. S., G. LASZLO, H. B. DICKLER, J. BRADSHAW, P. LINSLEY & R. J. HODES. 1993. Science **262:** 905–907.
21. BOSSHARDT, S. C., G. L. FREEMAN, JR., W. E. SECOR & D. G. COLLEY. 1996. IL-10 deficit correlates with chronic, hypersplenomegaly syndrome in male CBA/J mice infected with *Schistosoma mansoni.* Submitted.
22. COLLEY, D. G., A. A. GARCIA, J. R. LAMBERTUCCI, J. C. PARRA, N. KATZ, R. S. ROCHA & G. GAZZINELLI. 1986. Am. J. Trop. Med. Hyg. **35:** 793–802.
23. VILLANUEVA, P. O. F., H. REISER & M. J. STADECKER. 1994. J. Immunol. **153:** 5190–5199.
24. PEARCE, E. J., P. CASPAR, J.-M. GRZYCH, F. A. LEWIS & A. SHER. 1991. J. Exp. Med. **173:** 159–166.
25. GRZYCH, J.-M., E. PEARCE, A. W. CHEEVER, Z. A. CAULADA, S. HIENY, F. LEWIS & A. SHER. 1991. J. Immunol. **135:** 95–104.
26. BOSSIE, A. & E. S. VITETTA. 1991. Cell. Immunol. **135:** 95–104.
27. MOSSMANN, T. R. & R. L. COFFMAN. 1989. Ann. Rev. Immunol. **7:** 145–173.
28. LUKACS, N. W. & D. L. BOROS. 1993. Clin. Immunol. Immunopathol. **68:** 57–63.

29. WYNN, T. A., I. ELTOUM, I. P. OSWALD, A. W. CHEEVER & A. SHER. 1994. J. Exp. Med. **179:** 1551–1561.
30. HENDERSON, G. S., X. LU, T. L. MCCURLEY & D. G. COLLEY. 1992. J. Immunol. **148:** 2261–2269.
31. SHER, A., D. FIORENTINO, P. CASPAR, E. PEARCE & T. MOSMANN. 1991. J. Immunol. **147:** 2713–2716.
32. BLUESTONE, J. A. 1995. Immunity **2:** 555–559.

Long-Term Antibody Production Is Sustained by Antibody-Secreting Cells in the Bone Marrow following Acute Viral Infection[a]

MARK K. SLIFKA AND RAFI AHMED

Emory Vaccine Center and
Department of Microbiology and Immunology
Emory University School of Medicine
Atlanta, Georgia 30307

An important goal of vaccination is to induce long-term antibody production, since preexisting antibody typically provides the first line of defense against reinfection. It is well documented that a wide variety of acute viral infections induce long-term, potentially lifelong antibody responses.[1] For example, fully protective neutralizing antibody against yellow fever was demonstrated 75 years after infection.[2] Moreover, this impressive antiviral antibody response was sustained in the absence of any known reexposure to virus or virally infected mosquitoes. Although reexposure to a virus will undoubtedly boost an ongoing antibody response, several cases of long-term antibody production have been demonstrated in the absence of any known reexposure.[2–5] In addition, vaccination with nonreplicating antigens such as diptheria and tetanus toxoid induces antibody responses that are maintained for more than 20–30 years.[6–8]

One step towards understanding the nature of persistent serum antibody production is to identify the anatomic site of antibody-secreting cells (ASC) that actively secrete immunoglobulin. These experiments have been facilitated by the ELISPOT assay which allows direct quantitation of individual antigen-specific ASC from distinct anatomic locations such as the spleen and bone marrow. In the past, the bone marrow has been overlooked as a site of antibody production.[9] However, interest in bone marrow-derived antibody production has increased since the bone marrow was identified as the major site of antibody-secreting cells following acute viral infection. We previously demonstrated that long-term antibody production against the natural murine pathogen, lymphocytic choriomeningitis virus (LCMV), is maintained by antibody-secreting cells in the bone marrow compartment.[10] Long-term antibody production by virus-specific ASC in the bone marrow was also shown following other acute viral infections such as sendai virus, influenza, and vesicular stomatitis virus (VSV).[11,12]

To examine the anatomic site and duration of antibody production following an acute viral infection, we studied the humoral response of adult mice acutely infected with LCMV. LCMV causes a short-term viral infection in adult mice that is rapidly cleared in a $CD8^+$ T-cell–dependent manner[13–18] and induces lifelong virus-specific serum antibody production.[10,13,15,19]

Following LCMV infection, antiviral antibody responses in the spleen and bone marrow were compared at several timepoints ranging from 8–325 days after primary

---

[a]Tel: 404/727-3571; fax: 404/727-3722.

infection and from 3–30 days after secondary infection. Initially, the spleen was the major site of antibody production, but this response was transient and declined markedly after resolving the viral infection. As splenic ASC populations declined however, prolonged antibody production was maintained by a large population of virus-specific ASC located in the bone marrow.

MATERIALS AND METHODS

Mice. BALB/c Byj (H-2^d) mice were purchased from Jackson Laboratory, Bar Harbor, Maine or bred in our colony at the University of California at Los Angeles.

Virus. The Armstrong CA 1371 strain of LCMV was used in this study.[20] LCMV immune mice were obtained by injecting 5- to 8-week old mice intraperitoneally (ip) with 2×10^5 PFU of LCMV-Armstrong. For the secondary LCMV infection, mice were injected ip with 1×10^6 PFU of LCMV-Armstrong.

ELISPOT. LCMV-specific antibody-secreting cells were quantitated by the ELISPOT assay as previously described.[10]

Determination of Total Bone Marrow Cells. ^{59}Fe distribution studies have shown that ~12.6% of total mouse bone marrow is located in both femurs combined.[21] No differences have been detected between the ASC activity of bone marrow cells from femur, tibia, humerus, rib, or sternum.[21] Typically, two adult femurs yield between 2.0 and 2.5×10^7 bone marrow cells.

ELISA. LCMV-specific serum antibody was titered by a solid-phase enzyme-linked immunosorbent assay as described previously.[20,22] IgG subclass distribution patterns were determined by serial threefold dilutions of duplicate serum samples.

RESULTS

Acute LCMV Infection Induces Lifelong Virus-Specific Serum Antibody Production

Infection of adult BALB/c mice with LCMV-Armstrong results in an acute, systemic viral infection that is typically cleared within 10–15 days and induces lifelong T-cell and B-cell memory.[13–15,19] Likewise, high levels of LCMV-specific IgG were detected from day 8 to >300 days postinfection with little to no decline in antibody levels over this period of time (FIG. 1). Therefore, in accordance with previous work,[13,15,19] these results show that after clearing acute LCMV infection, antiviral serum antibody is maintained essentially for the lifespan of the mouse.

The Initial Antiviral ASC Response to Acute LCMV Infection Occurs in the Spleen, But after Resolving the Infection, Most ASC Localize in the Bone Marrow

To study the anatomic site of virus-specific antibody production, an LCMV-specific ELISPOT assay was developed (FIG. 2). This assay was used to quantitate virus-specific antibody-secreting cells directly *ex vivo*. Only virus-specific ASC that are spontaneously secreting antibody are detected by the ELISPOT assay, because this technique has only a 4-5–hour incubation period, a time interval too short for memory B cells to differentiate into antibody-secreting cells.[22] If the ELISPOT assay was performed on naive cells from uninfected mice, no spots were formed, indicating that only *in vivo*-generated LCMV-specific ASC were identified (FIG. 2). Using this

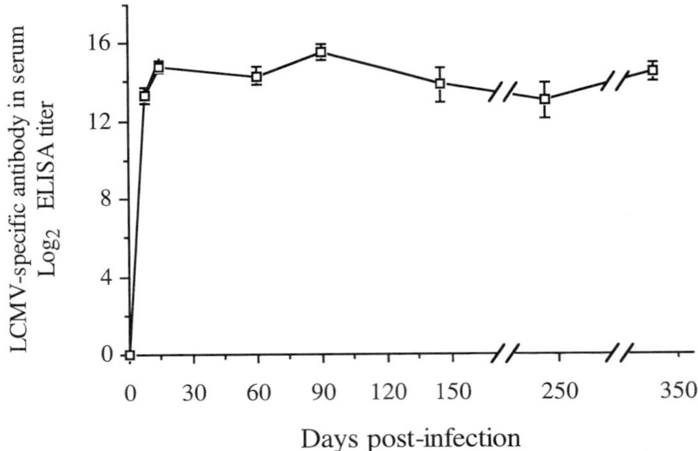

FIGURE 1. Acute infection with lymphocytic choriomeningitis virus (LCMV) induces life-long antiviral serum antibody. BALB/c micr were infected ip with 2×10^5 PFU of LCMV-Armstrong, and virus-specific serum antibody titers were calculated from the average of three to four mice for each timepoint by ELISA.

technique, antiviral ASC were quantitated in the spleen and bone marrow following acute LCMV infection.

The peak LCMV-specific ASC response in the spleen occurred at 8 days postinfection with a frequency of 580 ASC per 10^6 spleen cells. Splenic ASC numbers declined by day 15 to a frequency of about 200 ASC per 10^6 spleen cells. By 60 days postinfection, the frequency of antiviral ASC in the spleen declined to about 15 ASC per 10^6 spleen cells. Similar to the spleen, the lymph nodes had a high number of virus-specific ASC at 8 days postinfection with an average of ~ 140 ASC per 10^6 cells. At later timepoints (> 60 days), the lymph nodes averaged only 2–3 antiviral ASC per 10^6 cells, indicating ASC kinetics equivalent to those observed in the spleen.

During the course of infection, the kinetics of the antiviral ASC response in the bone marrow was strikingly different from that observed in the spleen. During the peak splenic ASC response at 8 days postinfection, no LCMV-specific ASC were identified in the bone marrow (<1 ASC per 5×10^6 bone marrow cells). However, as the splenic ASC populations declined, virus-specific ASC began to accumulate in the bone marrow with a frequency of 40 ASC per 10^6 bone marrow cells at 15 days postinfection. By 60 days postinfection and for the life of the animal, the virus-specific ASC populations in the bone marrow averaged about 150 ASC per 10^6 bone marrow cells and represented the major anatomic site of antiviral antibody production. It is unlikely that the migration of ASC to the bone marrow was due to prolonged viral infection of this site, because infectious virus is cleared from the bone marrow by day 8 postinfection with no viral RNA (as demonstrated by RT-PCR analysis) detected at this time.[10] Taken together, these results indicate that the humoral immune response against a virus first occurs in the spleen, but long-term production of antiviral antibody is sustained by ASC in the bone marrow (FIG. 3).

A phenotypic difference was observed between the rate of antibody secretion and/or general affinity of antibody secreted by ASC in the spleen at 8 days postinfection and the antibody produced by bone marrow localized ASC. Compared to the "spots" formed by antibody-secreting cells in the bone marrow, the relative size and intensity of the spots formed by splenic ASC at 8 days postinfection were considerably smaller and less intense in color (FIG. 4). Since the size of the spot is indicative of the rate of antibody secretion[23] and the color intensity gives an overall representation of binding affinity to antigen, this suggests that ASC may have undergone affinity maturation prior to migration to the bone marrow. The smaller, more diffusely staining spots obtained from ASC in the spleen at day 8 postinfection is not surprising because many of the splenic ASC at this early timepoint may be activated B cells that have not fully differentiated into mature plasma cells and therefore may secrete smaller amounts of antibody. In comparison to day 8 postinfection, most of the remaining splenic ASC observed at 100 days postinfection may be

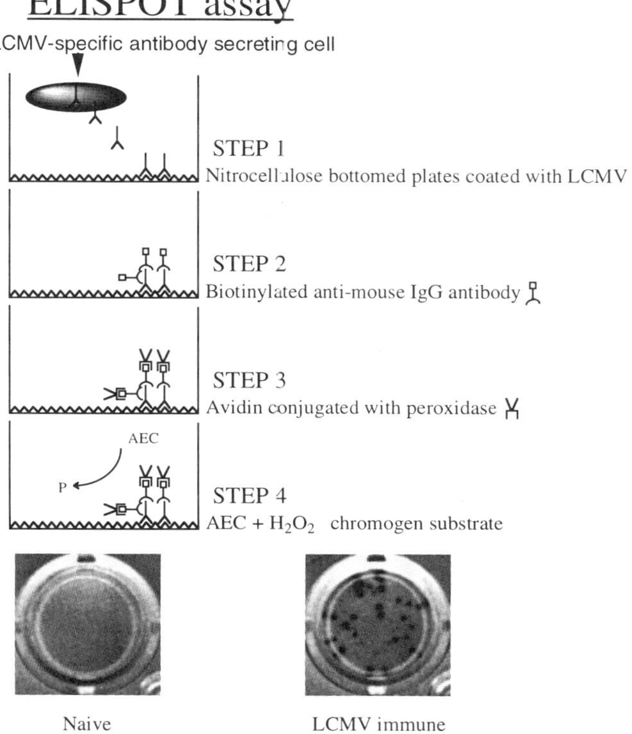

FIGURE 2. LCMV-specific ELISPOT assay. LCMV-specific antibody-secreting cells (ASC) were quantitated directly *ex vivo* by plating cells from the spleen or bone marrow into ELISPOT plates coated with virus. Performing the ELISPOT assay with cells from uninfected mice (naive) does not result in virus-specific spot formation. By contrast, cells from an LCMV-immune mouse (in this example, bone marrow cells taken at 84 days postinfection) yield many easily identified spots that result from the antibody secreted by LCMV-specific ASC during the 4–5–hour incubation period (step 1) of the ELISPOT assay.

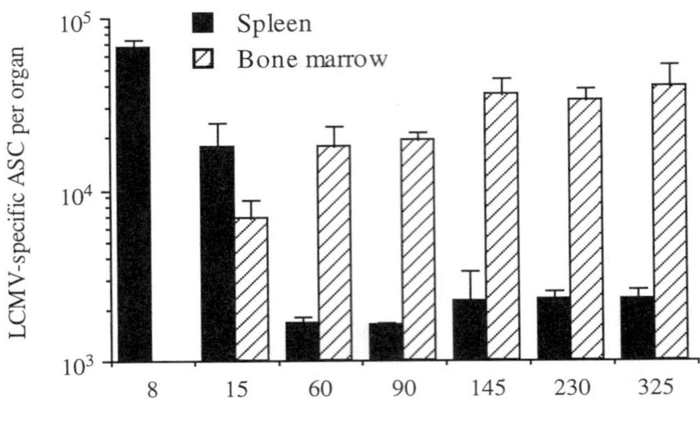

FIGURE 3. Initial antibody responses to acute viral infection occur in the spleen, but long-term antibody production occurs in bone marrow. The ELISPOT assay was used to quantitate individual LCMV-specific antibody-secreting cells (ASC) isolated from the spleen and bone marrow, and the data represent the average of 3–6 BALB/c mice assayed individually at the indicated timepoints after primary infection. The number of LCMV-specific ASC in bone marrow were below detection at 8 days postinfection (< 100 ASC per total bone marrow).

plasma cells since activated B cells are not likely to be present at this late timepoint, and these ASC demonstrate the phenotype of the ASC in the bone marrow, with a relatively high rate of antibody secretion (FIG. 4).

The IgG Subclass Profile of LCMV-Specific ASC in the Bone Marrow and Spleen Correlate with the IgG Subclass Distribution of LCMV-Specific Serum Antibody

Most viral infections induce an IgG response that is comprised mostly of IgG2a.[24,25] Following acute LCMV infection, the serum IgG subclass profile has been shown to be mostly IgG2a,[24-27] and we also found that IgG2a was the major IgG subclass produced following acute LCMV infection. This observation was further characterized by comparing the LCMV-specific IgG in the serum to the IgG subclasses being produced by antiviral ASC in the spleen and bone marrow (TABLE 1). The distribution of the IgG subclasses produced by antiviral ASC in both locations closely matched the LCMV-specific IgG in the serum at 8, 15, and 84 days postinfection.

Secondary LCMV Infection Results in a Transient Increase in Splenic ASC Numbers Followed by an Increased Population of Virus-Specific ASC in the Bone Marrow

The humoral response induced by secondary viral infection is quite different from that induced by primary viral infection for several reasons. During a primary infection, naive B cells are induced into antibody production, whereas during a secondary infection the more rapid anamnestic response is due mainly to restimulation of memory B cells. For this reason, it was of interest to examine the kinetics and anatomic location of virus-specific ASC formed during secondary viral infection. At

60 days after primary infection, LCMV-immune mice were challenged with virus, and the kinetics of the LCMV-specific ASC response were determined in the spleen and bone marrow (FIG. 5). As described previously,[10,19] the virus-specific ASC numbers in the spleen increased rapidly and peaked at day 5 postinfection (compared to day 8 after a primary LCMV infection) with a frequency of about 180 ASC per 10^6 cells. By 15 days postinfection, the splenic ASC response had declined by nearly 70%. LCMV-specific ASC numbers in the bone marrow remained virtually unchanged during the early stages of the secondary infection, but by 15 days after secondary infection, the ASC numbers increased by approximately twofold. This result was accompanied by a twofold increase in LCMV-specific serum antibody titers (FIG. 5). This indicates that the kinetics of the bone marrow-derived ASC response during the secondary infection were similar to the primary viral infection in that a delay of several days occurred between the peak ASC response in the spleen and the increase in ASC populations in the bone marrow. After a primary viral infection, virus-specific ASC in the bone marrow outnumbered those in the spleen by about 10 to 1, but at day 5 after secondary infection, the total number of antiviral

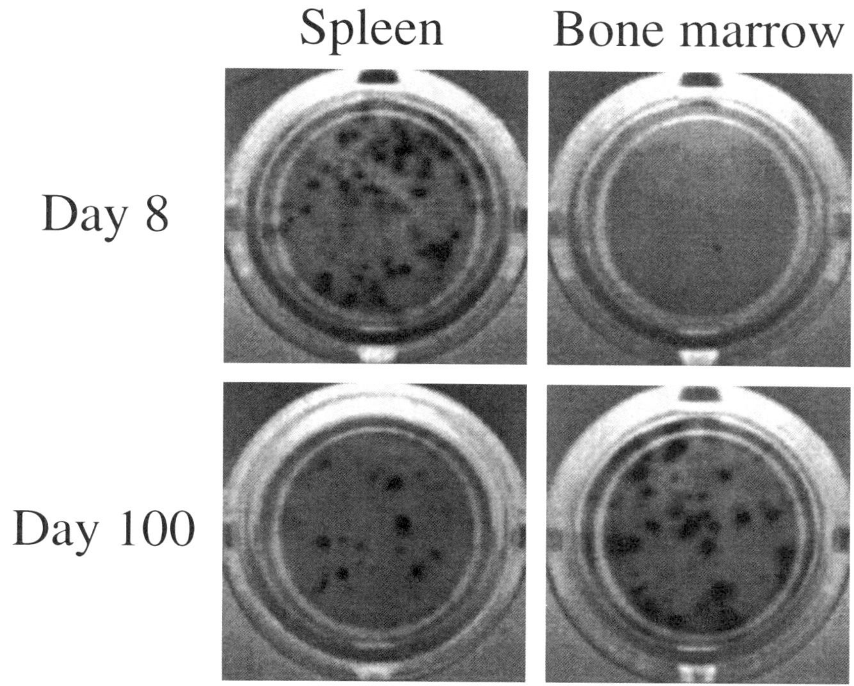

FIGURE 4. Representative ELISPOT showing size and color intensity of spots formed by LCMV-specific antibody-secreting cells (ASC) at different times postinfection. Equal numbers of bone marrow or spleen cells were added to each well, and the number of LCMV-specific ASC were quantitated by the ELISPOT assay using reagents specific for total IgG. The peak splenic ASC response occurred at 8 days postinfection, but no LCMV-specific ASC were detected in the bone marrow at this time. At 100 days postinfection, few LCMV-specific ASC remained in the spleen, whereas a large number of virus-specific ASC were found in the bone marrow.

TABLE 1. IgG Subclass Profile Following Acute LCMV Infection[a]

Days Postinfection	Sample	IgG Subclass			
		IgG1	IgG2a	IgG2b	IgG3
Day 8	Serum antibody	32%	55%	1%	12%
	Spleen ASC	30%	57%	1%	12%
	Bone marrow ASC	—	—	—	—
Day 15	Serum antibody	26%	70%	2%	2%
	Spleen ASC	24%	72%	4%	0%
	Bone marrow ASC	26%	69%	5%	0%
Day 84	Serum antibody	24%	75%	1%	0%
	Spleen ASC	24%	72%	2%	0%
	Bone marrow ASC	21%	77%	2%	0%

[a]IgG2a is the major IgG subclass produced after acute LCMV infection. BALB/c mice were infected with 2×10^5 PFU of LCMV-Armstrong ip and serum, spleen, and bone marrow samples were collected at 8, 15, and 84 days postinfection. Spleen and bone marrow data represent the average of three mice per group analyzed by the ELISPOT assay, and serum data represent the average of two mice per group analyzed by ELISA.

ASC in the spleen transiently surpassed the total number of ASC in the bone marrow. By day 30 however, the ratio of ASC in the bone marrow and the spleen returned to the ratio observed at late timepoints following primary viral infection with about 10-fold more ASC in the bone marrow. Therefore, the bone marrow remains the predominant source of virus-specific antibody-secreting cells following either primary or secondary viral infection.

DISCUSSION

Since the half-life of immunoglobulins in the serum ranges from only a few days to a few weeks,[28–31] a stable number of antigen-specific antibody-secreting cells is required to sustain serum antibody levels. Using the LCMV model system, we identified the anatomical site and duration of virus-specific ASC following acute viral infection. The initial antibody response occurred in the spleen and then declined over the next few weeks. As splenic ASC numbers decreased, virus-specific ASC began to accumulate in the bone marrow. After viral clearance, bone marrow was the major site of antiviral antibody production. Following secondary viral infection, the kinetics of the LCMV-specific ASC response were accelerated in comparison with the primary response. Again an initial rise in antiviral ASC numbers occurred in the spleen and was then followed by a delayed increase in LCMV-specific ASC in the bone marrow. These results indicate that after clearing either a primary or secondary viral infection, early antibody responses developed in the spleen, but long-term antibody production occurred in the bone marrow.

Our results and those of others have shown that the peak LCMV-specific ASC response in the spleen occurs at 8 days postinfection.[10,19] This timepoint has also been identified as the peak virus-specific effector cytolytic T-lymphocyte (CTL) response in the spleen.[14] This suggests that the effector phase of B cells (i.e., spontaneous *ex vivo* antibody production by ASC) and T cells (i.e., directly cytolytic CTL) in the spleen have comparable kinetics. However, it is intriguing that no LCMV-specific ASC were found in the bone marrow at 8 days postinfection, even though a direct *ex vivo* LCMV-specific CTL response is readily detectable in the bone marrow at this time (Slifka and Ahmed, manuscript in preparation). Because virus-specific B cells and T cells might be expected to have similar migratory patterns (homing to sites of inflammation or infection, for example), one can speculate that mechanism(s) may exist that influence ASC migration to the bone marrow. The observed delay in virus-specific ASC migration to the bone marrow (FIGS. 3 and 5) may allow time for somatic mutation and affinity maturation to occur. In accordance with this, the IgG subclass profile of bone marrow-derived ASC corresponded to the day-15 splenic IgG subclass profile and not to the day-8 IgG subclass profile (TABLE 1). Sequence analysis of the Ig V region of bone marrow-derived ASC versus splenic ASC may determine if affinity maturation occurs before ASC migrate to the bone marrow compartment. The possibility that newly generated ASC may be retained in the spleen and/or barred from the bone marrow during the initiation of primary and secondary humoral responses deserves further attention.

Antigenic stimulation of naive B cells and their subsequent differentiation into memory B cells and plasma cells take place in the germinal centers of the spleen and lymph nodes.[32] If plasma cells did not migrate out of these peripheral lymphoid organs, over the course of a lifetime, lymphoid follicles would need to allocate space for the many antigen-specific ASC that would have accumulated over this extended period of time. By targeting plasma cells to the bone marrow, peripheral lymphoid organs (spleen, lymph nodes, etc.) return to homeostasis, ready to mount new antibody responses upon the next antigenic encounter. Evidence supporting this

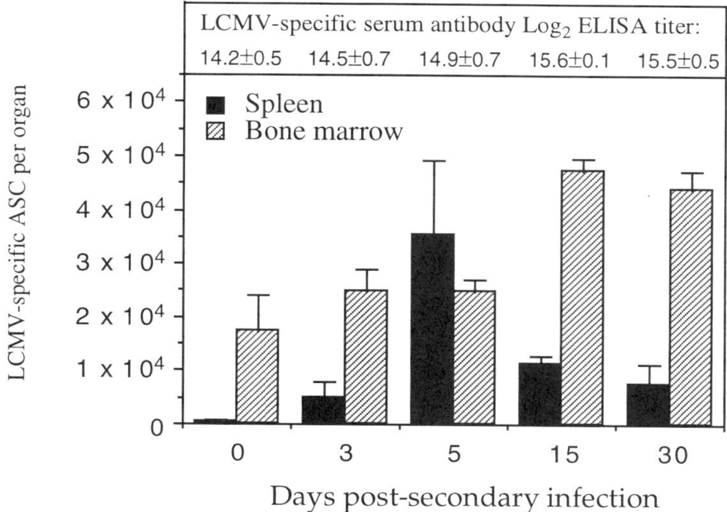

FIGURE 5. Secondary LCMV infection of immune mice induces a rapid, yet transient splenic antibody response followed by increased ASC numbers in bone marrow and higher LCMV-specific serum antibody. Adult BALB/c mice were first infected ip with 2×10^5 PFU of LCMV-Armstrong and were rechallenged 60 days later with 10^6 PFU of the same virus. The ELISPOT and ELISA data represent the average of three mice per group, except on day 15 which is an average of two mice. Primary response serum (pre-challenge) was assayed together with the corresponding secondary response (post-challenge) serum by LCMV-specific ELISA (represented on a $\log_2$ scale above each corresponding timepoint).

point of view includes studies showing that germinal centers recede within a few weeks after antigenic stimulation,[32] whereas antibody-secreting cells continue to accumulate in the bone marrow over time[9] (Slifka and Ahmed, unpublished results). Because memory B cells are rare or absent from the bone marrow[12,33] (Slifka and Ahmed, unpublished results), there may be an anatomic segregation of B-cell differentiation and long-term antigen-specific antibody production.

In these studies, we examined the humoral response against acute LCMV infection in terms of the number, duration, and anatomic site of antiviral antibody-secreting cells. Another essential aspect of humoral immunity is the development of memory B cells. Acute LCMV infection induces long-term B-cell memory. This was illustrated by the more rapid induction of the splenic antibody response following secondary viral infection (FIG. 5). We recently developed a limiting dilution assay for quantitating LCMV-specific memory B-cell precursors (MBCp).[22] Using this assay, we observed that LCMV-immune mice maintained a stable population of virus-specific MBCp for >300 days postinfection (Slifka and Ahmed, unpublished results). Therefore, both virus-specific memory B cells and antibody-secreting cells are maintained virtually for the lifespan of LCMV-immune mice.

The role of both plasma cells and memory B cells in maintaining continuous antibody production is an important consideration in studying long-term humoral immunity. The current notion is that plasma cells are short-lived, with a lifespan of 8 hours to 3 days.[34–38] This indicates the absolute necessity for memory B cells to replenish the rapidly disappearing plasma cell populations in order to maintain prolonged antibody production. A widely accepted theory of how long-term antibody production is maintained is that memory B cells are continually stimulated into antibody production by persisting antigen in the form of immune complexes on follicular dendritic cells (FDC).[39–41] Although antigen-antibody complexes may persist for several months or a few years, it is difficult to perceive how these complexes can support antibody production for greater than 25 years, as in diptheria vaccination,[6,7] or 75 years, as in the case of yellow fever infection.[2] It therefore is unlikely that this mechanism is the only one involved with maintaining serum antibody production. Another mechanism that may be involved with antibody maintenance is that some plasma cells may be long-lived. This hypothesis is supported by ^{3}H-incorporation studies showing that plasma cells may survive for several weeks to several months after antigenic stimulation.[42,43] In addition, we recently observed that antiviral antibody production can be sustained for at least 8 months after memory B cells are depleted (Slifka and Ahmed, manuscript in preparations), indicating that plasma cells may indeed have a much longer lifespan than previously believed. These results suggest a reevaluation of the current dogma concerning the mechanisms of persistent antibody production.

A fundamental difference appears to exist in the requirements for inducing long-term antibody responses after a live viral infection versus vaccination with nonreplicating antigens. For instance, a single acute viral infection often induces persistent antibody production,[1] whereas multiple immunizations with a nonreplicating antigen are typically required to generate long-term antibody responses.[9,44–46] Therefore, by studying viral infections that induce prolonged antibody production, we may gain a better understanding of the underlying mechanisms that determine the duration of humoral responses. This information may lead to the development of better adjuvants and vaccines that are more effective in inducing long-term antibody production.

SUMMARY

Acute viral infection of humans induces virus-specific serum antibody production that often persists for decades. To better understand the nature of this long-term antiviral antibody response, we studied antiviral antibody production of mice acutely infected with lymphocytic choriomeningitis virus (LCMV). Although this viral infection is resolved within 2 weeks, virus-specific serum antibody levels were maintained for > 300 days postinfection.

The anatomic site of long-term antibody production was identified using an ELISPOT assay to quantitate LCMV-specific antibody-secreting cells (ASC). The initial antiviral ASC response in the spleen peaked at 8 days postinfection and then declined sharply, with less than 10% of the day 8 ASC population remaining after 60 days. Although no LCMV-specific ASC were detected in the bone marrow at day 8, virus-specific ASC began accumulating in the bone marrow by 15 days postinfection. By day 60, approximately 10-fold more antiviral ASC were present in the bone marrow than in the spleen, and the bone marrow remained the major site of antibody production for > 10 months postinfection.

To further characterize the LCMV-specific antibody response, the relative percentage of each IgG subclass (IgG1, IgG2a, IgG2b, and IgG3) was determined. IgG2a was the predominant IgG subclass produced during LCMV infection, and the IgG subclass profile of virus-specific ASC in the spleen and bone marrow matched the IgG subclass profile of virus-specific IgG in the serum. Following a secondary infection with LCMV, splenic ASC numbers increased rapidly with a peak at 5 days after secondary infection. This was followed by a sharp decline in ASC numbers by day 15. In contrast, virus-specific ASC numbers in bone marrow remained essentially unchanged during the acute phase of the secondary infection but increased approximately twofold at day 15, corresponding to a twofold increase in virus-specific serum antibody levels.

These results indicate that following a primary viral infection or upon reexposure to a virus, the initial antibody response occurs in the spleen, but long-term antiviral antibody production is maintained in the bone marrow.

REFERENCES

1. SLIFKA, M. K. & R. AHMED. 1996. Trends Microbiol. **4:** 394–400.
2. SAWYER, W. A. 1931. J. Prev. Med. **5:** 413–428.
3. PANUM, P. L. 1847. Virchows Arch. **1:** 492.
4. PAUL, J. R., J. T. RIORDAN & J. L. MELNICK. 1951. Am. J. Hyg. **54:** 275–285.
5. COONEY, E. L., A. C. COLLIER, P. D., GREENBERG, *et al.* 1991. Lancet **337:** 567–572.
6. KJELDSEN, K., I. HERON & O. SIMONSEN. 1985. Lancet **1:** 900–902.
7. COHEN, D., M. S. GREEN, E. KATZENELSON, *et al.* 1994. Eur. J. Epidemiol. **10:** 267–270.
8. GOTTLIEB, S., F. X. MCLAUGHLIN, L. LEVINE, W. C. LATHAM & G. EDSALL. 1964. Am. J. Public Health **54:** 961–971.
9. BENNER, R., W. HIJMANS & J. J. HAAIJMAN. 1981. Clin. Exp. Immunol. **46:** 1–8.
10. SLIFKA, M. K., M. MATLOUBIAN & R. AHMED. 1995. J. Virol. **69:** 1895–1902.
11. HYLAND, L., M. SANGSTER, R. SEALY & C. COLECLOUGH. 1994. J. Virol. **68:** 6083–6086.
12. BACHMAN, M. F., T. M. KUNDIG, B. ODERMATT, H. HENGARTNER & R. M. ZINKERNAGEL. 1994. J. Immunol. **153:** 3386–3397.
13. AHMED, R. 1992. Sem. Immunol. **4:** 105–109.
14. LAU, L. L., B. D. JAMIESON, T. SOMASUNDARAM & R. AHMED. 1994. Nature **369:** 648–652.
15. BUCHMEIER, M. J., R. M. WELSH, F. J. DUTKO & M. B. A. OLDSTONE. 1980. Adv. Immunol. **30:** 275–331.

16. BYRNE, J. A. & M. B. A. OLDSTONE. 1984. J. Virol. **51:** 682–686.
17. LEHMANN-GRUBE, F., D. MOSKOPHIDIS & J. LOHLER. 1988. Ann. N.Y. Acad. Sci. **532:** 238–356.
18. ZINKERNAGEL, R. M. & P. C. DOHERTY. 1979. Adv. Immunol. **27:** 51–177.
19. MOSKOPHIDIS, D. & F. LEHMANN-GRUBE. 1984. J. Immunol. **133:** 3366–3370.
20. AHMED, R., A. SALMI, L. D. BUTLER, J. M. CHILLER & M. B. A. OLDSTONE. 1984. J. Exp. Med. **160:** 521–540.
21. BENNER, R., F. MEIMA, G. M. VAN DER MEULEN & W. VAN EWIJK. 1974. Immunology **27:** 747–760.
22. SLIFKA, M. K. & R. AHMED. 1996. J. Immunol. Methods. In press.
23. MOLLER, S. A. & C. A. BORREBAECK. 1985. J. Immunol. Methods **79:** 195–204.
24. COUTELIER, J.-P., J. T. M. VAN DER LOGT, F. W. A. HEESSEN, G. WARNIER & J. VAN SNICK. 1987. J. Exp. Med. **165:** 64–69.
25. COUTELIER, J.-P., J. T. M. VAN DER LOGT, F. W. A. HEESSEN, A. VINK & J. VAN SNICK. 1988. J. Exp. Med. **165:** 2373–2378.
26. THOMSEN, A. R., M. VOLKERT & O. MARKER. 1985. Immunology **55:** 213–223.
27. TISHON, A., A. SALMI, R. AHMED & M. B. A. OLDSTONE. 1991. Aids Res. Human Retroviruses **7:** 963–969.
28. FAHEY, J. L. & S. SELL. 1965. J. Exp. Med. **122:** 41–58.
29. TALBOT, P. J. & M. J. BUCHMEIER. 1987. Immunology **60:** 485–489.
30. VIEIRA, P. & K. RAJEWSKY. 1988. Eur. J. Immunol. **18:** 313–316.
31. CARAYANNOPOULOS, L. & J. D. CAPRA. 1993. *In* Fundamental Immunology. W. E. Paul, Ed.: 283–314. Raven Press, Ltd., New York.
32. MACLENNAN, I. C., Y. J. LIU & G. D. JOHNSON. 1992. Immunol. Rev. **126:** 143–161.
33. SHEPHERD, D. M. & R. J. NOELLE. 1991. Transplantation **52:** 97–100.
34. COOPER, E. H. 1961. Immunology **4:** 219–231.
35. SCHOOLEY, J. C. 1961. J. Immunol. **86:** 331–337.
36. NOSSAL, G. J. V. & O. MAKELA. 1962. J. Exp. Med. **115:** 209–230.
37. MAKELA, O. & G. J. V. NOSSAL. 1962. J. Exp. Med. **115:** 231–245.
38. LEVY, M., P. VIEIRA, A. COUTINHO & A. FREITAS. 1987. Eur. J. Immunol. **17:** 849–854.
39. GRAY, D. 1993. Annu. Rev. Immunol. **11:** 49–77.
40. MANDEL, T. E., R. P. PHIPPS, A. ABBOT & J. G. TEW. 1980. Immunol. Rev. **53:** 29–59.
41. SZAKAL, A. K., M. H. KOSCO & J. G. TEW. 1989. Annu. Rev. Immunol. **7:** 91–111.
42. HO, F., J. E. LORTAN, I. MACLENNAN & M. KHAN. 1986. Eur. J. Immunol. **16:** 1297–1301.
43. MILLER, J. J. 1964. J. Immunol. **92:** 673–681.
44. BENNER, R., A. VAN OUDENAREN & G. KOCH. 1981. *In* Immunological Methods. B. Pernis & I. Lefkovits, Eds.: 247–262. Academic Press. New York.
45. HILL, S. W. 1976. Immunology **30:** 895–906.
46. TEW, J. G., R. M. DiLOSA, G. F. BURTON, *et al.* 1992. Immunol. Rev. **126:** 99–112.

Bacterial Adherence and Mucosal Cytokine Responses

Receptors and Transmembrane Signaling[a]

CATHARINA SVANBORG,[b,c] MARIA HEDLUND,[b]
HUGH CONNELL,[b] WILLIAM AGACE,[b] RUI-DONG DUAN,[d]
ÅKE NILSSON,[d] AND BJÖRN WULLT

*Departments of [b]Medical Microbiology
(Section for Clinical Immunology),
[d]Medicine (Section for Gastroenterology),
and [e]Urology
Lund University
Lund, Sweden*

Receptors for nonmicrobial ligands such as hormones, growth factors, and cytokines are commonly defined by at least two features, specificity for the ligand and activation of effectors, which are responsible for the cellular and biologic consequences of the ligand-receptor interaction. The ligand binding site (receptor epitope) determines the specificity and affinity of the interaction with the ligand. The biologic effects result from activation of receptor-associated signaling pathways. For example, the cytoplasmic tail of a membrane-spanning receptor may be phosphorylated subsequent to cross-linking of the receptor by the ligand. Ligand-receptor interaction can also change the conformation of the receptor, leading to intracellular signals (see ref. 1 for review).

Microbial attachment to host cells or tissue surfaces is characterized by a high degree of specificity. Surface ligands on viruses, bacteria, or parasites recognize specific receptor epitopes on host cells. The molecular mechanisms of these interactions have been defined in a number of systems. Gram-negative bacteria carry surface lectins that specifically recognize oligosaccharide receptor epitopes expressed on glycolipids or glycoproteins.[2] The lectins are often associated with surface fimbriae, located at the tip and/or along the fimbrial rod. Other lectins occur in nonfimbrial form. Adherence can also be mediated by the host cell lectins that bind to carbohydrate epitopes on bacterial cell surface glycoconjugates (Virij *et al.,* this issue) or by protein-protein interactions (Tuomanen *et al.,* this volume).

The receptor molecules recognized by the bacterial ligands fulfill one of the two receptor criteria; they bind the ligand with a high degree of specificity. Binding may

[a]These studies were supported by: the Swedish Medical Research Council; the Medical Faculty, University of Lund; the Swedish Medical Society; the Royal Physiographical Society of Lund; and the Österlund, Crafoord, and Lundberg Foundations.

[c]Address for correspondence: Prof. C. Svanborg, Department of Medical Microbiology (Section for Clinical Immunology), Lund University, Sölvegatan 23, S-223 62 Lund, Sweden (tel: +46-46-173972; fax: +46-46-137468 e-mail: catharina.svanborg@mmb.lu.se).

result in attachment to the cell surface and may facilitate the action of bacterial toxins or invasins. Attaching bacteria may also activate the receptor-bearing cell to produce cytokines.[3] Whether the receptors for the bacterial adhesins per se are altered as a consequence of the ligand interaction and if they participate in signaling events that lead to activation of the host response has been discussed. This chapter summarizes our attempts to understand the molecular links between fimbriae-mediated attachment to glycoconjugate receptors, transmembrane signaling, and cytokine production and disease using P-fimbriated uropathogenic *Escherichia coli* as a model.

THE MODEL SYSTEM

Uropathogenic *E. coli* strains overcome the defenses that normally keep the urinary tract sterile and establish bacteriuria. The bacteria can cause symptomatic disease or be carried asymptomatically. The severity of infection depends, to a large extent, on the magnitude and characteristics of the inflammatory response. Patients with acute cystitis have an inflammatory reaction in the lower urinary tract, but no involvement of other tissue compartments. Acute pyelonephritis is an inflammatory process of the kidney that also activates systemic inflammation. Patients with acute pyelonephritis have fever, elevated acute phase reactants, and circulating leukocytes in addition to inflammatory changes in the urinary tract.[4]

The severity of infection depends on the virulence of the infecting strain. Uropathogenic *E. coli* that cause acute pyelonephritis possess an array of properties that are rare or absent in the strains that cause asymptomatic bacteriuria or are carried in the fecal flora. These virulence-associated traits include adherence factors, certain types of lipopolysaccharides and capsules, iron-binding proteins, and hemolysin.[5–7] Attachment shows the most clear-cut association with disease; tissue-specific adhesins are expressed by 90–95% of acute pyelonephritis strains compared with less than 20% by non-uropathogens. Thus, it may be inferred that adherence enhances the virulence of the infecting strain through a direct effect on the inflammatory processes that characterize acute pyelonephritis.[8]

Uropathogenic *E. coli* attach to epithelial cells lining the urinary tract. Molecular mechanisms of attachment have been characterized. Fimbriae-associated surface lectins bind to oligosaccharide receptor sequences in cell surface glycoconjugates.[2] Early epidemiologic studies showed disease severity to be associated with one specific adhesive interaction, that of P-fimbriae binding to the globoseries of glycolipids.[2,9,10] Subsequent studies in animal models showed that P-fimbriae–negative mutants have reduced ability to survive in the urinary tract and to cause inflammation.[11–15]

The receptors for *E. coli* P-fimbriae are Galα1-4Galβ-containing oligosaccharide sequences bound to ceramide in the globoseries of glycolipids.[2,16] These glycolipids occur in urinary tract epithelial cells and kidney tissue.[2,17] Individual variation in receptor expression influences the susceptibility to infection with P-fimbriated *E. coli*.[18,19] The receptor-specific recognition is mediated by the *pap*G-encoded adhesin located at the tip of the fimbriae.[20] There are *pap*G adhesin variants that recognize different Galα1-4Galβ-oligosaccharide isoreceptors,[21–24] and that differ in disease association.[21,25,26] The mechanisms underlying these differences have not been clarified, but they may relate to the propensity of these P-fimbriated strains to induce a mucosal and systemic inflammatory response.

BACTERIA ACTIVATE MUCOSAL CYTOKINE RESPONSES

The inflammatory response to infection is initiated when bacteria trigger the production of proinflammatory mediators at the local site of infection. We have shown that uropathogenic *E. coli* activate mucosal cytokine production in the urinary tract.[26,27] Proinflammatory cytokines such as interleukin-6 (IL-6) and IL-8 are secreted into the urine shortly after intravesical instillation of bacteria in mice and in patients. The magnitude of the response shows an association with disease severity.[27–30] It has been speculated, but not demonstrated, that the spread of cytokines from the site of production in the urinary tract such as IL-6 causes fever and acute phase responses in patients with acute pyelonephritis.[29,30]

We have studied the influence of bacterial adherence on the mucosal cytokine response in the human urinary tract. Colonizations with nonvirulent bacteria were performed to protect special patient groups from recurrent, symptomatic infections. This strategy was based on clinical observations in children and adults with asymptomatic bacteriuria.[31–33] Those who were untreated had a lower frequency of symptomatic recurrences than did patients who were given antibiotics to eliminate the bacteriuria. Follow-up of these patients did not reveal adverse effects of bacteriuria on renal function, suggesting that bacteriuria with a nonvirulent strain may protect against infection.

Patients with recurrent acute pyelonephritis due to neurogenic bladder disorders were enrolled in the colonization study. The role of bacterial adherence in human urinary tract cytokine responses was studied using isogenic *E. coli* strains that differ in the expression of fimbriae. Patients were injected intravesically with *E. coli* 83972 and P-fimbriated derivatives of this strain. *E. coli* 83972 *pap*$_{IA2}$ had received *pap*$_{IA2}$ DNA sequences in the single-copy plasmid pREG153. The *pap*$_{IA2}$ type of P-fimbriae predominates among uropathogenic *E. coli* that cause acute pyelonephritis.[25] *E. coli* 83972 was selected for these studies because of its documented ability to persist in the human urinary tract.[34] It was originally isolated from a young girl with asymptomatic bacteriuria who had carried it for 3 years without symptoms or adverse effects. The strain lacked the virulence traits that characterize acute pyelonephritis strains and had been shown to colonize several human hosts without causing symptoms.[34]

Results in one patient who received *E. coli* 83972 *pap*$_{IA2}$ are shown in FIGURE 1. The *E. coli* strain rapidly established a population of $\geq 10^7$ cfu/ml of urine and was maintained for several months. The P-fimbriated phenotype was detected for 5 days, but thereafter the strain became phenotypically negative for P-fimbriae. It still carried the plasmid with the *pap*$_{IA2}$ DNA sequences.

The cytokine response to colonization is shown in FIGURE 1. Instillation of *E. coli* 83972 *pap*$_{IA2}$ in the bladder was followed by an interleukin-6 (IL-6) response that lasted for the first 5 days and then subsided. Peak neutrophil counts in urine were registered during the first few days after colonization. The cytokine response coincided in time with expression of the P fimbriae and waned when the strains switched to a nonfimbriated phenotype. In a subsequent colonization with a P-fimbriae–negative variant of *E. coli* 83972, low cytokine responses were observed. These observations suggested that the fimbriae played an important role in the induction of cytokine responses *in vivo*.

BACTERIAL ADHERENCE ENHANCES EPITHELIAL CELL CYTOKINE RESPONSES

Epithelial cells predominate in the mucosal lining of the human urinary tract. Cellular elements such as M cells, goblet cells, and intraepithelial lymphocytes which occur at other mucosal sites are absent or less abundant in the urinary tract. Epithelial cells are the targets for attaching bacteria; they express glycolipid recep-

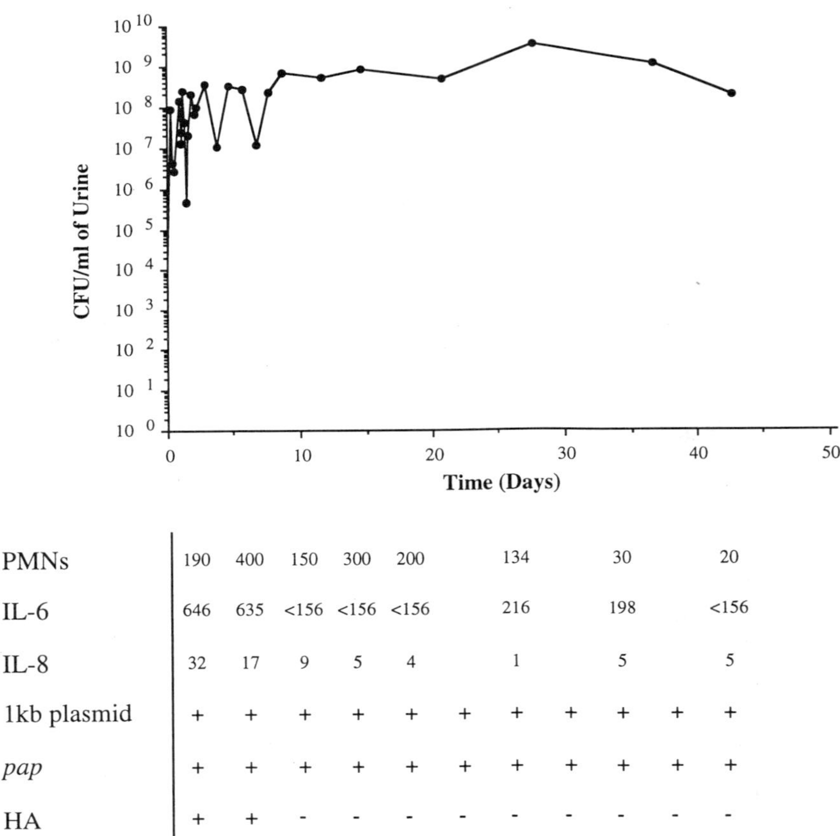

PMNs	190	400	150	300	200		134		30		20
IL-6	646	635	<156	<156	<156		216		198		<156
IL-8	32	17	9	5	4		1		5		5
1kb plasmid	+	+	+	+	+	+	+	+	+	+	+
pap	+	+	+	+	+	+	+	+	+	+	+
HA	+	+	-	-	-	-	-	-	-	-	-

FIGURE 1. Urinary tract colonization with *E. coli* 83972 *pap*$_{\text{IA2}}$. At time 0, the patient was colonized with the bacteria, which established a population of ~ 10^8 cfu/ml. Strain identity was controlled by detection of a 1.2-kb plasmid and the *pap* genotype using DNA-DNA hybridization. The fimbrial phenotype was assessed on bacteria harvested directly from urine without subculture by hemagglutination of human A_7P_7 erythrocytes in the presence of 2.5% α-D-mannose. Neutrophils were counted microscopically on uncentrifuged urine, and IL-6 and IL-8 were quantitated by ELISA. Bacteria expressed the P-fimbriae for 5 days after colonization. Subsequently the fimbriated phenotype was lost, but the strains remained *pap*$_{\text{IA2}}$ positive. Colonization caused a local urinary inflammatory response with increased levels of IL-6, IL-8, and neutrophils in urine. The inflammatory response waned after the P-fimbrial phenotype was switched off.

tors and bind P-fimbriated *E. coli*. We therefore explored the possibility that inflammatory mediators such as cytokines are produced by epithelial cells on contact with bacteria.[3] The initial study used epithelial cell lines from the urinary tract and demonstrated that epithelial cells produce cytokines and that bacteria can stimulate cytokine production in those cells.[35,36] Epithelial cell cytokine mRNA levels increased after bacterial stimulation as did the intracellular cytokine content and the secretion of cytokines. The cytokine repertoire of epithelial cells differed from that of macrophages exposed to *E. coli*. IL-6, IL-8, and IL-1, but not TNF, predominated in the epithelial cells.

Bacterial adherence enhances the bacterially induced epithelial cell cytokine response. Evidence may be summarized as follows:

1. P-fimbriated and type 1-fimbriated *E. coli* strains elicited higher cytokine responses than did isogenic, nonfimbriated strains.[35,37,38]
2. Isolated P-fimbriae elicited epithelial cell cytokine responses. Activation required a functionally active G adhesin; fimbriae lacking the receptor-binding domain did not elicit a cytokine response.[35]
3. Inhibition of epithelial cell glycolipid expression reduced both the adherence and the cytokine response to P-fimbriated *E. coli*, but it had no effect on the cytokine response to type 1-fimbriated *E. coli* that bind other glycoconjugate receptors.[38]
4. Receptor analogs (globotetraosylceramide for P-fimbriae and α-methyl-D-mannoside for type 1-fimbriae) inhibited bacterial adherence and epithelial cell cytokine responses.[13,37]

These observations suggest that fimbriae receptor interactions activate epithelial cell cytokine responses and that the receptor specificity of the fimbriae helps direct these responses.

P-FIMBRIATED *E. COLI* ACTIVATE THE
CERAMIDE SIGNALING PATHWAY

P-fimbriae bind Galα1-4Galβ–containing receptor epitopes on the globoseries of glycolipids. The globoseries of glycolipids consists of an oligosaccharide chain bound to ceramide that is localized in the outer leaflet of the lipid bilayer of the epithelial cell membrane.[9,16] Ceramide was recently identified as a second messenger in cell signaling. Exogenous ligands such as TNF, FAS, and IL-1 bind to their respective receptors and activate endogenous sphingomyelinases that release ceramide from sphingomyelin.[39–41] Ceramide can, in turn, activate the Ser/Thr family of protein kinases and phosphatases with Ser/Thr specificity.[42,43] Down-stream signaling results in cell activation and cytokine production or alternatively in apoptotic cell death. The ceramide signaling pathway in response to such ligands is summarized in FIGURE 2.

We tested the hypothesis that P-fimbriated *E. coli* might release ceramide and that the ceramide signaling pathway may be involved in epithelial cell cytokine responses.[44] For these experiments, we used a human kidney epithelial cell line, A498, that expresses the globoseries of glycolipids, binds P-fimbriated *E. coli*, and responds with cytokine production to stimulation with P-fimbriated *E. coli*.

Released ceramide was detected in lipid extracts of A498 cells by *in vitro* phosphorylation using the diacylglycerolkinase assay. The labeled product was run on thin layer chromatogram plates and quantitated by autoradiography. The P-fimbriated strains caused ceramide release that peaked after approximately 20 minutes of stimulation. The isogenic nonfimbriated control strain did not cause detectable ceramide release in the A498 cells.

The phosphorylation of ceramide to ceramide-1-phosphate was quantitated in cells that had been prelabeled with $^{32}P_i$ for 72 hours. P-fimbriated bacteria caused an increase in ceramide-1-phosphate that peaked around 20 minutes after stimulation. Increases in ceramide-1-phosphate levels were not detected in cells exposed to nonfimbriated strains.

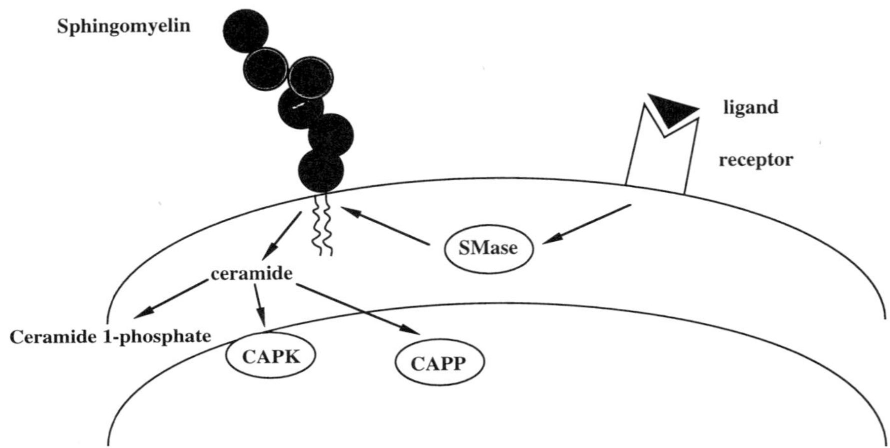

FIGURE 2. The ceramide signaling pathway. Ligands such as FAS, IL-1α, and TNF bind their respective cell surface receptor and activate endogenous sphingomyelinases that cleave sphingomyelin into ceramide and phosphocholine. The released ceramide activates protein kinases and protein phosphatases with Ser/Thr specificity. Down-stream activation includes upregulation of NF-κB and may lead to cytokine production by the activated cells.

Ceramide-activated protein kinases are Ser/Thr kinases with specificity for proline.[42] We tested the effects of protein kinase inhibitors on the IL-6 response of A498 cells to P-fimbriated *E. coli*. Staurosporin and K252-a (inhibitors of Ser/Thr kinases) inhibited the IL-6 response to P-fimbriated *E. coli* and PMA (positive control), but had no effect on the IL-6 response to the non-fimbriated *E. coli* control. Genestein and tyrphostin (inhibitors of tyrosine kinase) had no effect on the PMA or P-fimbriae–induced response.

These results demonstrate that P-fimbriated *E. coli* fimbriae caused the release of ceramide and suggest that the ceramide signaling pathway participates in the cytokine responses in epithelial cells. The mechanism(s) of the P-fimbriae–induced ceramide release need to be defined, and the origin of the ceramide involved in the induction of the IL-6 response needs to be established. Several hypotheses may be discussed and tested (FIG. 3). Studies to examine the hypotheses are ongoing.

1. Binding of P-fimbriae to the oligosaccharide portion of globotetraosylceramide or other Galα1-4Galβ–containing glycolipids may cause the release of ceramide from those molecules (FIG. 3A).

2. Binding of P-fimbriae to the globoseries of glycolipids may activate endogenous sphingomyelinases that cleave ceramide from sphingomyelin (FIG. 3B). Activation of endogenous sphingomyelinase activity was therefore examined using A498 cell ex-

tracts obtained 20 minutes after exposure to the bacteria (TABLE 1). Acid and neutral sphingomyelinase activity was tested as described.[45] The A498 cells had low endogenous sphingomyelinase activity in the acid and neutral pH ranges. Exposure to P-fimbriated *E. coli* and the nonfimbriated control strain caused an increase in neutral sphingomyelinase activity above the medium control. P-fimbriated *E. coli* activated higher sphingomyelinase levels than did the nonfimbriated strain. A similar trend was observed for acid sphingomyelinase. Acid sphingomyelinases are considered to be localized to the lysozomal compartment. Neutral sphingomyelinases are primarily localized to the plasma membrane, but their exact cellular distribution remains unclear.[46] These results establish that bacteria influenced the sphingomyelinase activity of the A498 cells.

3. Binding of P-fimbriae to the glycolipid receptors may increase the concentration of other bacterial components at the cell surface. Cytokine responses may be activated through these components rather than or in addition to the adhesin-receptor interaction.

A. Bacteria may produce sphingomyelinases that cleave ceramide from sphingomyelin other than from the receptor glycolipid. We have shown that exogenous sphingomyelinase can activate IL-6 production in the A498 cells. A dose-dependent increase in IL-6 secretion was noted with kinetics similar to those observed with bacterial stimulation (FIG. 4). We analyzed the sphingomyelinase activity of the *E. coli* strains in cell culture medium and in medium obtained after 20 minutes of incubation of the bacteria with the A498 cells (TABLE 1). Bacterial sphingomyelinase production was not evident.

B. Lipopolysaccharide was recently shown to be a structural analog of ceramide.[47] LPS might bypass ceramide and directly activate CAPK involved in the down-stream activation of the cytokine response. This pathway was shown to exist in CD-14–positive cells and to require LPS binding protein (FIG. 3B). We have shown that purified LPS is a poor activator of epithelial cell cytokine responses.[26,35,48] This may be secondary to the lack of LPS receptors in the epithelial cells. Epithelial cells and cell lines from the urinary tract are surface CD-14 negative. Reports, however, indicate that cells lacking surface CD-14 can be reconstituted using soluble CD-14 from human serum. We therefore tested LPS activation of A498 cells in the presence of human serum that contains soluble CD-14, but found no effect of human serum on the LPS responsiveness of the A498 cells. This suggests that the reconstitution of CD-14 was not sufficient to make those cells LPS responsive (TABLE 2) and that LPS was not the principal activator of the cytokine response.

P-fimbriae are proposed to contain LPS as an integral part of the pap_{IA2} adhesin adjacent to the receptor-binding domain.[13,49] If so, cells may see the bacterial lectin and LPS at the same time, and a dual signal may be delivered. The fimbriae may compensate for the lack of an LPS receptor on epithelial cells by delivering LPS to the epithelial cell surface in a molecular context that leads to cell activation.

TYPE 1 AND P-FIMBRIATED *E. COLI* ACTIVATE EPITHELIAL CELL CYTOKINE RESPONSES VIA DIFFERENT TRANSMEMBRANE SIGNALING PATHWAYS

A498 cells express receptors for *E. coli* type 1 fimbriae. Type 1 fimbriated strains attach to these cells and elicit higher cytokine responses than do nonfimbriated controls (FIG. 5). The receptor has not been identified, but the attachment is inhibited by α-methyl-D-mannoside, suggesting that the fimbriae recognize manno-

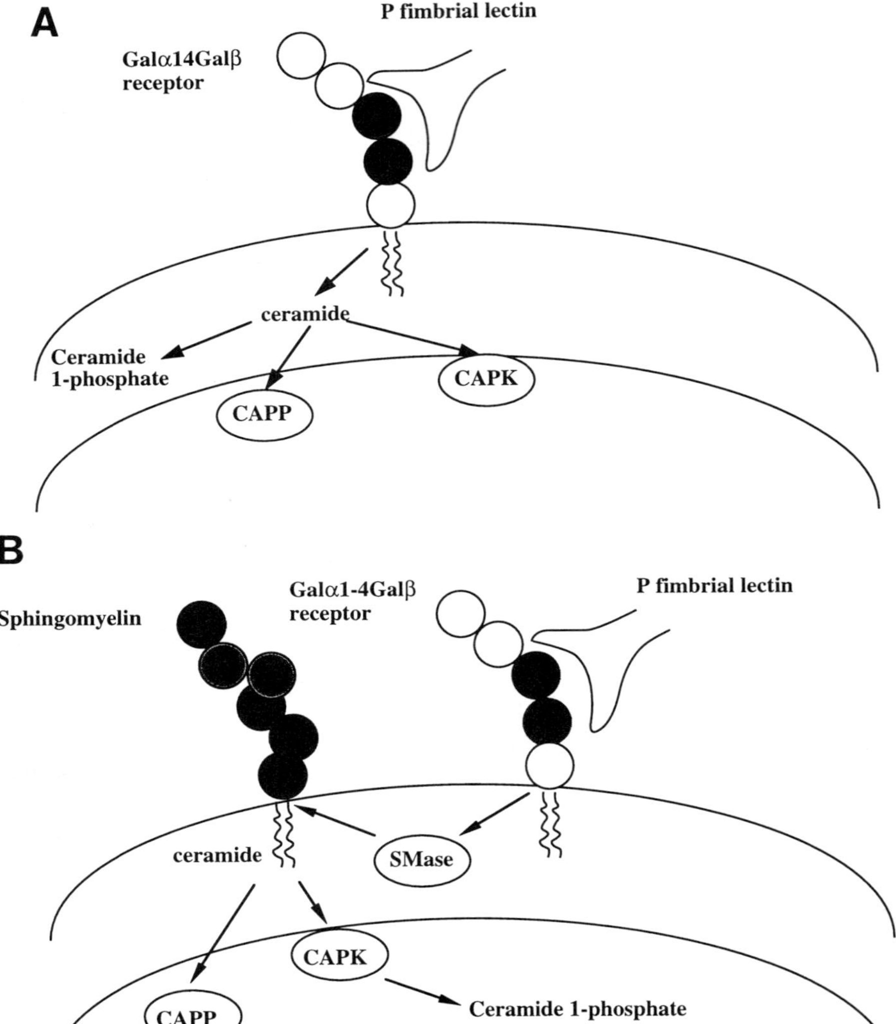

A
Galα14Galβ
receptor
P fimbrial lectin
ceramide
Ceramide
1-phosphate
CAPP
CAPK
B
Sphingomyelin
Galα1-4Galβ
receptor
P fimbrial lectin
ceramide
SMase
CAPP
CAPK
Ceramide 1-phosphate

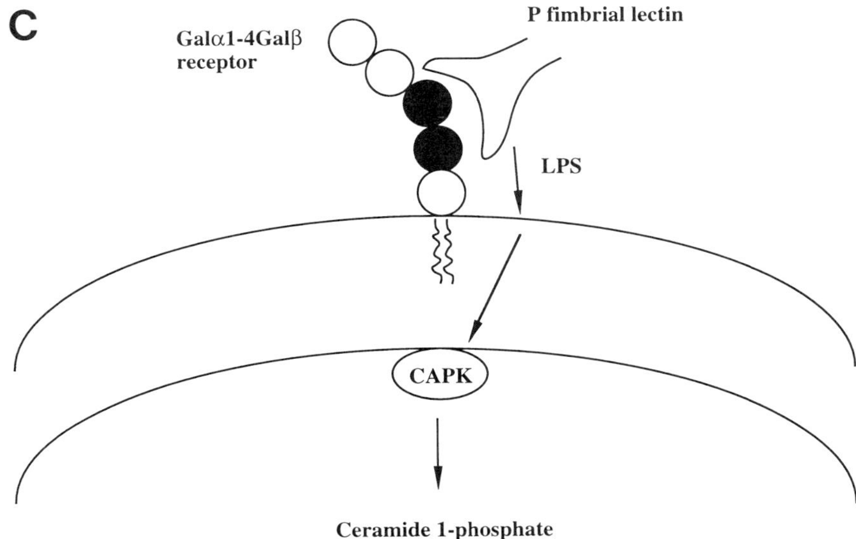

FIGURE 3. Hypothetical mechanisms by which P-fimbriated *E. coli* may activate the ceramide signaling pathway. (**A**) P-fimbriated *E. coli* bind the oligosaccharide portion of the globoseries of glycolipids and cause the release of ceramide from this molecule. (**B**) P-fimbriated *E. coli* activate endogenous sphingomyelinase activity. Ceramide is cleaved from sphingomyelin rather than from receptor glycolipids. (**C**) P-fimbrial lectin approximates LPS to the cells. LPS bypasses ceramide as an activator of CAPK and causes a cytokine response.

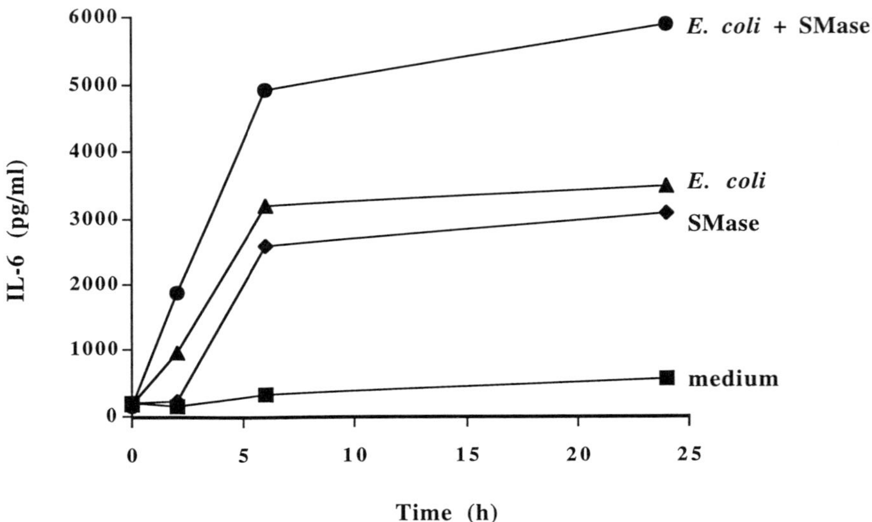

FIGURE 4. Sphingomyelinase induces an IL-6 response in A498 cells.

sylated glycoprotein(s). Mannose residues occur on glycoproteins rather than glyco-lipids. Consequently, type 1 fimbriated bacteria did not bind to glycolipid extracts from A498 cells. There was no evidence of ceramide release or phosphorylation of ceramide in cells exposed to type 1-fimbriated bacteria. Furthermore, type 1 fimbriated *E. coli*–induced cytokine response was insensitive to treatment with inhibitors of Ser/Thr kinases. These results strongly support the notion that fimbrial receptor specificity directs the transmembrane signaling pathways involved in cell activation.

SUMMARY

By attaching to cells or secreted mucosal components, microbes are thought to avoid elimination by the flow of secretions that constantly wash mucosal surfaces. The attached state enhances their ability to trap nutrients and allows the bacteria to multiply more efficiently than do unattached bacterial cells. Attachment is therefore

TABLE 1. Sphingomyelinase Activity (pmol/h/mg protein) of Cells, Cells Exposed to Bacteria, and Bacteria

	Acid Sphingomyelinase	Neutral Sphingomyelinase
A498 cells	1,189	248
+*E. coli*		
AD110	1,740	724
+*E. coli*		
HB101	1,338	578
E. coli AD110	190	29
E. coli HB101	58	0

TABLE 2. Interleukin-6 Secretion by Human Kidney A498 Cells in Response to LPS

	Interleukin-6 (pg/ml)	
	⁻Human serum	⁺Human serum
Medium control		
0 h	10	21
2 h	23	43
6 h	15	33
24 h	60	111
Lipopolysaccharide (1 mg/ml)		
0 h	23	17
2 h	59	87
6 h	154	185
24 h	340	248

regarded as an end result in itself, and emphasis has been placed on the role of adherence for colonization of mucosal surfaces. Specific adherence was shown to be essential for the tissue tropism that is to guide microbes to their respective sites of colonization/infection.

Attachment is not only a mechanism of tissue targeting but also a first step in the pathogenesis of many infections. The attaching bacteria engage in a "cross-talk" with the host cells through the mutual exchange of signals and responses. Enteropatho-

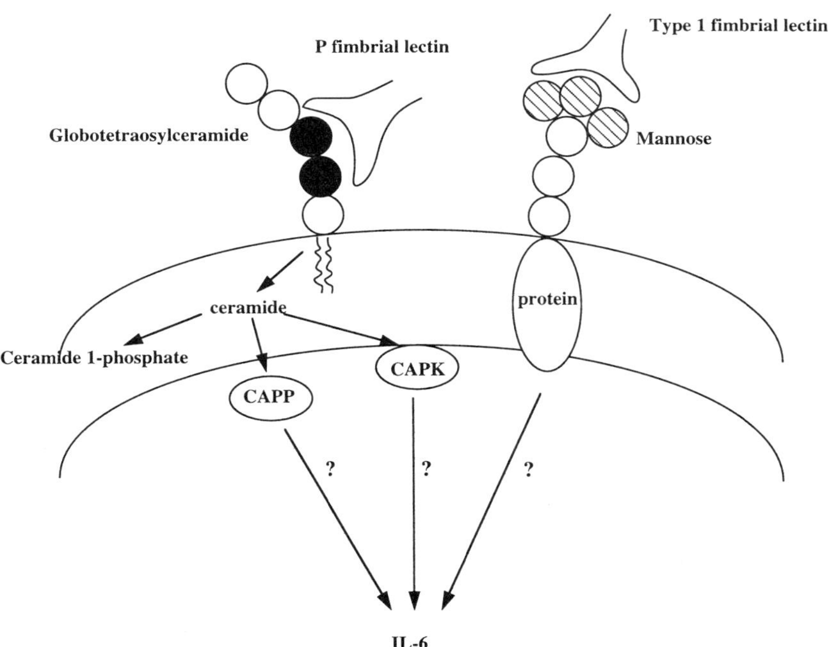

FIGURE 5. P-fimbriated and type 1 fimbriated *E. coli* activate epithelial cell cytokine production via different signaling pathways.

genic *E. coli* induce attaching and effacing lesions (Finley *et al.*, this issue). *Shigella* and *Listeria* sp. invade the cells and cause actin polymerization (Sansonetti *et al.*, this issue).

This review describes the ability of bacteria to trigger mucosal inflammation through activation of cells in the mucosal lining. The results suggest that receptors for bacterial adhesins bind their ligands with a high degree of specificity and that ligand-receptor interactions trigger transmembrane signaling events that cause cell activation. Receptors for microbial ligands thus appear to fulfill also the same criteria as those used to define receptors for other classes of ligands such as hormones, growth factors, and cytokines.

REFERENCES

1. 1995. Signal transduction. Science **268**: 221–251.
2. LEFFLER, H. & C. SVANBORG-EDÉN. 1980. Chemical identification of a glycosphingolipid receptor for *Escherichia coli* attaching to human urinary tract epithelial cells and agglutinating human erythrocytes. FEMS Microbiol. Lett. **8**: 127–134.
3. HEDGES, S., W. AGACE & C. SVANBORG. 1995. Epithelial cytokine responses and mucosal cytokine networks. Trends Microbiol. **3**: 266–270.
4. AGACE, W., H. CONNELL & C. SVANBORG. 1996. Host resistance to urinary tract infection. *In* Urinary Tract Infection: Molecular Pathogenesis and Clinical Management. H. Mobley & J. Warren, Eds.: 221–243. American Society for Microbiology. Washington.
5. SVANBORG-EDÉN, C., L. HANSON, U. JODAL, U. LINDBERG & A. SOHL-ÅKELUND. 1976. Variable adherence to normal human urinary-tract epithelial cells of *Escherichia coli* strains associated with various forms of urinary-tract infection. Lancet 490–492.
6. MABECK, C., F. ØRSKOV & I. ØRSKOV. 1971. *Escherichia coli* serotypes and renal involvement in urinary-tract infection. Lancet **1**: 1312–1314.
7. JOHNSON, J. 1991. Virulence factors in *Escherichia coli* urinary tract infection. Clin. Microbiol. Rev. **4**: 80–128.
8. DE MAN, P., U. JODAL, K. LINCOLN & C. SVANBORG-EDÉN. 1988. Bacterial attachment and inflammation in the urinary tract. J. Infect. Dis. **158**: 29–35.
9. LEFFLER, H. & C. SVANBORG-EDÉN. 1981. Glycolipid receptors for uropathogenic *Escherichia coli* on human erythrocytes and uroepithelial cells. Infect. Immun. **34**: 920–929.
10. VÄISÄNEN, R., J. ELO, L. TALLGREN, A. SIITONEN, P. MÄKELÄ, C. SVANBORG-EDÉN, G. KÄLLENIUS, S. SVENSON, H. HULTBERG & T. KORHONEN. 1981. Mannose resistant haemagglutination and P antigen recognition characteristics of *Escherichia coli* causing primary pyelonephritis. Lancet **ii**: 1366–1369.
11. HAGBERG, L., R. HULL, S. HULL, S. FALKOW, R. FRETER & C. SVANBORG-EDÉN. 1983. Contribution of adhesion to bacterial persistence in the mouse urinary tract. Infect. Immun. **40**: 265–272.
12. SVANBORG-EDÉN, C., L. HAGBERG, R. HULL, S. HULL, K.-E. MAGNUSSON, L. ÖHMAN. 1987. Bacterial virulence versus host resistance in the urinary tracts of mice. Infect. Immun. **55**: 1224–1232.
13. LINDER, H., I. ENGBERG, H. HOSCHÜTZKY, I. MATTSBY BALTZER & C. SVANBORG-EDÉN. 1991. Adhesin dependent activation of mucosal IL-6 production. Infect. Immun. **59**: 4357–4362.
14. ROBERTS, J., B.-I. MARKLUND, D. ILVER, M. HASLAM, G. KAAK, G. BASKIN, R. MÖLLBY, J. WINBERG & S. NORMARK. 1994. The Galα(1-4)Gal specific tip adhesin of *Escherichia coli* P-fimbriae is needed for pyelonephritis to occur in the normal urinary tract. Proc. Natl. Acad. Sci. USA **91**: 11889–11893.
15. WINBERG, J., R. MÖLLBY, J. BERGSTRÖM, K.-A. KARLSSON, I. LEONARDSSON, M. MILH, S. TENEBERG, D. HASLAM, B.-I. MARKLUND & S. NORMARK. 1995. The PapG-adhesin at the tip of P-fimbriae provides *Escherichia coli* with a competitive edge in experimental bladder infections of Cynomolgus monkeys. J. Exp. Med. **182**: 1695–1702.
16. BOCK, K., M. BREIMER, A. BRIGNOLE, G. HANSSON, K.-A. KARLSSON, G. LARSSON, H.

LEFFLER, B. SAMUELSSON, N. STRÖMBERG, C. SVANBORG-EDÉN & J. THURIN. 1985. Specificity of binding of a strain of uropathogenic *Escherichia coli* to Galα1-4Galβ containing glycosphingolipids. J. Biol. Chem. **260:** 8545–8551.

17. BREIMER, M., G. HANSSON & H. LEFFLER. 1985. The specific glycosphingolipid composition of human urethral epithelial cells. J. Biochem. **98:** 1169–1180.

18. LOMBERG, H., B. CEDERGREN, H. LEFFLER, B. NILSSON, A.-S. CARLSTRÖM & C. SVANBORG-EDÉN. 1986. Influence of blood group on the availability of receptors for attachment of uropathogenic *Escherichia coli.* Infect. Immun. **51:** 919–926.

19. LINDSTEDT, R., G. LARSON, P. FALK, U. JODAL, H. LEFFLER & C. SVANBORG. 1991. The receptor repertoire defines the host range for attaching *E. coli* recognizing globo-A. Infect. Immun. **59:** 1086.

20. LINDBERG, F., B. LUND, L. JOHANSSON & S. NORMARK. 1987. Localization of the receptor-binding protein adhesin at the tip of the bacterial pilus. Nature **328:** 84–87.

21. LUND, B., B.-I. MARKLUND, N. STRÖMBERG, F. LINDBERG, K. KARLSSON & S. NORMARK. 1988. Uropathogenic *Escherichia coli* can express serologically identical pili of different receptor binding specificities. Mol. Microbiol. **2:** 255–263.

22. STRÖMBERG, N., B.-I., MARKLUND, B. LUND, D. ILVER, A. HAMERS, W. GAASTRA, K.-A. KARLSSON & S. NORMARK. 1990. Host-specificity of uropathogenic *Escherichia coli* depends on differences in binding specificity to Galα-4Galβ-containing isoreceptors. EMBO J. **9:** 2001–2010.

23. LINDSTEDT, R., P. FALK, R. HULL, S. HULL, H. LEFFLER, C. SVANBORG-EDÉN & G. LARSON. 1989. Binding specificities of wild-type and cloned *Escherichia coli* strains that recognize globo-A. Infect. Immun. **57:** 3389–3394.

24. JOHANSON, I., R. LINDSTEDT & C. SVANBORG. 1992. The role of the *pap* and *prs* encoded adhesins in *Escherichia coli* adherence to human epithelial cells. Infect. Immun. **60:** 3416–3422.

25. PLOS, K., T. CARTER, S. HULL, R. HULL & C. SVANBORG-EDÉN. 1990. Frequency and organisation of *pap* homologous DNA in relation to clinical origin of uropathogenic *Escherichia coli.* J. Infect. Dis. **161:** 518–524.

26. JOHANSON, I.-M., K. PLOS, B.-I. MARKLUND & C. SVANBORG. 1993. *Pap, papG* and *prsG* DNA sequences in *Escherichia coli* from the fecal flora and the urinary tract. Microbial Path. **15:** 121–129.

27. DE MAN, P., C. VAN KOOTEN, L. AARDEN, I. ENGBERG & C. SVANBORG-EDÉN. 1989. Interleukin-6 induced by Gram-negative bacterial infection at mucosal surfaces. Infect. Immun. **57:** 3383–3388.

28. HEDGES, S., P. ANDERSON, G. LIDIN-JANSON, P. DE MAN & C. SVANBORG. 1991. Interleukin-6 response to deliberate colonization of the human urinary tract with gram-negative bacteria. Infect. Immun. **59:** 421–427.

29. HEDGES, S., K. STENQUIST, G. LIDIN-JANSON, J. MARTINELL, T. SANDBERG & C. SVANBORG. 1992. Comparison of urine and serum concentrations of interleukin-6 in women with acute pyelonephritis or asymptomatic bacteriuria. J. Infect. Dis. **166:** 653–656.

30. BENSON, M., U. JODAL, W. AGACE, M. HELLSTRÖM, S. MARILD, S. ROSBERG, M. SJÖSTRÖM, B. WETTERGREN, S. JONSON & C. SVANBORG. 1996. J. Infect. Dis., Nov. issue. In press.

31. LINDBERG, U. 1975. Asymptomatic bacteriuria in school girls. V. The clinical course and response to treatment. Acta Paediatr. Scand. **64:** 718–724.

32. HANSSON, S., D. CAUGANT, U. JODAL & C. SVANBORG-EDÉN. 1989. Untreated asymptomatic bacteriuria in girls. I. Stability of urinary isolates. Brit. Med. J. **298:** 853–855.

33. HAGBERG, L., A. BRUCE, G. REID, C. SVANBORG-EDÉN, K. LINCOLN & G. LIDIN-JANSON. 1986. Colonisation of the urinary tract with bacteria from the normal fecal and urethral flora in patients with recurrent urinary tract infections. *In* Host-Parasite Interactions in Urinary Tract Infections. E. Kass & C. Svanborg-Edén, Eds.: 194–297. Chicago Press. Chicago.

34. ANDERSON, P., I. ENGBERG, G. LIDIN-JANSON, K. LINCOLN, R. HULL, S. HULL & C. SVANBORG-EDÉN. 1991. Persistence of *Escherichia coli* bacteriuria not determined by bacterial adherence. Infect. Immun. **59:** 2915–2921.

35. HEDGES, S., M. SVENSSON & C. SVANBORG. 1992. Interleukin-6 response of epithelial cell lines to bacterial stimulation *in vitro.* Infect. Immun. **60:** 1295–1301.
36. HEDGES, S., P. DE MAN, H. LINDER, C. VAN KOOTEN & C. SVANBORG-EDÉN. 1990. Interleukin-6 is secreted by epithelial cells in response to Gram-negative bacterial challenge. *In* Advances in Mucosal Immunology, International Conference of Mucosal Immunity. T. MacDonald, Ed.: 144–148. Kluwer. London.
37. AGACE, W., S. HEDGES, M. CESKA & C. SVANBORG. 1993. IL-8 and the neutrophil response to mucosal Gram negative infection. J. Clin. Invest. **92:** 780–785.
38. SVENSSON, M., R. LINDSTEDT, N. RADIN & C. SVANBORG. 1994. Epithelial glucosphingolipid expression as a determinant of bacterial adherence and cytokine production. Infect. Immun. **62:** 4404–4410.
39. SCHÜTZE, S., K. POTTHOFF, T. MACHLEIDT, C. BERKOVIC, K. WIEGMAN & M. KRÖNKE. 1992. TNF activates NK-κB by phosphatidylcholine-specific phospholipase C-induced "acidic" sphingomyelin breakdown. Cell **71:** 765–776.
40. MATHIAS, S., A. YOUNES, C. KAN, I. ORLOW, C. JOSEPH & R. KOLESNICK. 1993. Activation of the sphingomyelin signaling pathway in intact EL4 cells and in a cell-free system by IL-1β. Science (Wash., DC). **259:** 519–522.
41. CIFONE, M., R. DE MARIA, P. RONCAIOLI, M. RIPPO, M. AZUMA, L. LANIER, A. SANTINI & R. TESTI. 1993. Apoptotic signaling through CD95 (Fas/Apo-1) activates an acidic sphingomyelinase. J. Exp. Med. **177:** 1547–1552.
42. MATHIAS, S., K. DRESSLER & R. KOLESNICK. 1991. Characterization of a ceramide-activated protein kinase: Stimulation by tumor necrosis factor α. Proc. Natl. Acad. Sci. USA **88:** 10009–10013.
43. DOBROWSKY, R. & Y. HANNUN. 1993. Ceramide-activated protein phosphatase: Partial purification and relationship to protein phosphatase 2A. Adv. Lipid Res. **25:** 91–104.
44. HEDLUND, M., M. SVENSSON, Å. NILSSON, R.-D. DUAN & C. SVANBORG. 1996. Role of the ceramide signalling pathway in cytokine responses to P fimbriated *Escherichia coli.* J. Exp. Med. **183:** 1–8.
45. GATT, S. 1976. Magnesium-dependent sphingomyelinase. Biochem. Biophys. Acta **68:** 235–241.
46. KOLESNICK, R. 1991. Sphingomyelin and derivatives as cellular signals. Prog. Lipid. Res. **30:** 1–38.
47. JOSEPH, C., S. WRIGHT, W. BORNMANN, J. RANDOLPH, E. KUMAR, R. BITTMAN, J. LIU & R. KOLESNICK. 1994. Bacterial lipopolysaccharide has structural similarity to ceramide and stimulates ceramide-activated protein kinase in myeloid cells. J. Biol. Chem. **269:** 17606–17610.
48. LINDER, H., I. ENGBERG, I. MATTSBY BALTZER, K. JANN & C. SVANBORG-EDÉN. 1988. Induction of inflammation by *Escherichia coli* on the mucosal level: Requirement for adherence and endotoxin. Infect. Immun. **56:** 1309–1313.
49. HOSCHÜTZKY, H., F. LOTTSPEICH & K. JANN. 1989. Isolation and characterization of the alpha-galactosyl-1,4-beta-galactosyl-specific adhesin (P-adhesin) from fimbriated *Escherichia coli.* Infect. Immun. **57:** 76–81.

Development of an Antipathology Vaccine for Schistosomiasis

THOMAS A. WYNN

Immunobiology Section
Laboratory of Parasitic Diseases
National Institutes of Health
Building 4/126
Bethesda, Maryland 20892

Schistosomiasis is a chronic and debilitating disease that affects over 200 million people in tropical countries. The pathology resulting from infection with the helminth parasite *Schistosoma mansoni* is predominantly due to the host reaction to parasite eggs that become trapped in the liver and intestine. The associated fibrosis leads to portal hypertension which causes much of the morbidity and mortality associated with this disease.

The inflammatory process initiated by the trapped eggs depends on CD4[+] T cells[1] and was classically described as a delayed type hypersensitivity (DTH) reaction.[2] Thus, because of their association with DTH responses,[3] the Th1-associated cytokines (gamma interferon [IFN-γ]/interleukin-2 [IL-2]) were expected to be critical to the formation of granulomas. Nevertheless, Th2-type cytokines (IL-4, IL-5, and IL-13) have been implicated as the major mediators of egg-induced granuloma formation,[4–6] whereas IFN-γ is believed to play an antiinflammatory role.[7–10]

Although relatively little is known about the immediate cellular response to deposited eggs or the particular components of the eggs that drive Th2 cell differentiation, recent studies suggest that through cytokine-induced immunomodulation it may be possible to block the development of pathogenic Th2 responses. Although numerous factors influence CD4[+] T cell differentiation, the cytokine milieu present during the initial phase of an immune response appears to play a dominant role in Th subset selection. IL-4 and IL-10 together promote Th2 cell differentiation, while IFN-γ and IL-12 are the primary cytokines stimulating Th1-type responses.[11] Based on this information, it has been possible to modulate the immune response to a variety of infectious agents by depleting or adding specific cytokines during initial exposure to the pathogen.[12,13] We have attempted to exploit this strategy to develop a vaccination approach that will reduce or eliminate the Th2 cell-dependent pathology seen during infection with *S. mansoni*.

TH2-TYPE CD4[+] T-CELL RESPONSES INDUCE GRANULOMA FORMATION

Cytokine neutralization experiments have been particularly informative in dissecting the contribution of Th1 and Th2 cytokines to schistosome egg-induced granuloma formation. In one study of primary granuloma formation in mice, neutralizing IL-4 at the time of intravenous egg injection blocked lesion formation and nearly completely suppressed *in vivo* Th2-associated cytokine mRNA expression.[14] In two related studies, repeated injections of anti-IL-4 monoclonal antibodies given to acutely (8-week) infected mice suppressed hepatic granuloma formation[15] while also markedly decreasing hepatic collagen deposition.[16] Again, the reduced inflammation and fibrosis were associated with significant decreases in liver IL-5 and IL-13 mRNA expression. Splenic IL-4 production in response to *in vitro* antigenic stimulation was also reduced in mice treated with anti-IL-4 monoclonal antibodies. As in pulmonary granuloma studies,[6,14] neutralization of IL-4 enhanced the production of Th1 cytokines.[16] Interestingly, administration of rIL-4 to chronically infected animals reversed the downregulated granulomatous response seen during the latter stages of infection.[15] Together, these findings demonstrate that Th2-type cytokines are critical in the genesis and maintenance of schistosoma egg-induced granulomatous inflammation and hepatic fibrosis.

ANTI-INFLAMMATORY ROLE OF IFN-γ IN GRANULOMA FORMATION

Recent studies suggest that the development of egg-specific Th2 responses is preceded by a Th0 phase of differentiation.[17] This was also demonstrated *in vivo* by examination of the evolution of cytokine mRNA expression in the lungs of mice injected intravenously with eggs.[14] The initial response to injected eggs, seen as early as day 1, is the expression of IFN-γ, followed on days 3–6 by both Th1- and Th2-type cytokines. After 7–10 days, Th2 cytokines become dominant in the response. A question that arose from these observations is, what role does IFN-γ play in granuloma formation and in Th cell differentiation given the known downregulatory role of this cytokine in Th2-type responses?[18] By using the pulmonary granuloma model, it was confirmed that IFN-γ plays an antiinflammatory role in egg-induced granuloma formation. Neutralization of endogenous IFN-γ with monoclonal antibodies significantly increased lesion size while simultaneously increasing the local production of several Th2-associated cytokine mRNAs.[7] Moreover, administering IFN-γ to mice at 6–8 weeks of infection decreased pulmonary granuloma formation.[9] Recently, the suppressive role of IFN-γ in granuloma formation and Th2 cytokine development was confirmed using IFN-γ gene knockout mice.[8] Thus, the early appearance of IFN-γ following exposure to parasite eggs seems to suppress the development of Th2 cells, resulting in reduced granuloma size.

Cells staining positive for asialo GM_1, a marker on natural killer (NK) cells, have been observed in pulmonary granulomas.[19] Thus, the rapid appearance of IFN-γ following egg deposition suggested that NK cells might be a source of this early IFN-γ. This hypothesis was confirmed by NK cell depletion studies which demonstrated that the increase in IFN-γ mRNA seen on day 1 was highly dependent on the presence of NK cells.[7] As observed in anti-IFN-γ monoclonal antibody-treated animals, NK cell depletion increased granuloma size while increasing Th2-like cytokine responses. Thus, the accumulated evidence supports an antiinflammatory role for NK cells and IFN-γ in schistosome egg-induced granuloma formation.

REGULATORY ROLE OF IL-12 IN GRANULOMA FORMATION

Natural killer cell stimulatory factor (IL-12) plays an important role in the induction of IFN-γ synthesis by NK cells as well as activated T cells and selectively stimulates Th1 cell differentiation.[11] Interestingly, a small but significant increase in IL-12 p40 mRNA expression was detected in the lungs of mice injected with schistosome eggs.[7] Similar to previous IFN-γ and NK cell depletion experiments, neutralization of IL-12 increased granuloma formation and enhanced Th2 cytokine responses, arguing for an endogenous downregulatory role for IL-12. Not surprisingly, administration of IL-12 nearly completely suppressed Th2 responses and primary schistosome granuloma formation in intravenously challenged mice.[7] A marked increase in IFN-γ, IL-2, IL-12, and IL-10 mRNA expression was detected *in vivo*, and lymph node cultures restimulated *in vitro* with soluble egg antigen (SEA) or mitogen produced elevated quantitites of IFN-γ.[7,20]

The increased IL-10 in IL-12–treated animals suggested that IL-10, a potent downregulatory cytokine, might contribute to the suppressed granulomatous response. However, depletion of IFN-γ, but not IL-10, restored Th2 mRNA responses in IL-12–treated mice, arguing that the major suppressive effects of IL-12 on granuloma formation and Th2 cytokine expression were mediated through IFN-γ.[7] This finding was recently confirmed in egg-injected IFN-γ knockout mice which showed exaggerated rather than suppressed inflammatory reactions when treated with IL-12.[8]

In addition to affecting primary granuloma formation, IL-12 profoundly inhibited the vigorous anamnestic granulomatous response seen in animals presensitized with eggs, and this suppression correlated with a modest decrease in the Th2 cytokine mRNA expression profile.[7] The latter observations are of basic interest, because they indicate that IL-12 may be used to alter established Th2 responses. In the granuloma model the mechanism of this reversal is unclear. One possibility is that IL-12 alters cytokine expression of Th2 cells *in vivo*, causing them to shift to a Th1- or Th0-like pattern. This explanation is consistent with data showing that IL-12 can induce IFN-γ production in human Th2 cell lines and clones.[21,22] A more likely alternative is that *in vivo* IL-12 treatment drives the differentiation of egg-specific Th0 lymphocytes in the sensitized animals into Th1- rather than Th2-type secreting cells. These findings are important, because they may have an impact on the feasibility of using IL-12 therapeutically to suppress pathogenic Th2-type inflammatory responses.

DEVELOPMENT OF AN ANTIPATHOLOGY VACCINE FOR SCHISTOSOMIASIS BASED ON IL-12 IMMUNOREGULATION

The ability of IL-12 to suppress both primary and secondary egg-induced Th2 responses suggested the possibility of prophylactically immunizing mice against granulomatous inflammation by sensitizing them to egg antigens in the presence of exogenous IL-12. This method of sensitization resulted in nearly complete inhibition of granuloma formation after challenge with eggs in the absence of additional IL-12. As predicted, pulmonary cytokine responses showed a reversal in the Th expression pattern similar to that observed in animals treated with IL-12 during primary egg injection.[7] These results suggest that if given during priming, IL-12 redirects Th differentiation so that a Th1 rather than a Th2 response dominates subsequent secondary antigenic stimulation.

We recently extended these studies to investigate whether this antipathology approach would protect animals from granuloma formation and fibrosis resulting from natural schistosome infections. Indeed, although this vaccination protocol appears to have no effect on worm or egg burden, it has dramatic effects on fibrosis, reducing both collagen mRNA levels and liver hydroxyproline (a chemical measure of collagen).[23] Again, the reduced pathology, previously observed in the pulmonary model,[7] was associated with a marked increase in Th1-associated cytokines including IFN-γ, tumor necrosis factor-alpha, and IL-12 and a significant reduction in Th2-type cytokine mRNA expression. We hypothesized that the reduction in fibrosis may result from both the reduced expression of collagen-inducing cytokines such as TGF-β and IL-4[24] and a corresponding increase in cytokines (IFN-γ and TNF-α) known to inhibit collagen mRNA synthesis.[25,26] Together, these data suggest that

IL-12 may be important as an immunomodulatory agent during vaccination, altering both the quality and the quantity of protective cell-mediated responses.

SUMMARY

The data presented here clearly demonstrate that IL-12 can act as an adjuvant, suppressing both granuloma formation and fibrosis induced after natural schistosome infection. Recently, we showed that IL-12 can increase protective immunity provided by an attenuated larval schistosome vaccine as well.[27] In both cases the vaccines appear to suppress in large part the parasite-induced Th2 responses. Thus, the use of cytokines as adjuvants offers a rational approach for immunomodulation when the effector mechanism of a particular vaccine is known. Clearly, IL-12 has enormous potential for modulating the outcome of immunization and may have broad application in preventing a variety of different infectious diseases.

ACKNOWLEDGMENTS

I would like to thank Joe Sypek and Stan Wolf of Genetics Institute for the kind gift of IL-12 and Paula Jardieu and Kim Zioncheck at Genentech for providing the INF-γ knockout mice. I would also like to acknowledge the support of Alan Sher and Allen Cheever in this work.

REFERENCES

1. MATHEW, R.C. & D. L. BOROS. 1986. Anti L3T4 antibody treatment suppresses hepatic granuloma formation and abrogates antigen-induced interleukin 2 production in *Schistosoma mansoni* infection. Infect. Immun. **54:** 820–826.
2. WARREN, K. S., E. S. DOMINGO & R. B. T. COWAN. 1967. Granuloma formation around schistosome eggs as a manifestation of delayed hypersensitivity. Am. J. Pathol. **51:** 735–756.
3. MOSMANN, T. R. & R. L. COFFMAN. 1989. Th-1 and Th-2 cells: Different patterns of lymphokine secretion lead to different functional properties. Ann. Rev. Immunol. **7:** 145–173.
4. GRZYCH, J. M., E. J. PEARCE, A. CHEEVER, Z. A. CAULADA, P. CASPAR, S. HEINY, F. LEWIS & A. SHER. 1991. Egg deposition is the major stimulus for the production of Th2 cytokines in murine *Schistosomiasis mansoni*. J. Immunol. **146:**1322–1327.
5. PEARCE, E. J., P. CASPAR, J. M. GRZYCH, F. A. LEWIS & A. SHER. 1991. Downregulation of Th1 cytokine production accompanies induction of Th2 responses by a parasitic helminth, *Schistosoma mansoni*. J. Exp. Med. **173:** 159–166.
6. CHENSUE, S. W., P. D. TEREBUH, K. S. WARMINGTON, S. D. HERSHEY, H. L. EVANOFF, S. L. KUNKEL & G. I. HIGASHI. 1992. Role of interleukin-4 and gamma-interferon in *Schistosoma mansoni* egg-induced hypersensitivity granuloma formation. Orchestration, relative contribution, and relationship to macrophage function. J. Immunol. **148:** 900–906.
7. WYNN, T. A., I. ELTOUM, I. P. OSWALD, A. W. CHEEVER & A. SHER. 1994. Endogenous interleukin-12 (IL-12) regulates granuloma formation induced by eggs of *Schistosoma mansoni* and exogenous IL-12 both inhibits and prophylactically immunizes against egg pathology. J. Exp. Med. **179:** 1551–1561.
8. WYNN, T. A., D. JANKOVIC, S. HIENY, K. ZIONCHECK, P. JARDIEU P., A. W. CHEEVER & A. SHER. 1995. IL-12 exacerbates rather than suppresses T helper 2-dependent pathology in the absence of endogenous IFN-γ. J. Immunol. **154:** 3999–4009.
9. LUKACS, N. W. & D. L. BOROS. 1993. Lymphokine regulation of granuloma formation in murine *Schistosomiasis mansoni*. Clin. Immunol. Immunopathol. **68:** 57–63.

10. CHENSUE, S. W., K. S. WARMINGTON, J. RUTH, P. M. LINCOLN & S. L. KUNKEL. 1994. Cross-regulatory role of interferon-gamma (IFN-gamma), IL-4, and IL-10 in schistosome egg granuloma formation: *In vivo* regulation of Th activity and inflammation. Clin. Exp. Immunol. **98:** 395–400.

11. TRINCHIERI, G. 1995. Interleukin-12: A proinflammatory cytokine with immunoregulatory functions that bridge innate resistance and antigen-specific adaptive immunity. Annu. Rev. Immunol. **13:** 251–276.

12. HEINZEL, F. P., D. S. SCHOENHAUT, R. M. RERKO, L. E. ROSSER & M. K. GATELY. 1993. Recombinant interleukin-12 cures mice infected with *Leishmania major.* J. Exp. Med. **177:** 1505–1509.

13. SYPEK, J. P., C. L. CHUNG, S. E. H. MAJOR, J. M. SUBRAMANYAM, S. J. GOLDMAN, D. S. SIEBURTH, S. F. WOLF & R. G. SCHAUB. 1993. Resolution of cutaneous leishmaniasis: Interleukin 12 initiates a protective T helper type 1 immune response. J. Exp. Med. **177:** 1797–1800.

14. WYNN, T. A., I. ELTOUM, A. W. CHEEVER, F. A. LEWIS, W. C. GAUSE & A. SHER. 1993. Analysis of cytokine mRNA expression during primary granuloma formation induced by eggs of *Schistosoma mansoni.* J. Immunol. **151:** 1430–1440.

15. YAMASHITA, T. & D. L. BOROS. 1992. IL-4 influences IL-2 production and granulomatous inflammation in murine *Schistosomiasis mansoni.* J. Immunol. **149:** 3659–3664.

16. CHEEVER, A. W., M. E. WILLIAMS, T. A. WYNN, F. D. FINKELMAN, R. A. SEDER, T. M. COX, S. HIENY, P. CASPAR & A. SHER. 1994. Anti-IL-4 treatment of *Schistosoma mansoni*-infected mice inhibits development of T cells and non-B, non-T cells expressing Th2 cytokines while decreasing egg-induced hepatic fibrosis. J. Immunol. **153:** 753–759.

17. VELLA, A. T. & E. J. PEARCE. 1992. CD4$^+$ Th2 response induced by *Schistosoma mansoni* eggs develops rapidly, through an early, transient, Th0-like stage. J. Immunol. **148:** 2283–2290.

18. GAJEWSKI, T. F., J. JOYCE & F. W. FITCH. 1989. Anti-proliferative effect of IFN-γ in immune regulation. I. IFN-γ inhibits the proliferation of Th2 but not Th1 murine helper T lymphocyte clones. J. Immunol. **140:** 4245–4252.

19. REMICK, D. G., S. W. CHENSUE, J. C. HISERODT, G. I. HIGASHI & S. L. KUNKEL. 1988. Flow-cytometric evaluation of lymphocyte subpopulations in synchronously developing *Schistosoma mansoni* egg and sephadex bead pulmonary granulomas. Am. J. Pathol. **131:** 298–307.

20. OSWALD, I. P., P. CASPAR, D. JANKOVIC, T. A. WYNN, E. J. PEARCE & A. SHER. 1994. IL-12 inhibits Th2 cytokine responses induced by eggs of *Schistosoma mansoni.* J. Immunol. **153:** 1707–1713.

21. YSSEL, H., S. FASLER, J. E. DE VRIES & R. DE WAAL MALEFYT. 1994. IL-12 transiently induces IFN-gamma transcription and protein synthesis in human CD4$^+$ allergen-specific Th2 T cell clones. Int. Immunol. **6:** 1091–1096.

22. MANETTI, R., F. GEROSA, M. G. GIUDIZI, R. BIAGIOTTI, P. PARRONCHI, M.-P. PICCINNI, S. SAMPOGNARO, E. MAGGI, S. ROMAGNANI & G. TRINCHIERI. 1994. Interleukin 12 induces stable priming for interferon-γ (IFN-γ) production during differentiation of human T helper (Th) cells and transient IFN-γ production in established Th2 cell clones. J. Exp. Med. **179:** 1273–1280.

23. WYNN, T. A., A. W. CHEEVER, D. JANKOVIC, R. W. POINDEXTER, P. CASPAR, F. A. LEWIS & A. SHER. 1995. An IL-12-based vaccination method for preventing fibrosis induced by schistosome infection. Nature **376:** 594–597.

24. KHALIL, N., O. BEREZNAY, M. SPORN & A. H. GREENBERG. 1989. Macrophage production of transforming growth factor β and fibroblast collagen synthesis in chronic pulmonary inflammation. J. Exp. Med. **170:** 727–737.

25. CZAJA, M. J., F. R. WEINER, S. TAKAHASHI, M.-A. GIAMBRONE, P. H. VAN DER MEIDE, H. SCHELLEKENS, L. BIEMPICA & M. A. ZERN. 1993. γ-interferon treatment inhibits collagen deposition in murine schistosomiasis. Hepatology **10:** 795–800.

26. KOVACS, E. J. 1991. Fibrogenic cytokines: The role of immune mediators in the development of scar tissue. Immunol. Today **12:** 17–22.

27. WYNN, T. A., D. JANKOVIC, S. HIENY, A. W., CHEEVER & A. SHER. 1995. IL-12 enhances vaccine-induced immunity to *Schistosoma mansoni* in mice and decreases T helper 2 cytokine expression, IgE production, and tissue eosinophilia. J. Immunol. **154:** 4701–4709.

Proteins Expressed by DNA Vaccines Induce Both Local and Systemic Immune Responses[a]

J. LINDSAY WHITTON[b] AND MASAYUKI YOKOYAMA

Department of Neuropharmacology, CVN-9
The Scripps Research Institute
10550 N. Torrey Pines Rd.
La Jolla, California 92037

Although some 200 years in the making, the revolution spawned by Jenner's experiment remains remarkable. Antiviral vaccination has, of course, allowed eradication of smallpox, and extermination of poliomyelitis virus, the childhood plague of the middle part of this century, is on the horizon. Although eradication is not in sight, nevertheless control of measles, mumps, and rubella viruses has been relatively well achieved, particularly in the developed countries. Nevertheless, significant virus-induced diseases remain to torment mankind. Rotavirus-induced diarrheal disease is responsible for approximately 1,000,000 childhood deaths per year in Africa, and for significant morbidity and hospitalization in the developed countries.[1] Although several rotavirus vaccines have entered clinical trials, they have not been outstandingly successful. Indeed, development of an effective rotaviral vaccine may be particularly difficult, because even wild-type infection renders only 60–70% of survivors resistant to subsequent rotavirus challenge. Influenza remains a leading cause of lost work hours in the United States, despite the availability of a vaccine. Respiratory syncytial virus is a major cause of morbidity and mortality in infancy and no vaccine is available. HIV remains a growing specter for which no vaccine has been developed despite a full decade of intensive research. Finally, there are no vaccines against newly emerging viral agents such as Ebola and Marburg viruses. Thus, improvement of traditional vaccines and the emergence of new challenges are sufficient to justify significant attempts to develop new modalities of immunization. To date, all antiviral vaccines have been one of two classes. Most vaccines consist of attenuated live viruses that replicate in the host to induce long-lasting cross-reactive immunity, but they are of such diminished pathogenicity as to represent an extremely minor risk to the vaccinee. Secondly, killed viral vaccines (or recombinant proteins) have been used; these are nonreplicating agents, and their protein constituents directly induce the antiviral immune state. Over the last several years, a new approach to vaccination has been developed. Nucleic acid vaccines, most often using plasmid DNA but occasionally RNA, have been shown to induce biologically effective antiviral responses. The benefits, real and potential, of nucleic acid immunization (hereinafter referred to as DNA immunization) in comparison to those of the live virus and killed virus counterparts are summarized in TABLE 1. DNA vaccines may be produced inexpensively, in great quantity, and at high purity. As they are produced in bacteria, there is no risk of contamination by eukaryotic viruses; this had

[a]This work was supported by Public Health Service grant R-01AI 37186 from the National Institutes of Health. This is manuscript number 9670-NP from The Scripps Research Institute.
[b]Tel: 619-784-7090; fax: 619-784-7380; e-mail: lwhitton@scripps.edu

previously presented a problem because a batch of polio virus propagated in cells of simian origin was contaminated with monkey virus SV40. DNA vaccines should not be pathogenic to the host. Although studies have clearly demonstrated that injected plasmid DNA may remain in host tissues for many months, all evidence suggests that it does so in an episomal state, rather than integrating into the host genome. Thus, concern that the DNA may integrate into the host chromosome, potentially altering gene expression, is probably inapposite. By contrast, live virus vaccines may themselves be dangerous. Vaccinia virus may cause severe systemic disease and may even be fatal in immunosuppressed individuals.[2] Poliovirus vaccine, when given orally to an infant, rapidly reverts to a more virulent phenotype, and by 7 days postimmunization the infant's stool contains potentially virulent poliovirus[3]; this virulent virus is the cause of the few poliomyelitis cases current in Western society, which occur in

TABLE 1. Comparison of Salient Features of Three Classes of Vaccine

	Live Virus	Killed Virus	DNA Vaccine
Safety			
Risk of disease: vaccine may be pathogenic or may become so	+	$-^a$	$-^a$
Risk of adventitious agents contaminating vaccine	+	$-^a$	$-^a$
Can be given in pregnancy	−	$++^a$	?
Vaccination may exacerbate disease caused by pathogen	+	+++	?
Efficacy			
Proteins enter class I MHC pathway	$+++^a$	+/−	$+++^a$
Proteins enter class II MHC pathway	$+++^a$	$+++^a$	$++ (?)^a$
Induce long-lasting immunity without boosting	$+++^a$	+	?
Induced immunity is cross-reactive (combats various virus serotypes)	$+++^a$	+	$++ (?)^a$
Effective in infants carrying maternal antibodies	−	−	?
Ease of production/use			
Ease of production	+	+	$+++^a$
Stability/ease of handling and distribution	−	$+++^a$	$+++^a$

^{a}"Desirable" feature.

nonimmune caregivers exposed to this fecal material.[4] Although killed virus vaccines should carry no risk of disease, the infamous "Cutter incident," in which a batch of polio virus was inadequately inactivated, resulted in several cases of acute disease and paralysis in vaccinees,[5] and underscored the potential hazard of the killed vaccine approach. DNA vaccines, in contrast, should hold none of these disadvantages. DNA vaccines have other potential benefits which remain untested. For example, measles vaccine is safe and effective in all age groups, with the exception of children under 9 months of age. In this age group, maternal anti-measles antibody inactivates the measles virus vaccine, and vaccine recipients therefore remain unprotected and susceptible to wild-type measles infection (the maternal antibody seems less able to combat the wild-type pathogen). Measles virus takes full advantage of this window of opportunity and is directly or indirectly responsible for up to 1,000,000 deaths per year in third world countries. Administration of a DNA vaccine encoding measles virus protein should, in theory, circumvent this problem, because the maternal antibodies would not recognize the nucleic acid molecule. The measles proteins would therefore be synthesized within the infant's cells and would be presented, via the class I MHC pathway, to allow induction of antiviral cytotoxic T lymphocytes. It remains possible that induction of antibodies would be less effective, because introduction of the measles proteins into the class II MHC pathway would most probably require release of soluble protein into the extracellular fluids, thus potentially exposing them to inactivation by the maternal antibodies. (It could be argued, however, that this may allow access to the antigen to B cells, which can present antigen via the class II pathway.[6])

DNA vaccines have been effective in several animal model systems and against many families of viruses. They appear to be effective against orthomyxoviruses such as influenza,[7-9] herpesviruses,[10] arenaviruses,[11-13] and rhabdoviruses.[14] Immunity can be induced by either viral surface glycoproteins or "internal" viral proteins. In the latter case, protective immunity is most likely conferred by induction of antiviral cytotoxic T lymphocytes (CTL).[7] We[15-17] and others[18-20] clearly demonstrated in the lymphocytic choriomeningitis virus (LCMV) mouse model that vaccine-mediated induction of CTL alone, in the absence of vaccine-induced antibody, is sufficient to confer complete protection against subsequent viral challenge. This phenomenon is true for a wide variety of viruses. For example, it was demonstrated for influenza virus,[21] respiratory syncytial virus,[22] cytomegalovirus,[23] and vesicular stomatitis virus.[24]

DNA immunization has been effective when given through a variety of routes. Most commonly, nucleic acid is injected intramuscularly.[25] More recently, intradermal immunization has proven successful,[26] and a "gene gun" has been developed in which microscopic gold beads are coated with the nucleic acid and are impelled under pressure into the epidermis and dermis, where the encoded proteins are expressed[27] Following inoculation of DNA, regardless of route, expression of marker proteins is detectable in the target tissue; however, not all approaches are equally effective, as we demonstrate herein. Given expression of the encoded proteins, it is perhaps not surprising that immune responses ensue; however, in no case has the host cell responsible for the induction of immunity been identified. In this report we show that the DNA solvent used and the route of injection have major effects on the expression and immunogenicity of the encoded proteins. We confirm that immunization with DNA complexed with cationic lipids can induce systemic immunity, protecting against viral challenge. In addition, we evaluate the local immune response that follows intramuscular (im) injection of DNA; although myositis in naive mice is minimal, we show marked antigen-specific inflammatory responses in mice already immune to the encoded protein.

MATERIALS AND METHODS

Mice. BALB/cByJ (H-2^d) male mice were obtained from the breeding colony at the Scripps Research Institute. Mice were used at 8–12 weeks of age.

Cell Lines and Viruses. BALB C17 (H-2^d) cell line was maintained in Dulbecco's minimal essential medium (DMEM) supplemented with 10% fetal calf serum, penicillin G (50 units/L), and streptomycin (50 mg/L as streptomycin sulfate).

Plasmid DNAs. The gene encoding LCMV nucleoprotein (NP) was inserted into the NotI site of plasmid pCMV (derived by excision of the β-gal gene from pCMV-β (Clontec, Palo Alto, California) to generate pCMV-NP. For marker protein expression studies, the chloramphenicol acetyltransferase (CAT) gene was inserted into the NotI site, resulting in pCMV-CAT. Cloning, production in competent *Esch-*

erichia coli, and purification of plasmid DNAs were carried out by standard techniques. All DNAs were passed over endotoxin removal columns before use.

Preparation of DNA Complexed with Cationic Lipids. A cationic lipid reagent similar to the commercially available Lipofectin (Gibco/BRL) was prepared from 1,2-dioleoyl-*sn*-glycero-3-phosphoethanolamine (DOPE, Avanti polar-lipids, Inc., Alabaster, Alabama) and *N*-[1-(2,3-dioleoyloxy)propyl]-*N,N,N*,-trimethylammonium chloride (DOTMA), according to refs. 101 and 119. DOTMA was the generous gift of Syntex corp. Following filter sterilization using μStarLB model 8112 (0.45 mm, Costar), the reagent was stored at 4°C at a concentration of 12.3 mg lipids per milliliter in distilled water and was diluted to 5.7 mg/ml immediately before use. DNA was dissolved in Opti-MEM medium (Gibco BRL, New York) at a concentration of 1 mg/ml. Equal volumes of lipid and DNA were mixed (yielding a lipid:DNA ratio of 5.7:1 w/w). The DNA in Opti-MEM was added to the lipid solution, and this mixture was pipetted several times, followed by incubation at room temperature for 10 minutes. Then 200 μl of the mixture (100 μg DNA) was injected using a 28-gauge needle.

Preparation of "naked" DNA in Saline Solution. In some of the reported studies, DNA was injected im in saline solution. An appropriate amount of DNA was pelleted, air-dried, and resuspended in sterile 1 N saline solution to a final concentration of 1 mg/ml. Then 100 μl (100 μg DNA) was injected.

Routes of Injection. DNA (in saline solution or complexed with cationic lipids as described above) was injected by three routes. Intramuscular (im) injection was in the large (quadriceps) muscle of the leg. Intraperitoneal (ip) injection was carried out in mice pre-treated with thioglycollate (to induce peritoneal macrophages). Intravenous (iv) injection was into the tail vein.

Detection of Chloramphenicol Acetyltransferase (CAT) Expression. BALB/cByJ mice were injected with pCMV-CAT by the im, ip, or iv route. Mice were sacrificed 2 days postinjection. For im injection, muscle was harvested. For ip injection, macrophages were recovered by peritoneal lavage. For iv injection, several organs (spleen, lung, and heart) were harvested. Organs/cells were disrupted with a glass homogenizer (Wheaton tissue grinder model 357424) in 0.2M Tris buffer (pH 7.5, 250–750 ml) followed by two freeze-thaw cycles (−70°C for 10 minutes/37°C for 5 minutes) and centrifugation to remove cell debris. The resulting material was heated at 65°C for 15 minutes and following centrifugation the supernate was recovered. Forty microliters of the supernate was mixed with 57 μl of the Tris buffer, 1 μl of 50 mM acetyl coenzyme A solution (Sigma A-2056), and 2 μl of ^{14}C-chloramphenicol solution (25 μCi/ml, Amersham CFA 754). The reaction was allowed to proceed at 37°C for 14 hours, and following extraction with ethyl acetate, the reaction products were separated by thin layer chromatography on a silica gel plate before exposure to photographic film.

Evaluation of Local Immune Responses. LCMV-immune mice were obtained by inoculating adult BALB mice was 2×10^5 pfu of LCMV ip. These mice will clear the virus, and will retain LCMV memory CTL.[28] At least 6 weeks post-LCMV, mice were inoculated im with 100 μg of either pCMV or pCMV-NP in saline solution. To minimize variation between mice, individual mice received pCMV-NP in one limb and pCMV in the contralateral limb. Four days postinjection, mice were sacrificed, and muscles were harvested and processed for histologic analysis. Paraffin sections (4 μm) were cut, stained with hematoxylin and eosin, and evaluated for local inflammation.

In Vivo Protection Assay. Mice were immunized with pCMV-NP. Negative control mice received pCMV. In both cases, DNA was administered complexed with cationic lipid or in saline solution. Mice were given DNA by the iv or im route, as described in the legend to FIGURE 3. Positive controls received LCMV (live virus) by the intraperitoneal route; such mice clear the virus and are solidly immune to subsequent challenge. Six weeks following immunization, mice were challenged intracranially with a normally lethal dose of LCMV (20 LD_{50}, 25 pfu, in 50 μl). Mice were observed daily for 16 days for signs of sickness, and days of death were recorded. Negative control mice (pCMV) died 6–7 days after the LCMV intracranial injection.

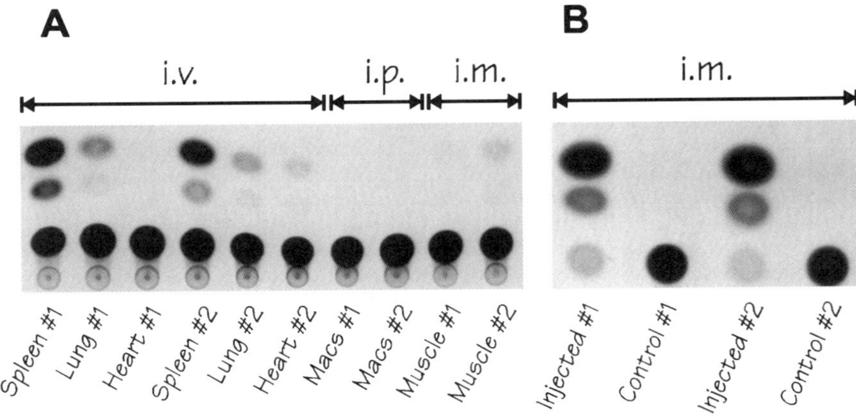

FIGURE 1. Protein expression varies with vehicle and route of delivery. pCMV-CAT DNA was administered complexed with cationic lipids (panel A) or dissolved in saline (panel B), and was introduced by the i.m. route (using both delivery vehicles) or by the i.v. or i.p. route (DNA/lipid only). Tissues were harvested 2 days post-injection, and were assayed for CAT activity. Tissue samples from two mice (labeled #1 or #2) were evaluated for each combination of vehicle & route. In panel B, 'control' is contralateral (non-injected) muscle.

RESULTS

Gene Expression Varies Depending on Route of DNA Inoculation

We compared a variety of routes of inoculation and of vehicles in which DNA is suspended. Only a subset of these data is presented here. In FIGURE 1 the comparison is presented of CAT activities following injection of pCMV-CAT DNA im, ip, or iv. DNA was complexed with cationic lipid (panel A) or "naked" in saline solution (panel B). In both panels, results from two mice are shown. Intravenous injection of DNA/lipids led to easily detectable levels of CAT expression in the three tissues shown, spleen > heart > lung. In contrast, iv injection of DNA in saline solution led to low or undetectable levels of activity in all tissues analyzed (spleen, lung, heart, liver, kidney, brain, and muscle; data not shown). Peritoneal macrophages showed no CAT activity following ip DNA/lipid injection. CAT was detectable in muscle following im injection of DNA/lipid (panel A), but, interestingly, enzymatic activity was very much lower than that in muscles that received the same amount of DNA dissolved in saline solution (panel B). This result was observed consistently. Thus, compared to DNA in saline solution, complexing DNA with cationic lipids appears to enhance expression following iv administration, but to inhibit expression following im delivery.

Local Response to Inoculated Plasmid DNA

The expression of encoded marker proteins in muscle cells following intramuscular administration of plasmid DNA has been described. Such protein expression, if responsible for induction of immunity, might also lead to marked inflammatory responses at and around the site of injection. Conversely, if muscle cells are unable to present the antigen to T cells, a low, or no, local inflammatory response might be engendered. We therefore investigated the degree of inflammation in LCMV-immune mice injected either with a control plasmid lacking any LCMV sequences or with pCMV-NP. As can be seen in FIGURE 2A, severe local myositis ensued when an LCMV-immune recipient was inoculated with pCMV-NP (saline, im). In contrast, no inflammatory reaction was seen in the contralateral limb of the same animal in response to pCMV injection. The immune response is, therefore, antigen-specific (i.e., LCMV NP-specific). The extent of the local cellular immune response in an LCMV immune animal suggests that the viral antigen may be presented at the site of injection. However, it remains possible that the local inflammation results from recognition of antigen presented by local macrophages, or similar cells, even though such cells are not plentiful in muscle tissue.

Protection Conferred by Viral Gene Correlates with Expression Levels of Marker Protein

To determine the efficacy of the pCMV-NP construct when delivered in different vehicles, by different routes, mice were immunized with pCMV-NP or pCMV in saline solution or with lipid, and im or iv. Six weeks postimmunization, mice were challenged with a normally lethal dose of LCMV. As shown in FIGURE 3, DNA in saline solution, when administered im, induced protection in 50% of mice, as we have previously shown.[29] In contrast, im administration of the same plasmid DNA complexed with cationic lipids resulted in no protection. However, the same DNA preparation, when given iv, protected 50% of challenged mice. Thus, the presence of protection (FIG. 3) correlates well with the level of CAT expression (FIG. 1). We have not evaluated the protective efficacy of DNA/saline solution given by the iv route.

DISCUSSION

In this study we confirm the importance of DNA delivery vehicles and routes. In addition, we demonstrate extensive myositis in animals receiving DNA encoding an antigen to which they are already immune. Finally, we show that the degree of protection appears to correlate with the level of gene expression achieved using a marker protein.

The route and vehicle of DNA administration both appear to be important. For example, cationic lipid enhances gene expression following iv inoculation, but

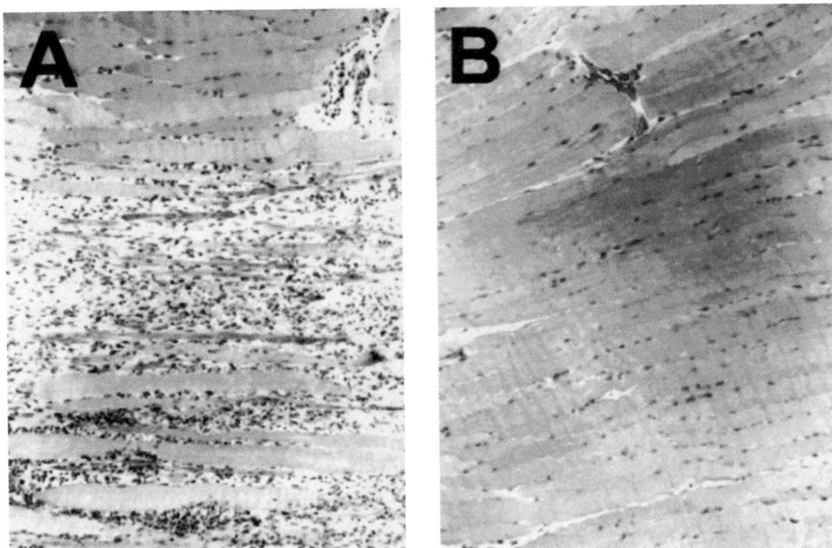

FIGURE 2. DNA inoculation induces an antigen-specific response in immune mice. An LCMV-immune mouse was injected (i.m. in saline) with pCMV-NP in one limb (**A**) or with pCMV in the opposite limb (**B**). Four days post-injection the mouse was sacrificed and the muscles harvested. Following paraffin embedding, 4 μm sections were cut, and stained with H & E.

expression is low when the im route is chosen (FIG. 1A). Conversely, DNA administered in saline solution is expressed efficiently in muscle after im injection (FIG. 1B), but it is not efficiently expressed following iv inoculation (data not shown). Thus, there is no simple equation for deciding the optimal route and delivery vehicle. The situation is further complicated by the availability of topical routes (intradermal injection,[26] "gene-gun" delivery,[9,27] and topical administration as a lipid/DNA solution[30]), all of which can lead to gene expression. Furthermore, there are circumstances in which DNA inoculation can predictably lead to good gene expression and outstanding immunogenicity. For example, we hypothesized that macrophages are cells that are efficient in uptake of extraneous materials and are highly effective in presenting antigen to T cells. For these reasons, we chose to induce activated peritoneal macrophages by ip injection of thioglycollate and, a few days later, to administer DNA by the same route. Although peritoneal lavage revealed many macrophages (data not shown), essentially no CAT activity was detectable (FIG. 1A). In addition, this route of administration resulted in little, if any, protective immunity (not shown). We have not further investigated the reasons for this outcome. It is conceivable that macrophages do not take up the DNA or that, if they do so, the DNA is not expressed, perhaps because of compartmentalization within the macrophage and/or degradation in this cell type.

The cell lineage(s) involved in inducing immunity following DNA immunization remains undefined. It is clear that following DNA immunization, muscle cells express the encoded proteins, but doubts remain about the ability of these cells to present antigen in a manner recognizable to T cells. In favor of a role of muscle cells

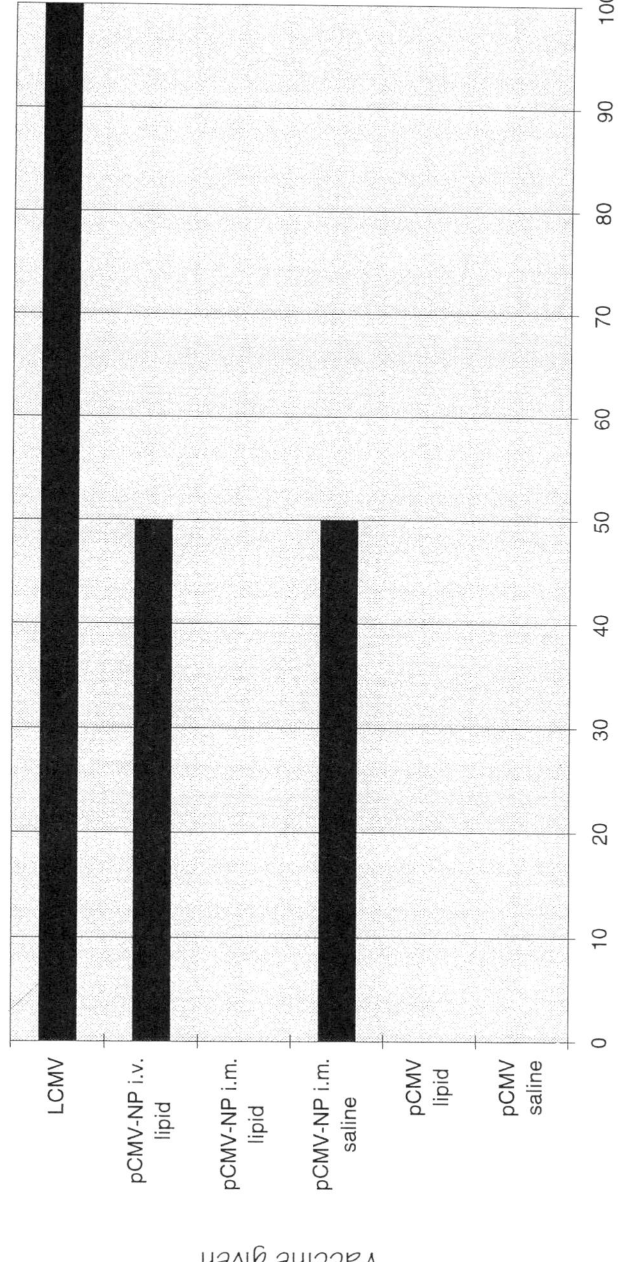

FIGURE 3. Effect of delivery vehicle and route upon establishment of protective immunity. Mice were inoculated with pCMV or pCMV-NP, in saline or in cationic lipid, i.v. or i.m. Positive control mice were immunized with LCMV. Six weeks postimmunization mice were challenged with LCMV intracranially and were observed daily for 16 days. All mice that succumbed to challenge did so on days 6 or 7 post-challenge.

in immune priming is the requirement for CD8[+] cells in the induction of viral myocarditis,[31] and the fact that muscle cells can be lysed by CD8[+] CTL *in vitro*.[32] However, under normal circumstances, muscle cells express low levels of MHC molecules. Furthermore, recent studies suggest that although other than specializing antigen-presenting cells appear able to induce immunity, this works well only if the cells are moved to an "immunologically enhanced" environment such as a lymph node.[33] It is difficult to see how this would apply to muscle cells following injection. In part to address this issue, we inoculated DNA into LCMV-immune mice. We observed a florid local myositis, and this inflammatory response was antigen specific, because the control plasmid, pCMV, induced no such reaction. The extent of the response suggests that muscle cells can indeed present antigen in a form recognizable to T cells. However, several caveats must be borne in mind. First, it remains possible that the inflammatory response results from antigen presentation by another cell type in the muscle, although any such cells (for example, specialized antigen-presenting cells) are infrequent (by histologic analysis) in the uninjected or pCMV-injected muscle. Second, even if antigen on muscle cells is being recognized by memory CTL in our study, this does not address the issue of induction of the primary response. It is possible that muscle cells are incapable of inducing an immune response, but once such a response is present, they can be recognized and killed. Third, we have not identified the cells that comprise the infiltrate. Identification of the inflammatory cells, allied with judicious depletion studies, may help determine the presentation pathway of the antigen recognized in the muscle. It is critical that the cell types responsible for induction of DNA-induced immunity be identified, because such knowledge would allow us to specifically target these cells, thus further increasing the efficiency of immunization using plasmid DNA.

Two conclusions may be drawn from the protection studies portrayed in FIGURE 3. First, the local immunity manifested in FIGURE 2 is demonstrably of biologic significance, conferring protection against a normally lethal viral challenge. Second, a correlation exists between the levels of CAT expression shown in FIGURE 1 and the levels of immunity demonstrated in FIGURE 3. Thus, DNA/lipid injected iv results in high levels of protein expression in several organs and protects 50% of animals. Conversely, the same material injected im leads to very poor protein expression and no detectable protection. However, the fault lies not in the im route per se, because DNA injected im in saline solution leads to excellent protein expression (FIG. 1B) and 50% protection (FIG. 3). The possible relation between expression levels and induced protection mandates a continued search for methods to optimize levels of expression of proteins encoded by, and injected, as nucleic acid vaccines.

ACKNOWLEDGMENT

We thank Terry Calhoun for excellent secretarial assistance.

REFERENCES

1. CONNER, M. E., D. O. MATSON & M. K. ESTES. 1994. Rotavirus vaccines and vaccination potential. Curr. Top. Microbiol. Immunol. **185:** 285–337.
2. FREED, E. R., R. J. DUMA & M. R. ESCOBAR. 1972. Vaccinia necrosum and its relationship to impaired immunologic responsiveness. Am. J. Med. **52:** 411–420.
3. EVANS, D. M., G. DUNN, P. D. MINOR, *et al.* 1985. Increased neurovirulence associated with a single nucleotide change in a noncoding region of the Sabin type 3 poliovaccine genome. Nature **314:** 548–550.

4. NKOWANE, B. M., S. G. WASSILAK, W. A. ORENSTEIN *et al.* 1987. Vaccine-associated paralytic poliomyelitis. United States: 1973 through 1984. JAMA **257:** 1335–1340.

5. NATHANSON, N. & A. D. LANGMUIR. 1995. The Cutter incident. Poliomyeliltis following formaldehyde-inactivated poliovirus vaccination in the United States during the spring of 1955. II. Relationship of poliomyelitis to Cutter vaccine. 1963 [classical article]. Am. J. Epidemiol. **142:** 109–140; discussion 107–108.

6. LANZAVECCHIA, A. 1987. Antigen uptake and accumulation in antigen-specific B cells. Immunol. Rev. **99:** 39–51.

7. ULMER, J. B., J. J. DONNELLY, S. E. PARKER, *et al.* 1993. Heterologous protection against influenza by injection of DNA encoding a viral protein. Science **259:** 1745–1749.

8. ROBINSON, H. L., L. A. HUNT & R. G. WEBSTER. 1993. Protection against a lethal influenza virus challenge by immunization with a haemagglutinin-expressing plasmid DNA. Vaccine **11:** 957–960.

9. FYNAN, E. F., R. G. WEBSTER, D. H. FULLER, J. R. HAYNES, J. C. SANTORO & H. L. ROBINSON. 1993. DNA vaccines: Protective immunizations by parenteral, mucosal, and gene-gun inoculations. Proc. Natl. Acad. Sci. USA **90:** 11478–11482.

10. COX, G. J. M., T. J. ZAMB & L. A. BABIUK. 1993. Bovine herpesvirus 1: Immune responses in mice and cattle injected with plasmid DNA. J. Virol. **67:** 5664–5667.

11. PEDROZA MARTINS, L., L. L. LAU, M. S. ASANO & R. AHMED. 1995. DNA vaccination against persistent viral infection. J. Virol. **69:** 2574–2582.

12. WHITTON, J. L., M. YOKOYAMA & J. ZHANG. 1995. DNA immunization in an arenavirus model. *In* Antiviral Immunity. M. Eibl & H. H. Peter, Eds.: 151–164. Springer-Verlag. New York.

13. ZAROZINSKI, C. C., E. F. FYNAN, L. K. SELIN, H. L. ROBINSON & R. M. WELSH. 1995. Protective CTL-dependent immunity and enhanced immunopathology in mice immunized by particle bombardment with DNA encoding an internal virion protein. J. Immunol. **154:** 4010–4017.

14. XIANG, Z. Q., S. SPITALNIK, M. TRAN, W. H. WUNNER, J. CHENG & H. C. ERTL. 1994. Vaccination with a plasmid vector carrying the rabies virus glycoprotein gene induces protective immunity against rabies virus. Virology **199:** 132–140.

15. WHITTON, J. L., N. SHENG, M. B. A. OLDSTONE & T. A. MCKEE. 1993. A "string-of-beads" vaccine, comprising linked minigenes, confers protection from lethal-dose virus challenge. J. Virol. **67:** 348–352.

16. WHITTON, J. L. 1990. Lymphocytic choriomeningitis virus CTL. Sem. Virol. **1:** 257–262.

17. KLAVINSKIS, L. S., M. B. A. OLDSTONE & J. L. WHITTON. 1989. Designing vaccines to induce cytotoxic T lymphocytes: Protection from lethal viral infection. *In* Vaccines 89. Modern Approaches to New Vaccines Including Prevention of AIDS. F. Brown, R. Chanock, H. Ginsberg & R. Lender, Eds.: 485–489. Cold Spring Harbor Laboratory. Cold Spring Harbor.

18. SCHULZ, M., R. M. ZINKERNAGEL & H. HENGARTNER. 1991. Peptide-induced antiviral protection by cytotoxic T cells. Proc. Natl Acad. Sci. USA **88:** 991–993.

19. HANY, M., S. OEHEN, M. SCHULZ, *et al.* 1988. Anti-viral protection and prevention of lymphocytic choriomeningitis or of the local footpad swelling reaction in mice by immunization with vaccinia recombinant virus expressing LCMV-we nucleoprotein or glycoprotein. Eur. J. Immunol. **19:** 417–424.

20. AHMED, R., B. D. JAMIESON & D. D. PORTER. 1987. Immune therapy of a persistent and disseminated viral infection. J. Virol. **61:** 3920–3929.

21. SCHEEPERS, K. & H. BECHT. 1994. Protection of mice against an influenza virus infection by oral vaccination with viral nucleoprotein incorporated into immunostimulating complexes. Med. Microbiol. Immunol. (Berl.) **183:** 265–278.

22. KULKARNI, A. B., P. L. COLLINS, I. BACIK, *et al.* 1995. Cytotoxic T cells specific for a single peptide on the M2 protein of respiratory syncytial virus are the sole mediators of resistance induced by immunization with M2 encoded by a recombinant vaccinia virus. J. Virol. **69:** 1261–1264.

23. DEL VAL, M., H. J. SCHLICHT, H. VOLKMER, M. MESSERLE, M. J. REDDEHASE & U. H. KOSZINOWSKI. 1991. Protection against lethal cytomegalovirus infection by a recombinant vaccine containing a single nonameric T-cell epitope. J. Virol. **65:** 3641–3646.

24. BACHMANN, M. F., T. M. KUNDIG, G. FREER, *et al.* 1994. Induction of protective cytotoxic T cells with viral proteins. Eur. J. Immunol. **24:** 2228–2236.

25. WOLFF, J. A., R. W. MALONE, P. WILLIAMS, *et al.* 1990. Direct gene transfer into mouse muscle in vivo. Science **247:** 1465–1468.

26. RAZ, E., D. A. CARSON, S. E. PARKER, *et al.* 1994. Intradermal gene immunization: The possible role of DNA uptake in the induction of cellular immunity to viruses. Proc. Natl. Acad. Sci. USA **91:** 9519–9523.

27. TANG, D. C., M. DEVIT & S. A. JOHNSTON. 1992. Genetic immunization is a simple method for eliciting an immune response. Nature **356:** 152–154.

28. AHMED, R. 1992. Immunological memory against viruses. Semin. Immunol. **4:** 105–109.

29. YOKOYAMA, M., J. ZHANG & J. L. WHITTON. 1995. DNA immunization confers protection against lethal lymphocytic choriomeningitis virus infection. J. Virol. **69:** 2684–2688.

30. LI, L. & R. M. HOFFMAN. 1995. The feasibility of targeted selective gene therapy of the hair follicle. Nature Med **1:** 705–706.

31. HENKE, A., S. A. HUBER, A. STELZNER & J. L. WHITTON. 1995. The role of CD8$^+$ T lymphocytes in coxsackie virus B3-induced myocarditis. J. Virol. **69:** 6720–6728.

32. ESTRIN, M. & S. A. HUBER. 1987. Coxsackie virus B3-induced myocarditis. Autoimmunity is L3T4$^+$ T helper cell and IL-2 independent in BALB/c mice. Am. J. Pathol. **127:** 335–341.

33. KUNDIG, T. M., M. F. BACHMANN, C. DEPAOLO, *et al.* 1995. Fibroblasts as efficient antigen-presenting cells in lymphoid organs. Science **268:** 1343–1347.

Protective Immunity to *Listeria monocytogenes* Elicited by Immunization with Heat-Killed *Listeria* and IL-12

Potential Mechanism of IL-12 Adjuvanticity[a]

MARK A. MILLER, MARIANNE J. SKEEN,
AND H. KIRK ZIEGLER[b]

Department of Microbiology and Immunology
Emory University School of Medicine
Atlanta, GA 30322

The development of effective vaccine strategies has been responsible for the elimination of some of the most challenging afflictions of mankind. The incidence of diseases such as measles, whooping cough (pertussis), rubella, polio, and tetanus has been reduced dramatically, whereas smallpox has been eradicated entirely as a result of vaccine development. However, successful vaccine strategies for many human pathogens have been elusive. Creating protective vaccines for most of these organisms as well as emerging infectious agents remains a primary frontier of immunology research.

Vaccine development involves the evaluation of numerous immunization parameters including choice of immunogen(s), dose, adjuvant, route of administration, and so on, to optimize the production of protective immune responses. Many possible forms of a given antigen can be used for the preparation of vaccines such as whole organisms that have been inactivated or attenuated (by a variety of methods), subunit preparations (purified macromolecules, recombinant antigens/vectors,[1,2] or synthetic peptide homologs), or multivalent subunit preparations. The type of adjuvant combined with the antigen preparation can dramatically affect the efficacy of any vaccine strategy. Some adjuvants, such as Freund's or alum, cause slow release of antigen, resulting in extended exposure to the immune system that typically results in increased immunogenicity of the antigen. Adjuvants that elicit fewer systemtic effects can be used to stimulate responsiveness of specific immune cell populations to generate the desired immune response. For instance, antigens can be coupled to ligands of (or antibodies specific for) class I[3] or class II MHC[4-6] molecules to enhance cytotoxic or helper T-cell responses, respectively, whereas other adjuvants potentiate isotype-specific antibody production and are potentially useful when antigen-specific antibodies of a particular isotype are desired.[7-10] During the last decade, as more was learned about the effects of many cytokines on a variety of cell types, many immunologists began to evaluate the potential utility of cytokines as adjuvant components of vaccines.[11-16]

Interleukin-12 (IL-12), a heterodimeric cytokine, is produced by monocyte/

[a]This work was supported in part by National Institute of Allergy and Infectious Disease grants F32 AI-09051 to M.A.M. and RO1 AI-25132, AI-35285, and AI-34065 to H.K.Z. and ACS grant IM-655 to H.K.Z.

[b]Corresponding author: H. Kirk Ziegler, Ph.D., Emory University School of Medicine, Department of Microbiology and Immunology, 1510 Clifton Road, Rollins Research Building, Atlanta, GA 30322 (tel: 404/727-5974; fax: 404/727-3659).

macrophages, B cells, and other accessory cells in response to bacteria, bacterial products, or parasites.[17,18] IL-12 has a broad range of stimulatory effects that generally act to promote cell-mediated immunity. IL-12 reportedly promotes the growth of activated T cells and NK cells,[19–22] stimulates the production of gamma interferon (IFN-γ) by αβ T cells and NK cells[18,23–26] and γδ T cells,[27,28] and enhances cytolytic T-lymphocyte (CTL) and natural killer cell activity.[17,20,29] IL-12 is also reportedly required for Th1 cell generation[30] and its exogenous addition to cell cultures *in vitro* can induce Th1 development, presumably by stimulating additional production of other cytokines such as IFN-γ.[31–33] Several studies have revealed the beneficial effects of rIL-12 as a therapeutic treatment for mice infected with the intracellular parasites *Leishmania major,*[34,35] *Plasmodium chabaudi,*[36] *Schistosoma mansoni,*[37] and *Toxoplasma gondii*[25] as well as with several viral systems including murine cytomegalovirus[38] and HIV.[39] In fact, depletion of IL-12 *in vivo* can exacerbate disease progression in infection models such as listeriosis,[40] malaria,[36] and leishmaniasis.[35] Additionally, the utility of IL-12 as a vaccine component was demonstrated in a murine model system in which a soluble leishmanial antigen preparation (SLA), which alone elicited a nonprotective Th2-type response, induced a protective Th1-type response when administered along with rIL-12.[41] These reports have all revealed that the use of IL-12 as a component of therapeutic or vaccine strategies induces a shift from Th2- to Th1-type responses that correlates with clearance/protection. Because the development of Th1-mediated responses is particularly important for the production of protective cellular immune responses against intracellular and viral pathogens, and because intracellular pathogens account for a large percentage of infectious disease experienced by humans, the potential for IL-12 as a vaccine component for these types of pathogens is obvious.

We began to study the adjuvant effects of IL-12 using the murine listeriosis system. *Listeria monocytogenes* is a ubiquitous gram-positive, facultative intracellular bacterium that can be a human pathogen associated with severe infections of newborns, elderly, or immunocompromised individuals.[42–46] The murine model of *Listeria* infection has been well developed in the last several decades and has been a powerful tool for the study of basic immunologic processes.[47–53] In the murine infection model, ip inoculation of mice with viable *Listeria* is initially followed by rapid but incomplete clearance of bacteria by phagocytes and by antigen-specific T cells (if present), γδ T cells, and/or NK cells. The remaining viable *Listeria* grow exponentially in the spleen and liver for the next 2–3 days, reaching 10^6–10^8 CFU/organ in susceptible mice;[48] death typically occurs between days 4 and 10. Inoculation of mice with sublethal doses of viable *Listeria* elicits a cell-mediated immune response that protects the mice from subsequent challenge with lethal doses of the bacteria.[42,48,54–56] Specific immunity to *Listeria* results in a 2–4 $\log_{10}$ decrease in organ colony-forming units with respect to immunologically naive or otherwise nonimmune mice, and because bacterial growth *in vivo* correlates directly with survival following challenge with a large dose of viable *L. monocytogenes,*[55] immunity to *Listeria* can be monitored by enumeration of colony-forming units in homogenates of the spleen or liver of mice that have been challenged with a large dose of *L. monocytogenes.* Thus, the murine *Listeria* infection model offers an ideal system for testing candidate vaccines or immunotherapy strategies.

It has been well documented that experimental infection of mice with sublethal doses of *L. monocytogenes* generates a protective Th1-type immune response,[31,57,58] whereas immunization with HKLM or viable bacteria that lack expression of listeriolysin O (LLO; *hly⁻*) does not elicit a protective immune response.[57,59,60] In fact, ip, immunization of mice with HKLM alone or *hly⁻ Listeria* typically fails to elicit detectable *Listeria*-specific T-cell responses.[57,59–63] In the current study, the effectiveness of IL-12 as an adjuvant was investigated by coinjecting HKLM and IL-12 into the peritoneal cavity of female C3HeB/FeJ mice (unless otherwise indicated) followed by evaluation of either the immune responsiveness of peritoneal exudate T cells (termed nonchallenge experiments) or the protective capacity of the vaccine upon challenge with a typically lethal dose of live *L. monocytogenes* (termed challenge experiments). Importantly, we observed no apparent toxicity of IL-12 during the course of these studies. Portions of the findings reported here were presented in greater detail in a previous publication.[66]

RESULTS AND DISCUSSION

Adjuvant Effects of IL-12 as a Component of a HKLM-Based Vaccine as Measured by T-Cell Responsiveness

Initially, the efficacy of IL-12 as a potentiator of T-cell responses was evaluated. Groups of mice (3 per group) were immunized intraperitoneally with either phosphate-buffered saline solution (PBS) only, 0.5 μg murine rIL-12 + PBS, HKLM (10^9) + PBS, or HKLM (10^9) + 0.5 μg murine rIL-12 on day 0. An identical booster dose was administered on day 5. Another group of mice received a single sublethal dose of viable *L. monocytogenes* (*Listeria*-infected; positive control) on day 0. On day 10 following primary immunization, the mice were sacrificed, and peritoneal cells were collected by lavage and pooled, and plastic nonadherent cell (PNA) populations were prepared. PNA cultures were stimulated *in vitro* with a series of stimuli, at predetermined optimal doses, for 24 hours at 37°C. Cell-free supernatants from these cultures were analyzed to quantitate IL-2 production in response to *in vitro* restimulation as an indication of antigen-specific T-cell responsiveness.

As detailed in FIGURE 1A, the pattern of reactivity of peritoneal T cells from mice immunized with HKLM + IL-12 was remarkably similar to that of cells from *Listeria*-infected/immune mice. Although T cells from all of the test groups responded to the polyclonal stimulator concanavalin A (Con A), only the *Listeria*-infected/immune and HKLM + IL-12–injected mice specifically reacted to HKLM. Restimulation with other listerial antigen preparations (soluble listerial protein [SLP][64] or crude listeriolysin O [cLLO][63]) yielded similar results (data not shown). Neither the *Listeria*-infected/immune or HKLM + IL-12–immunized mice produced IL-2 in response to *in vitro* restimulation with heat-killed *Salmonella typhimurium* SL1004 (HKST; FIG. 1A), suggesting that the immune responses mounted by these mice were specific for listerial components. In addition, inoculation of mice with live *Salmonella typhimurium*[65] or HKST (10^9) + IL-12 (FIG 1B) elicited T cells that produced IL-2 in response to HKST but not to HKLM, confirming the antigen specificity of the response. The data shown in FIGURE 1 are representative of results obtained in several different experiments (data not shown). Similar studies with the soluble listerial antigens cLLO and SLP or a synthetic peptide homolog of an immunodominant T-cell epitope (defined by residues 203–226 of LLO[63]) revealed that IL-12 effectively potentiated specific T-cell immune responses when coinjected (ip) along with these listerial antigen preparations, whereas when injected alone, each of these antigens failed to elicit detectable T-cell responses following *in vitro* restimulation with any of the listerial antigens tested (data not shown). Because of well-documented general immune stimulatory effects of lipopolysaccharide (LPS), similar studies were also performed in C3H/HeJ mice (LPS low-responder strain), and it was determined that the *Listeria*-specific T-cell responses elicited by the IL-12 and HKLM combination were independent of LPS effects (data not shown). It is also important to note that no antigen-specific IL-4 production was detected in supernatants of PNA cultures from any of the described test groups following restimulation *in vitro* (data not shown). Together, these results demonstrated that the combination of IL-12 and HKLM (or the soluble antigen preparations cLLO, SLP, or LLO P203–226) elicited a potent Th1-type T-cell response that was remarkably similar in both intensity and specificity to the protective immune response elicited by sublethal infection with viable *Listeria* organisms.

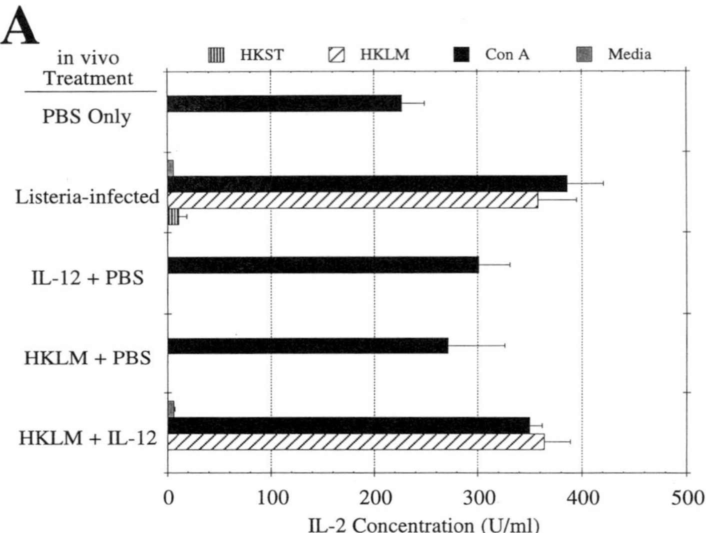

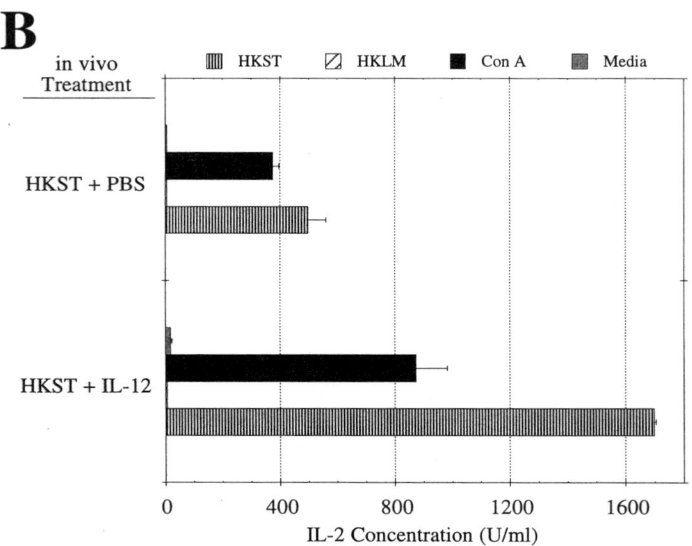

FIGURE 1. Legend is on facing page.

TABLE 1. Phenotyping of Peritoneal Lymphocytes from Vaccine Recipients

Vaccine Administered	Phenotype of Peritoneal Lymphocytes (PNA)[a]							
	% CD3[+] Lymphocytes in PNA				% $\alpha/\beta/\gamma/\delta$ T Cells in PNA Lymphocytes			
PBS	13 ± 8 $(n = 25)$[b]				$83 \pm 5/17 \pm 7$ $(n = 15)$[b]			
Listeria-infected	50 ± 10 $(n = 25)$[b]				$65 \pm 7/35 \pm 6$ $(n = 15)$[b]			
	1	2	3	4	1	2	3	4
IL-12 + PBS	18	—	—	12	72/27	—	—	75/17
HKLM + PBS	29	22	15	24	71/32	78/32	70/10	59/37
HKLM + IL-12	62	53	32	49	90/12	87/24	88/9	81/9

[a]On day 10 postimmunization, mice were sacrificed and plastic nonadherent peritoneal cells (PNA) were prepared from peritoneal lavage pooled from all mice within each of the immunization groups (from four independent experiments); $1–5 \times 10^5$ cells from each PNA pool were stained with anti-CD3 and either anti-α/β TCR or anti-γ/δ TCR and FACS analysis was performed. Experiments 1, 2, and 4 employed five, three, and three female C3H/FeJ mice, respectively, while experiment 3 employed three male C3H/HeJ mice. Groups that were not tested are indicated with a dash (−).

[b]These values represent the mean (±SD) of results from many independent experiments $(n = x)$.

Induction of CD3[+] Cells in the Peritoneal Cavity by HKLM + IL-12

Previously, this laboratory has reported that infection of C3HeB/FeJ mice with sublethal doses of *Listeria* results in pronounced induction of CD3[+] T cells in the peritoneal cavity.[52] Therefore, in addition to analysis of the cytokine profiles of PNA from each of the immunization groups just described, flow cytometric analysis was performed to characterize the cell populations induced/recruited into the peritoneal cavity by the various immunogens. As shown in TABLE 1, a marked increase in the percentage of cells that were CD3[+] was observed in peritoneal exudate from *Listeria*-infected/immune mice and HKLM + IL-12–immunized mice compared to the other test groups. In addition, the actual number of total cells collected from the peritoneal cavity of the *Listeria*-infected/protected and HKLM + IL-12–immunized mice was typically two to fourfold higher than the number of cells recovered from the PBS only, IL-12 + PBS, and HKLM + PBS injected animals (data not shown). It should also be pointed out that no difference in natural killer (NK) cell frequency was apparent in any of the test groups studied; NK cells represented <1% of the peritoneal cells in all test groups (data not shown). Thus, administration of HKLM +

←

FIGURE 1. *Listeria*-specific T-cell responses of peritoneal T cells from immunized mice. **(A)** Mice (3 per group) were immunized intraperitoneally with either PBS only, 0.5 μg rIL-12 + PBS, HKLM (10^9) + PBS, or HKLM (10^9) + 0.5 μg IL-12 on days 0 and 5. A single sublethal dose of live *L. monocytogenes* was administered to one group of mice on day 0., **(B)** In addition, mice (5 per group) were immunized with either HKST (10^9) + PBS or HKST (10^9) + 0.5 μg IL-12 on days 0 and 5. On day 10 following primary immunization the mice were sacrificed and PEC were collected by peritoneal lavage and pooled, and PNA were prepared. PNA cell cultures (1.5×10^6 cells/ml) were stimulated *in vitro* with culture medium, Con A (2 μg/ml), HKLM (10^7/ml), or HKST (10^7/ml) for 24 hours at 37°C. Cell-free supernatants from these cultures were analyzed via bioassay[66] to quantitate the concentration of IL-2 produced in response to the indicated *in vitro* stimuli as a measure of specific T-cell activation. Each assay was performed in triplicate, and results were expressed as units of IL-2 per milliliter (±SD). Data were adapted from previously published work.[66]

IL-12 resulted in an increase in CD3$^+$ cells similar to that observed following immunization with viable *Listeria*. In contrast to the induction of αβ T cells and the preferential induction of γδ T cells typically observed after infection with live *Listeria*,[52] the HKLM + IL-12 combination appeared to preferentially augment the αβ T-cell population (TABLE 1).

IL-12 Production and Class II MHC Expression by Macrophages from Mice Injected with HKLM and IL-12

As additional measures of the immune status of mice injected with the various immunogen/cytokine mixtures, IL-12 production and class II MHC expression by peritoneal macrophages were monitored. Peritoneal macrophages obtained on sacrifice of the mice from each of the previously described groups were cultured for 24 hours at 37°C with medium alone or with known inducers of IL-12 to monitor both basal and *in vitro* restimulation-induced release of IL-12. IL-12 was quantitated by an IL-12 ELISA as described previously.[66] These analyses revealed that peritoneal macrophages from *Listeria*-infected/immune and HKLM + IL-12–immunized mice produced very large amounts of IL-12 compared to the levels produced by the macrophages from mice injected with PBS only, IL-12 + PBS, or HKLM + PBS (FIG. 2). Macrophages from both *Listeria*-infected and HKLM + IL-12–treated mice also experienced significant upregulation of class II MHC expression (IE^K ELISA assay) as compared to the other treatment groups (FIG. 3A). Similar results were observed when soluble listerial antigen preparations (cLLO and SLP) were coinjected with IL-12, but not when either of these antigen preparations was administered alone (FIG. 3B). Thus, upregulation of class II MHC expression, IL-12 elaboration, and *Listeria*-specific T-cell responses occurred in HKLM + IL-12–treated mice to a similar extent as observed in *Listeria*-infected/immune mice.

Coinjection of HKLM and IL-12 Elicits Immunity to Challenge with a High Dose of Listeria

Intraperitoneal inoculation of naive mice with sublethal does of *Listeria* results in relatively rapid clearance of bacteria and the development of strongly protective T–cell mediated immune responses.[42,48,52,54–56] Conversely, ip inoculation of naive mice with larger doses of *Listeria* (LD$_{50}$ in C3HeB/FeJ mice is 4–6 × 10^4) yields a systemic infection characterized by large numbers of viable bacteria in the spleen and liver for 2–4 days, followed by death approximately 4–10 days postinfection.[48,67] Because the level of *Listeria* replication ongoing in the spleen (or liver) is related to the immune status of the infected mouse and correlates with survival,[55] quantitation of the colony-forming units of *Listeria* present in these organs 2–4 days postchallenge is a valid method for evaluating the effectiveness of vaccine strategies in the murine *Listeria* model.

To determine if the impressive *Listeria*-specific T-cell responses (FIG. 1) elicited by the HKLM + IL-12 mixture (just described) correlated with resistance to infection, groups of mice (5 per group) were immunized ip with either PBS only, 0.5 μg murine rIL-12 + PBS, HKLM (10^9) + PBS, or HKLM (10^9) + 0.5 μg murine rIL-12 on days 0 and 5. A single sublethal dose of live *L. monocytogenes* (6 × 10^3) was administered to one group of mice (*Listeria*-infected/immune) on day 0; this test group was used as the benchmark for the typical specific acquired immunity that results following recovery from infection. A large challenge dose of viable *L.*

monocytogenes (5×10^5/mouse) was administered on day 27. The mice were sacrificed 4 days later, and the colony-forming units of *Listeria* in spleens and livers were determined. As detailed in FIGURE 4, the *Listeria*-infected/immune mice and the HKLM + IL-12–immunized mice experienced greater than a 3 $\log_{10}$ reduction in *Listeria* colony-forming units in both spleens (FIG. 4) and livers (data not shown) compared to the mice given PBS, IL-12 + PBS, or HKLM + PBS. A series of protection experiments, with minor differences in the timing of challenge dose administration, confirmed these results. It should be noted that specific immunity was apparent as long as 41 days following vaccination. Furthermore, immunization

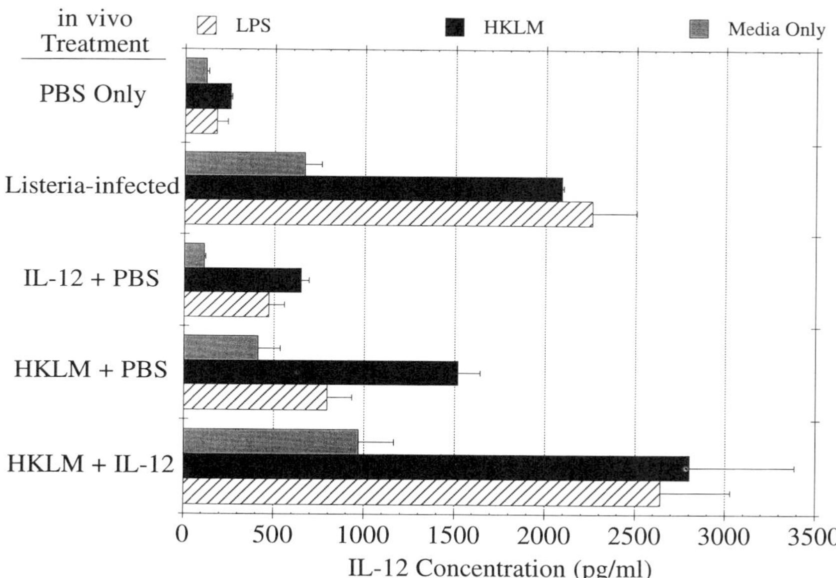

FIGURE 2. IL-12 production by *in vitro* restimulated peritoneal macrophages from mice immunized with HKLM + IL-12. Mice (3 per group) were immunized ip with the indicated antigen preparations on days 0 and 5. On day 10 the mice were sacrificed and PEC were collected by peritoneal lavage. Macrophages from the peritoneal exudate were isolated by incubation (2.0×10^6 cells/well) in 24-well tissue culture plates for 2 hours at 37°C; nonadherent cells were removed by washing. Macrophages were stimulated *in vitro* with culture medium, HKLM (10^8/ml), or lipopolysaccharide (1 µg/ml) for 24 hours at 37°C. Cell-free supernatants from these cultures were analyzed by ELISA[66] to quantitate the concentration of IL-12 produced in response to the indicated *in vitro* stimuli. All assays were performed in triplicate and results were expressed in picograms of IL-12 per milliliter (±SD). Data were adapted from previously published work.[66]

with a cocktail of IL-12 and two synthetic peptides, which correspond to immunodominant epitopes of listeriolysin O, has also been shown to elicit protective responses that protect mice against high dose *Listeria* challenge (M. A. Miller *et al.*, manuscript in preparation).

There have been previous reports that immunization with killed *L. monocytogenes,* when administered along with immunosuppressive agents (dextran sulfate 500, suramin)[68] or in a specific strain of mice,[69] resulted in immunity to *Listeria.* However,

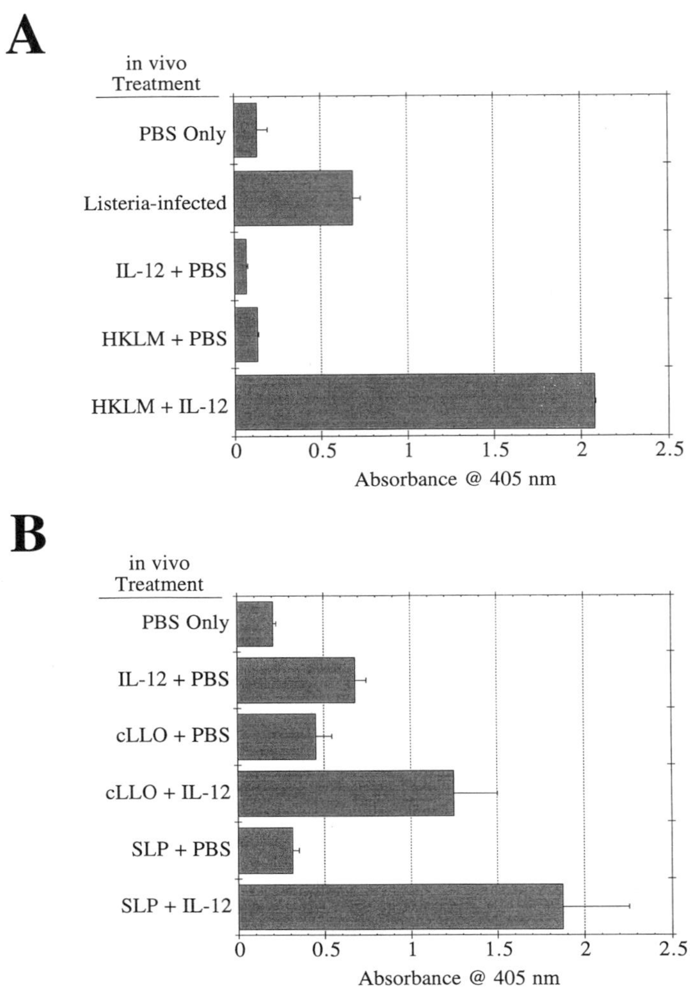

FIGURE 3. Class II MHC expression by peritoneal macrophages from mice immunized with particulate and soluble *Listeria* antigens + IL-12. Mice (5 per group) were immunized with the indicated antigen preparations on days 0 and 5. Mice were challenged ip on day 27 with a large dose of live *L. monocytogenes* (5×10^5; $LD_{50} = 4$–6×10^4) and sacrificed (4 days postchallenge) on day 31 (**A**) or sacrificed on day 10 (**B**). Macrophages were isolated by incubating peritoneal exudate cells (1.5×10^5 cells/well) in 96-well tissue culture plates for 2 hours at 37°C; nonadherent cells were removed by washing. Cells were fixed with paraformaldehyde and expression of class II MHC was measured by ELISA.[66] All assays were performed in triplicate, and results were expressed as relative expression of I-E^K (absorbance at 405 nm ± SD). Data were adapted from previously published work.[66]

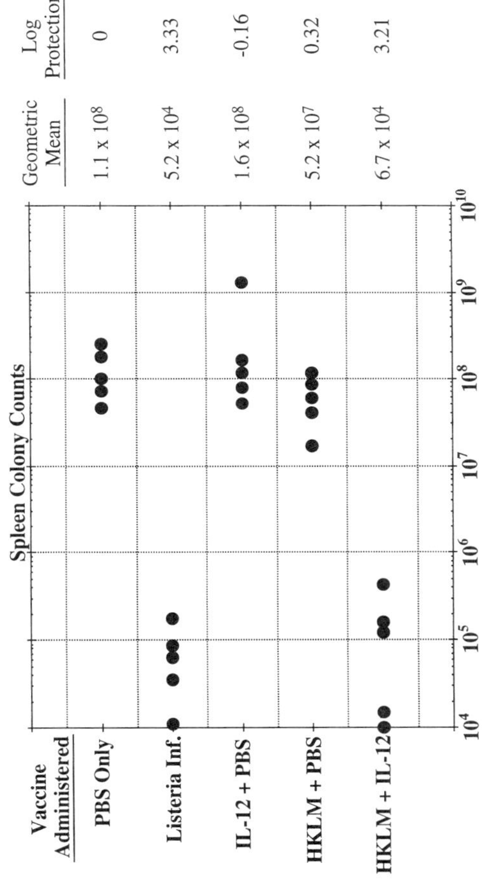

FIGURE 4. Protection of mice from large dose *Listeria* challenge by immunization with HKLM + IL-12. Mice (5 per group) were immunized with the indicated antigen preparations on days 0 and 5. On day 27 the mice were challenged ip with a large dose of live. *L. monocytogenes* (5×10^5; $LD_{50} = 4$–6×10^4). On day 31 (4 days postchallenge), the mice were sacrificed, spleens were removed via sterile dissection, and colony-forming units of *Listeria* in the spleen of each mouse were quantitated. Data were adapted from previously published work.[66]

these results were later shown to be compromised due to contamination of HKLM preparations with viable *Listeria*.[61] Furthermore, many subsequent studies have confirmed that immunization with killed or replication-incompetent *L. monocytogenes* fails to induce acquired immunity to *Listeria* infection.[57,59–61,70,71] Therefore, to date, this is the first vaccine strategy employing nonviable *Listeria* (or perhaps any nonviable intracellular bacterium) that can be shown to effectively elicit a protective immune response. Moreover, the protective T-cell responses resulting from coinjection of HKLM and IL-12 do not appear to result from a switch from Th2- to Th1-type responses (because viable *Listeria* induces a Th1-type response and HKLM fails to elicit any detectable response), but instead indicate that IL-12 has profound adjuvant effects *in vivo*.

TABLE 2. *In Vivo* Activation of Peritoneal Macrophages from Lipopolysaccharide Low-Responder Mice for Increased Interleukin-12 Production

	In Vitro Restimulation with:		
In Vivo Injection:[a]	Medium	HKLM (10^8/ml)	POLY I:C (50 μg/ml)
PBS (1 ml)	17 (9)[b]	248 (20)	116 (8)
Con A (100 μg)	167 (17)	4,263 (117)	2,158 (86)
Peptone (1.5 ml)	9 (5)	166 (13)	75 (9)
Thioglycollate (2.5 ml)	68 (28)	19,288 (546)	10,225 (546)
Poly I:C (100 μg)	19 (7)	5,651 (403)	NT
$NaIO_4$ (1 mg)	38 (12)	10,161 (720)	8,580 (935)
HKLM (10^9)	9 (14)	2,042 (232)	1,827 (327)
HKST (10^9)	16 (14)	1,335 (90)	834 (75)
Latex beads (10^9)	65 (21)	597 (36)	379 (33)
IL-12 (0.5 μg)	170 (2)	6,095 (579)	4,784 (375)
HKLM (10^9) + IL-12 (0.5 μg)	58 (16)	50,786 (4,652)	49,525 (1,953)
HLY + LM (1 × 10^4)	680 (135)	96,986 (1,394)	18,237 (769)
HLY − LM (1 × 10^4)	57 (16)	1228 (104)	3,331 (123)

[a]C3H/HeJ mice were injected ip. Peritoneal macrophages were incubated with *in vitro* stimuli for 24 hours.

[b]Values are means of triplicate samples in an ELISA with standard deviations in parentheses. NT = not tested.

Regulation of IL-12 Production by Macrophages in Vivo

Although a relatively large database describing the effects of IL-12 *in vitro* and *in vivo* has formed rapidly, comparatively little is known about the regulation of its production. As detailed here, we examined IL-12 production by murine peritoneal macrophages from two perspectives: (1) macrophage activation *in vivo*, and (2) stimulation of IL-12 secretion *in vitro*. Portions of the findings reported here were presented in greater detail in a previous publication.[72]

Initially we investigated the ability of a wide variety of stimulatory agents as well as bacteria or bacterial products to activate macrophages for IL-12 production. C3H/HeJ mice (LPS low-responder strain) were injected ip with the indicated *in vivo* stimulant (TABLE 2) on day 0. On day 3, mice were sacrificed and peritoneal macrophages were isolated in 24-well tissue culture plates and then incubated with the indicated stimulants *in vitro* for 24 hours; these stimulants included media alone (no further stimulation), HKLM, and polyinocynic-polycytidylic acid (poly I:C;

served as a stimulus unrelated to bacteria to avoid any potential elements of antigen specificity). IL-12 was measured in cell-free supernatants from each culture by ELISA. Injection of general peritoneal inflammatory agents yielded differing and somewhat surprising results. Stimulation of macrophages to produce IL-12 was greatest after injection of thioglycolate, whereas moderate stimulation was elicited by injection of Con A (a polyclonal stimulator of T cells), poly I:C (which recruits NK cells), or $NaIO_4$ (a macrophage-stimulating agent). To our surprise, injection of peptone failed to activate macrophages with respect to their ability to produce IL-12 in response to *in vitro* restimulation. Interestingly, injection of killed bacteria, viable *hly⁻ Listeria,* or IL-12 alone activated macrophages to produce only minimal levels of IL-12 upon restimulation *in vitro,* whereas HKLM + IL-12 and viable *hly⁺ Listeria* stimulated dramatic activation of macrophages; these results are consistent with those detailed in FIGURE 2. Together, these findings demonstrated that general inflammation of the peritoneal cavity was not necessarily sufficient to activate macrophages to produce IL-12 and that while killed or replication-incompetent bacteria were also insufficient, HKLM injected along with IL-12 was sufficient to dramatically influence the ability of macrophages to produce IL-12.

Regulation of IL-12 Production by Macrophages in Vitro

Studies to evaluate the ability of various agents to stimulate production of IL-12 by macrophages *in vitro* were performed using thioglycolate-elicited peritoneal macrophages from C3H/HeJ mice in order to eliminate any potential effects of LPS contamination and to provide a maximum dynamic range for detection of changes in IL-12 production; the enhanced ability of thioglycolate-elicited macrophages to produce IL-12 (TABLE 2) provided a sensitive system in which even small changes induced by weak stimuli were detectable. Both HKLM (FIG. 5) and viable hly⁺ *Listeria* (data not shown) induced IL-12 production in a dose-dependent manner upon *in vitro* restimulation of macrophages. Interestingly, latex beads of comparable size (to bacteria) failed to induce production of IL-12 (FIG. 5), even when used at concentrations 100-fold higher than the highest concentration of HKLM tested (data not shown). These observations suggested that bacterial products were necessary for induction of IL-12 production and that phagocytosis alone was an insufficient stimulus.

Upon extending these studies to investigate the potential of a diverse array of microbial products to induce IL-12 production *in vitro,* we found that the universal ability of microbial products to stimulate IL-12 production was striking. In addition to the ability of HKLM to stimulate IL-12 elaboration (FIG. 5), souble listerial protein preparations (SLP and cLLO) were effective as stimulators of IL-12 production (data not shown). Preparations from other microbial sources, including yeast extracts, double-stranded RNA (poly I:C), and staphylococcal superantigens, were also effective to varying degrees. Studies with LPS revealed that it was a strong stimulus for *in vitro* production of IL-12 in LPS responder mice, but it had no effect on macrophages isolated from LPS-nonresponder mice (data not shown). Another "family" of molecules that can be broadly associated with bacteria are heat shock proteins (HSPs). As demonstrated in FIGURE 6, IL-12 production by peritoneal macrophages was stimulated in a dose-dependent manner on the addition of *Mycobacteria*-derived HSPs. Because HSPs are highly conserved phylogenetically, and because mammalian cells produce HSPs in response to heat or other stress signals, including infection by microbial agents, it seemed possible that upregulation of mammalian HSPs could contribute to increased IL-12 production by host macro-

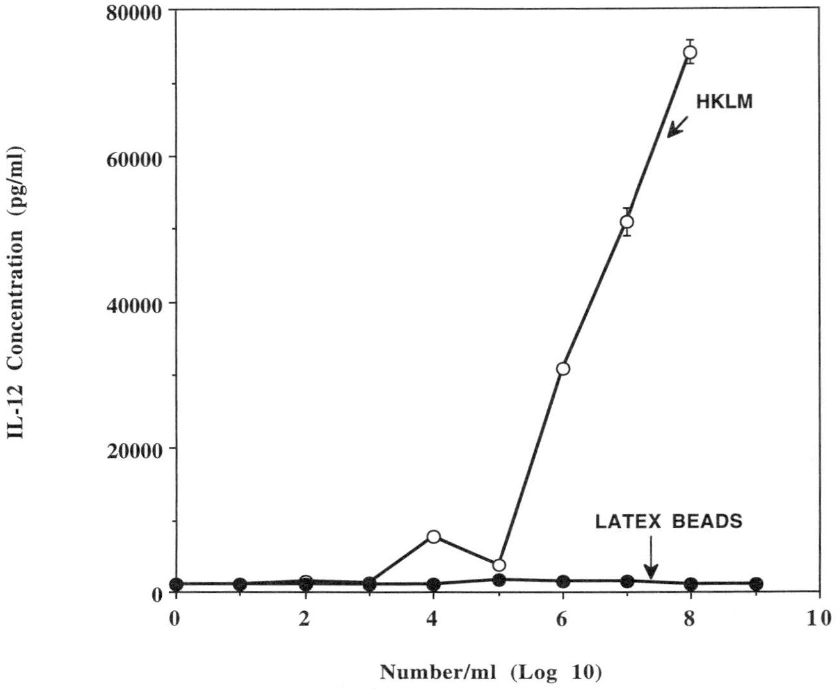

FIGURE 5. *In vitro* activation of macrophages by HKLM but not inert latex beads. C3HeB/FeJ mice were injected ip with 2.5 ml of thioglycolate broth 3 days before harvest of PEC. PEC (2.0×10^6) were added to wells of a 24-well tissue culture plate, incubated for 2 hours at 37°C, and nonadherent cells were removed. The resulting adherent population was then incubated for 24 hours with either HKLM or latex beads of equivalent size (1.1 μM average diameter) at the indicated concentrations. IL-12 was measured in cell-free culture supernatants by ELISA.[66] Values represent the mean (±SD) of triplicate samples. Data were adapted from previously published work.[72]

phages. To our surprise, however, only moderate stimulation was observed when mammalian HSPs were added at relatively high doses or when macrophages were heat-shocked; overall, they were far less stimulatory than the microbial HSPs (data not shown). Similar results were obtained using the continuous macrophage-like cell line J774 (data not shown), suggesting that the stimuli act directly on macrophages and require no "helper" cells. Taken together, these results suggest that peritoneal macrophages that have been stimulated *in vivo* are particularly sensitive to stimulation by microbial products *in vitro*.

What Is the Mechanism of IL-12 Adjuvanticity?

The observed difference in responsiveness of peritoneal macrophages to viable, replication-competent bacteria and killed or replication-deficient bacteria or bacterial products *in vivo* coupled with the ability to induce protective immunity by injecting HKLM along with the macrophage-derived cytokine IL-12 is intriguing. The results described here (and elsewhere[66,72]) demonstrate that actively replicating bacteria are required for macrophage activation *in vivo*. The difference(s) between replication-competent *Listeria* and killed or replication-incompetent *Listeria* which relate to their relative ability (or inability) to induce protective immunity remains mechanistically undefined. Several explanations have been offered: (1) antigen dose was insufficient or antigen lacked persistence; (2) epitopes that elicit protective antigen-specific T cells are either destroyed by heat treatment or are present in insufficient quantity because they are primarily produced *in vivo* or are encoded by genes that are specifically upregulated *in vivo* or in response to the host environment during infection; (3) lack of LLO production prevents cytoplasmic localization of listerial antigens which is required for entrance into the MHC class I presentation pathway, thus preventing the development of *Listeria*-specific CD8+ T cells; (4) absence of secreted or specifically upregulated listerial gene products that may have unique biological properties (e.g., signal transducing activity) that affect function of

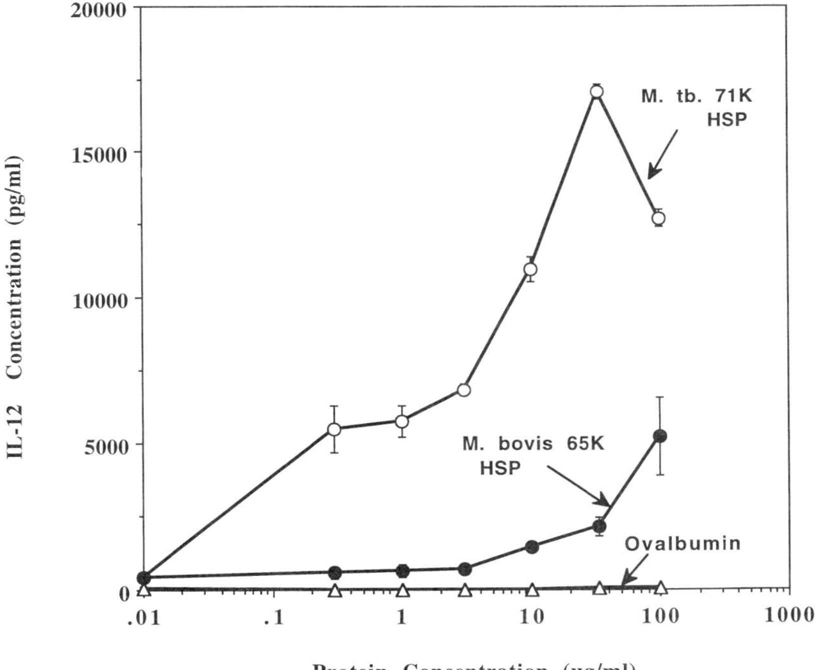

FIGURE 6. Prokaryotic HSPs stimulate peritoneal macrophages from LPS-low-responder mice to produce IL-12 *in vitro*. C3H/HeJ mice were injected ip with 2.5 ml of thioglycolate broth 3 days before harvest of PEC. PEC (2.0 × 10^6/well) were incubated in 24-well tissue culture plates for 24 hours at 37°C, and nonadherent cells were removed. The resulting adherent population was then incubated for 24 hours with the indicated concentrations of recombinant HSP or ovalbumin (control). IL-12 concentration in cell-free supernatants was determined by ELISA,[66] and results reflect the mean (± SD) of triplicate test samples. Data were adapted from previously published work.[72]

immune cells, and/or (5) differences in the local production of cytokines in response to HKLM vs viable *Listeria* (may relate to number 4). The studies just described demonstrated conclusively that HKLM retains epitopes that are capable of eliciting protective responses and that coinjection of one cytokine (IL-12) with HKLM overcomes the apparent immunogenic deficiency(s) of HKLM, resulting in specific acquired immunity to *Listeria* infection. Therefore, these studies imply that the differential abilities of live and killed *Listeria* to stimulate macrophages in a manner that leaves them poised to produce IL-12 and possibly other cytokines may correlate with their contrasting abilities to elicit a protective T-cell response.

To more precisely define the effects of the HKLM + IL-12 combination on macrophages *in vivo* and how these effects may influence development of a protective cellular immune response, we performed a kinetic analysis of the production of IL-12 by peritoneal macrophages isolated from mice from each of the test groups just described above (FIGS. 1–4). Mice were immunized with either IL-12 + PBS, HKLM + PBS, or HKLM + IL-12 on days 0 and 5 or injected with a nonlethal dose of viable *Listeria* on day 0. Peritoneal macrophages from each immunization group were isolated and cultured *in vitro* for 24 hours with HKLM (10^8/ml) at the indicated timepoints. As detailed in FIGURE 7, *Listeria* infection resulted in a rapid increase in the ability of macrophages to produce IL-12, with peak production 2 days after injection. Immunization with HKLM + IL-12 resulted in a similar kinetic profile of IL-12 production initially, and then another peak of IL-12 production occurred between days 4 and 6 presumably in response to the booster immunization on day 5. Interestingly, peritoneal macrophages isolated from mice injected with either HKLM + PBS or IL-12 + PBS were not primed to produce high levels of IL-12 at any timepoint that was examined. These results demonstrated that although neither IL-12 nor HKLM alone, when injected ip, was capable of "priming" macrophages for IL-12 production, when injected together, the antigen (HKLM) and IL-12 synergize to heighten the ability of macrophages to produce IL-12 in a manner consistent with that observed in *Listeria*-infected mice.

These results suggest that another cytokine or network of cytokines may be operative and that exogenous addition of IL-12 (along with HKLM or other bacterial antigens) is involved in the initiation of the operative cytokine cascade. As a first step in defining additional cytokines that may be involved, we investigated the ability of many cytokines (IL-1, IL-2, IL-4, IL-7, IL-10, IL-12, IL-13, IFN-γ, TNF-α, TGF-β, and GM-CSF) and combinations of cytokines (IL-1 + IL-7, IL-1 + IL-12) to influence IL-12 production by macrophages *in vitro*. Except for modest increases following the addition of 10–1,000 U/ml of IFN-γ, none of the cytokines or combinations of cytokines tested elicited increased ability of macrophages to produce IL-12 (data not shown). However, when added along with HKLM, several of these cytokines synergized with HKLM, resulting in either marked upregulation or profound inhibition of IL-12 production by peritoneal macrophages. IFN-γ, a Th1 cytokine, acted in synergy with HKLM to induce a dramatic upregulation of IL-12 production (FIG. 8A). By contrast, IL-2 (another TH1 cytokine) failed to influence IL-12 production even when added along with HKLM (FIG. 8A). Interestingly, the addition of the Th2 cytokines IL-4 and IL-10 along with HKLM profoundly inhibited the production of IL-12 by peritoneal macrophages (FIG. 8B). These results are consistent with the well described ability of IL-12 to promote the development of Th1-type immune responses.

Based on these results, our speculative working model to explain the adjuvant activity of IL-12 relates to amounts of IL-12 and IFN-γ that are produced by a positive regulatory loop involving the interaction of macrophages, $\gamma\delta$ T cells, NK

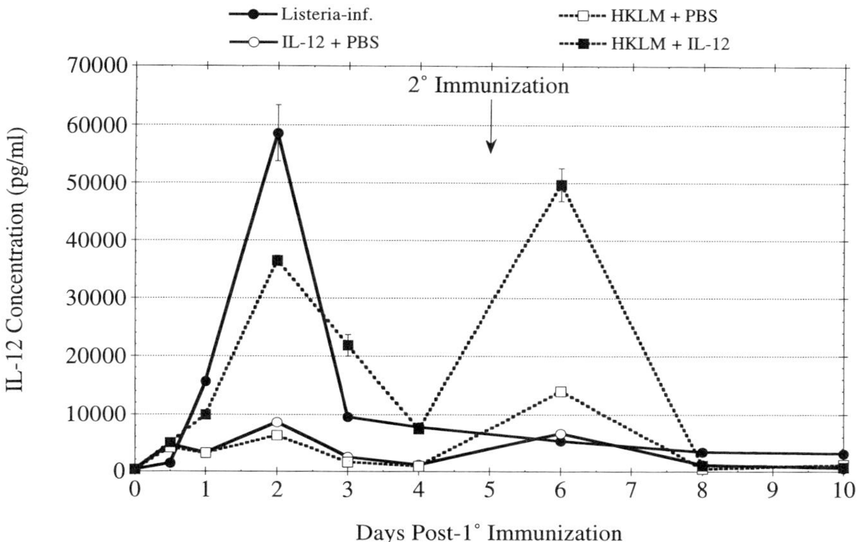

FIGURE 7. Kinetic analysis of IL-12 production by peritoneal macrophages from *Listeria*-immunized mice. C3HeB/FeJ mice (19/group) were injected ip on days 0 and 5 with either 0.5 μg IL-12 + PBS, HKLM (10^9) + PBS, or HKLM (10^9) + 0.5 μg IL-12. Another group of 19 mice were injected ip with a sublethal dose of viable *L. monocytogenes* (6×10^3/mouse). At the indicated timepoints postimmunization either two mice per group (12 hours, 24 hours, 2 days, 3 days, and 4 days) or three mice per group (days 6, 8, and 10) were sacrificed, and PEC were harvested by lavage. PEC (2×10^6/well) were incubated in 24-well tissue culture plates for 2 hours at 37°C. Nonadherent cells were removed, and the adherent cell populations were restimulated *in vitro* with 10^8 HKLM for 24 hours. IL-12 concentration in cell-free supernatant from each culture was determined by ELISA.[66] Values represent the mean (±SD) of triplicate samples. Data were adapted from previously published work.[72]

cells, and ultimately αβ T cells. This model is based on the assumption that IL-12 production is rate limiting *in vivo*. Several activation events are known: (1) IL-12 + IL-1 activates γδ T cells and IL-12 + TNF-α activates NK cells for IFN-γ production; (2) IFN-γ (in the presence of bacterial products) activates macrophages in terms of increased IL-12 and possibly IL-1 and TNF production; and (3) antigen presentation by macrophages can occur more efficiently via upregulation of class I and class II MHC expression caused by IFN-γ and is important for optimal development of antigen-specific αβ T cells. Therefore, HKLM (or other bacterial products) supplies sufficient antigen to drive the αβ T-cell response and possibly provides sufficient signals for production of IL-1 and TNF-α that would in turn act synergistically with exogenously added IL-12. This combination sets into motion the positive regulatory loop as follows: HKLM causes IL-1 and TNF-α production; IFN-γ is produced by γδ T cells and NK cells in response to IL-1/IL-12 and TNF-α/IL-12, respectively; IFN-γ not only augments the production of cytokines by macrophages which drive the positive regulatory loop, but also induces MHC expression (and cell surface accessory molecules) which augments antigen presentation to αβ T cells. Studies designed to further examine this hypothetical model of IL-12 adjuvanticity are ongoing.

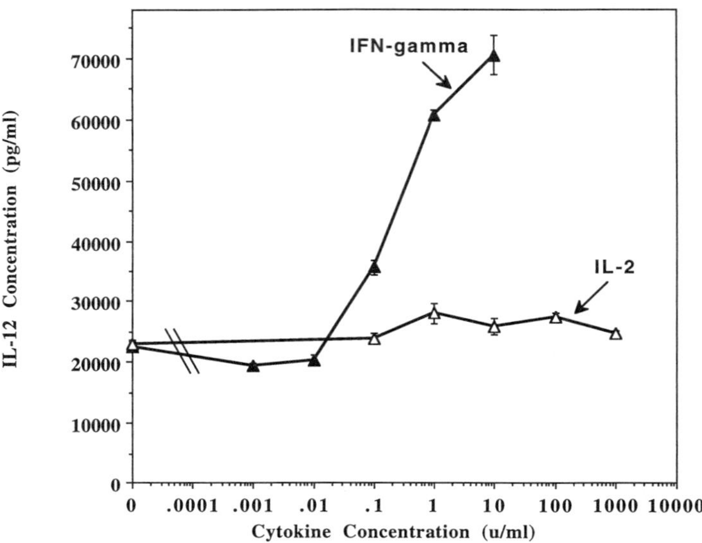

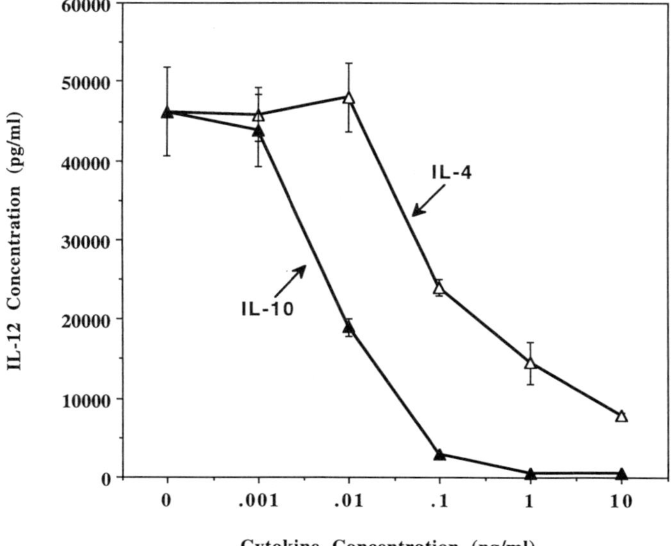

FIGURE 8. Legend is on facing. page.

SUMMARY

The results presented here demonstrate the striking potentiating effects of IL-12 when it is combined with listerial immunogens. Although HKLM alone does not elicit strong T-cell responses,[57,59–61] the results presented here demonstrate that the combination of HKLM and IL-12 elicited vigorous *Listeria*-specific Th1-type T-cell responses when administered intraperitoneally. The intensity of these responses, as well as the cytokine profiles of the *Listeria*-specific peritoneal T cells and macrophages, was remarkably similar to that of *Listeria*-infected/immune mice. These studies also revealed that typically nonimmunogenic forms of soluble listerial antigen preparations (cLLO, SLP) and LLO peptide homologs (M. A. Miller *et al.*, manuscript in preparation) elicited intense *Listeria*-specific T-cell responses when administered with IL-12. In conjunction with the generation of specific T-cell responses following injection of IL-12 in combination with either killed *Listeria* or soluble listerial antigen preparations, macrophages from these mice expressed upregulated quantities of class II MHC and produced increased amounts of IL-12 following restimulation *in vitro*. Protection studies established that the *Listeria*-specific T-cell responses elicited by the HKLM + IL-12 mixture conferred protective immunity of mice to a lethal dose of viable *L. monocytogenes*.

Studies designed to investigate the regulation of IL-12 production by peritoneal macrophages revealed that activated macrophages are particularly sensitive to bacterial products. However, nonviable or replication-incompetent bacteria or bacterial products injected alone were unable to influence the ability of macrophages to produce IL-12. The ability of activated macrophages to respond to HKLM was dramatically upregulated upon addition of IFN-γ and markedly downregulated in the presence of the Th2 cytokines, IL-4 and IL-10. In light of what is known about the ability of IL-12 to induce IFN-γ production by NK cells and $\gamma\delta$ T cells, these results suggest that the exogenous addition of IL-12 may help initiate a cytokine cascade which enables the immune system to interact productively with an antigen that is typically nonimmunogenic when administered alone. These findings demonstrate that IL-12 may prove to be a powerful and broadly useful adjuvant component of particulate and soluble antigen-based vaccines directed towards many types of intracellular pathogenic microorganisms. Studies aimed at determining the generality of these findings in other infectious disease models as well as experiments designed to further elucidate the mechanism(s) of IL-12 adjuvanticity are continuing.

ACKNOWLEDGMENTS

The data presented here were adapted from data previously published in the Journal of Immunology, refs. 66 and 72. The authors would like to thank Drs. Leo

---

FIGURE 8. Production of IL-12 by macrophages *in vitro* can be modulated by exogenous addition of Th1 or Th2 cytokines. C3H/HeJ mice were injected ip with 2.5 ml of thioglycolate broth 3 days before harvest of PEC. Macrophages were isolated by incubating PEC (2.0×10^6/ well) in 24-well tissue culture plates for 2 hours at 37°C, and nonadherent cells were removed. The resulting adherent population was then incubated for 24 hours with the indicated concentrations of recombinant Th1 (**A**) or Th2 (**B**) cytokines + HKLM (10^8). IL-12 was measured in cell-free culture supernatants by ELISA,[66] and results were expressed as the mean ($\pm$ SD) of triplicate samples. Data were adapted from previously published work.[72]

Francois, Ralph Kubo, and Giorgio Trinchieri for providing hybridoma cell lines for monoclonal antibodies. We thank Immunex Corp. and Hoffman-LaRoche, Inc. for kindly providing recombinant cytokines. We particularly wish to thank Dr. Maurice Gately for his contribution to this work. We would also like to acknowledge the excellent technical assistance of Edna Scott.

REFERENCES

1. BURKE, K. L., G. DUNN, M. FERGUSON, P. D. MINOR & J. W. ALMOND. 1988. Antigen chimeras of poliovirus as potential new vaccines. Nature **332:** 81.
2. CURTISS, R. I., S. M. KELLY, P. A. GULIG & K. NAKAYAMA. 1989. Selective delivery of antigens by recombinant bacteria. Curr. Top. Micriobiol. Immunol. **146:** 45.
3. CASTEN, L. A., P. KAUMAYA & S. K. PIERCE. 1988. Enhanced T cell responses to antigenic peptides targeted to B cell surface Ig, Ia, or class I molecules. J. Exp. Med. **168:** 171.
4. CARAYANNIOTIS, G. & B. H. BARBER. 1987. Adjuvant-free IgG responses induced with antigen coupled to antibodies against class II MHC. Nature **327:** 59.
5. CARAYANNIOTIS, G., E. VIZI, J. M. PARKER, R. S. HODGES & B. H. BARBER. 1988. Delivery of synthetic peptides by anti-class II MHC monoclonal antibodies induces specific adjuvant-free IgG responses *in vivo.* Molec. Immunol. **25:** 907.
6. CARAYANNIOTIS, G. & B. H. BARBER. 1990. Characterization of the adjuvant-free serological response to protein antigens coupled to antibodies specific for class II MHC determinants. Vaccine **8:** 137.
7. COOPER, P. D. 1985. Complement and cancer: Activation of the alternative pathway as a theoretical basis for immunotherapy. Adv. Immunol. Cancer Therapy **1:** 125.
8. COOPER, P. D. & E. J. STEELE. 1988. The adjuvanticity of gamma-inulin. Immunol. Cell Biol. **66:** 345.
9. MCGHEE, J. R., J. MESTECKY, C. O. ELSON & H. KIYONO. 1989. Regulation of IgA synthesis and immune response by T cells and interleukins. J. Clin. Immunol. **9:** 175.
10. MCGHEE, J. & J. MESTECKY. 1990. In defense of mucosal surfaces. Development of novel vaccines for IgA responses at the portals of entry of microbial pathogens. Infect. Dis. Clin. North Am. **4:** 315.
11. KAWAMURA, H., S. A. ROSENBERG & J. A. BERZOFSKY. 1985. Immunization with antigen and interleukin 2 *in vivo* overcomes Ir gene low responsiveness. J. Exp. Med **162:** 381.
12. LEBMAN, D. A., F. D. LEE & R. L. COFFMAN. 1990. Mechanism for transforming growth factor B and IL-2 enhancement of IgA expression in lipopolysaccharide-stimulated murine B lymphocytes. J. Immunol. **144:** 952.
13. MEUER, S. C., H. DUMANN, K. H. MEYER ZUM BUSCHENFELD & H. KOHLER. 1989. Low-dose interleukin 2 induces systemic immune responses against HBsAg in immuno-deficient non-responders to hepatitis B vaccination. Lancet **1:** 15.
14. MURRAY, P. D., D. T. MCKENZIE, S. L. SWAIN & M. F. KAGNOFF. 1987. Interleukin 5 and interleukin 4 produced by Peyer's patch T cells selectively enhance immunoglobulin A expression. J. Immunol. **139:** 2669.
15. ROUSE, B. T., L. S. MILLER, L. TURTINEN & R. N. MOORE. 1985. Augmentation of immunity to herpes simplex virus by *in vivo* administration of interleukin 2. J. Immunol. **134:** 926.
16. SNAPPER, C. M. & W. E. PAUL. 1987. Interferon-gamma and B cell stimulatory factor-1 reciprocally regulate Ig isotype production. Science **236:** 944.
17. KOBAYASHI, M., L. FITZ, M. RYAN, R. M. HEWICK, S. C. CLARK, S. CHAN, R. LOUDON, F. SHERMAN, B. PERUSSIA & G. TRINCHIERI. 1989. Identification and purification of natural killer cell stimulatory factor (NKSF), a cytokine with multiple biological effects on human lymphocytes. J. Exp. Med. **170:** 827.
18. D'ANDREA, A., M. RENGARAJU, N. M. VALIANTE, J. CHEHIMI, M. KUBIN, M. ASTE, S. H. CHAN, M. KOBAYASHI, D. YOUNG, E. NICKBARG, R. CHIZZONITE, S. F. WOLF & G. TRINCHIERI. 1992. Production of natural killer cell stimulatory factor (interleukin-12) by peripheral blood mononuclear cells. J. Exp. Med. **176:** 1387.
19. GATELY, M. K., B. B. DESAI, A. G. WOLITZKY, P. M. QUINN, C. M. DWYER, F. J.

PODLASKI, P. C. FAMILLETTI, F. SINIGAGLIA, R. CHIZONNITE, U. GUBLER & A. S. STERN. 1991. Regulation of human lymphocyte proliferation by a heterodimeric cytokine, IL-12 (cytotoxic lymphocyte maturation factor). J. Immunol. **147:** 874.

20. ROBERTSON, M. J., R. J. SOIFFER, S. F. WOLF, T. J. MANLEY, C. DONAHUE, D. YOUNG, S. H. HERRMANN & J. RITZ. 1992. Response of human natural killer (NK) cells to NK cell stimulatory factor (NKSF): Cytolytic activity and proliferation of NK cells are differentially regulated by NKSF. J. Exp. Med. **175:** 779.

21. BERTAGNOLLI, M. M., B. Y. LIN, D. YOUNG & S. H. HERRMANN. 1992. IL-12 augments antigen-dependent proliferation of activated T lymphocytes. J. Immunol. **149:** 3778.

22. PERUSSIA, B., S. H. CHAN, A. D'ANDREA, K. TSUJI, D. SANTOLI, M. POSPISIL, D. YOUNG, S. F. WOLF & G. TRINCHIERI. 1992. Natural killer (NK) cell stimulatory factor or IL-12 has differential effects on the proliferation of TCR-alpha beta, TCR-gamma delta$^+$ T lymphocytes, and NK cells. J. Immunol. **149:** 3495.

23. CHAN, S. H., B. PERUSSIA, J. W. GUPTA, M. KOBAYASHI, M. POSPISIL, H. A. YOUNG, S. F. WOLF, D. YOUNG, S. C. CLARK AND G. TRINCHIERI. 1991. Induction of interferon gamma production by natural killer cell stimulatory factor: Characterization of the responder cells and synergy with other inducers. J. Exp. Med. **173:** 869.

24. CHAN, S. H., M. KOBAYASHI, D. SANTOLI, B. PERUSSIA & G. TRINCHIERI. 1992. Mechanisms of IFN-gamma induction by natural killer cell stimulatory factor (NKSF/IL-12). Role of transcription and mRNA stability in the synergistic interaction between NKSF and IL-2. J. Immunol. **148:** 92.

25. GAZZINELLI, R. T., S. HIENY, T. A. WYNN, S. WOLF & A. SHER. 1993. Interleukin-12 is required for the T-lymphocyte-independent induction of interferon gamma by an intracellular parasite and induces resistance in T-cell-deficient hosts. Proc. Natl. Acad. Sci. USA **90:** 6115.

26. TRIPP, C. S., S. F. WOLF & E. R. UNANUE. 1993. Interleukin-12 and tumor necrosis factor alpha are costimulators of interferon gamma production by natural killer cells in severe combined immunodeficiency mice with listeriosis, and interleukin 10 is a physiologic antagonist. Proc. Natl. Acad. Sci. USA **90:** 3725.

27. ZIEGLER, H. K., M. J. SKEEN & K. M. PEARCE. 1994. Role of α/β and γ/δ T cells in innate and acquired immunity. *In* Microbial Pathogenesis and Immune Response. E. W. Ades, R. F. Rest & S. A. Morse, Eds. Ann. N.Y. Acad. Sci. **730:** 53.

28. SKEEN, M. J. & H. K. ZIEGLER. 1994. Activation of γ/δ T cells for production of IFNγ is mediated by bacteria via macrophage-derived cytokines IL-1 and IL-12. J. Immunol. **154:** 5832.

29. GATELY, M. K., A. G. WOLITZKY, P. M. QUINN & R. CHIZZONITE. 1992. Regulation of human cytolytic lymphocyte responses by interleukin-12. Cell. Immunol. **143:** 127.

30. TRINCHIERI, G. 1993. Interleukin-12 and its role in the generation of Th1 cells. Immunol. Today **14:** 335.

31. HSIEH, C. S., S. E. MACATONIA, C. S. TRIPP, S. F. WOLF, A. O'GARRA & K. M. MURPHY. 1993. Development of TH1 CD4$^+$ T cells through IL-12 produced by *Listeria*-induced macrophages. Science **260:** 547.

32. SEDER, R. A., R. GAZZINELLI, A. SHER & W. E. PAUL. 1993. Interleukin-12 acts directly on CD4$^+$ T cells to enhance priming for interferon gamma production and diminishes interleukin-4 inhibition of such priming. Proc. Natl. Acad. Sci. USA **90:** 10188.

33. MANETTI, R., P. PARRONCHI, M. G. GIUDIZI, M. P. PICCINNI, E. MAGGI, G. TRINCHIERI & S. ROMAGNANI. 1993. Natural killer cell stimulatory factor (interleukin-12 [IL-12]) induces T helper type 1 (Th1)-specific immune responses and inhibits the development of IL-4-producing Th cells. J. Exp. Med. **177:** 1199.

34. HEINZEL, F. P., D. S. SCHOENHAUT, R. M. RERKO, L. E. ROSSER & M. K. GATELY. 1993. Recombinant interleukin-12 cures mice infected with *Leishmania major*. J. Exp. Med. **177:** 1505.

35. SYPEK, J. P., C. L. CHUNG, S. E. MAYOR, J. M. SUBRAMANYAM, S. J. GOLDMAN, D. S. SIEBURTH, S. F. WOLF & R. G. SCHAUB. 1993. Resolution of cutaneous leishmaniasis: interleukin-12 initiates a protective T helper type 1 immune response. J. Exp. Med. **177:** 1797.

36. STEVENSON, M. M., M. F. TAM, S. F. WOLF & A. SHER. 1995. IL-12 induced protection

against blood-stage *Plasmodium chabaudi* AS requires IFN-γ and TNF-α and occurs via a nitric oxide-dependent mechanism. J. Immunol. **155:** 2545.

37. WYNN, T. A., A. W. CHEEVER, D. JANKOVIC, R. W. POINDEXTER, P. CASPAR, F. A. LEWIS & A. SHER. 1995. An IL-12-based vaccination method for preventing fibrosis induced by schistosome infection. Nature **376:** 594.

38. ORANGE, J. S., S. F. WOLF & C. A. BIRON. 1994. Effects of IL-12 on the response and susceptibility to experimental viral infections. J. Immunol. **152:** 1253.

39. CLERICI, M., D. R. LUCEY, J. A. BERZOFSKY, L. A. PINTO, T. A. WYNN, S. P. BLATT, M. J. DOLAN, C. W. HENDRIX, S. F. WOLF & G. M. SHEARER. 1993. Restoration of HIV-specific cell-mediated immune responses by interleukin-12 *in vitro.* Science **262:** 1721.

40. TRIPP, C. S., M. K. GATELY, J. HAKIMI, P. LING & E. R. UNANUE. 1994. Neutralization of IL-12 decreases resistance to *Listeria* in SCID and C.B-17 mice. J. Immunol. **152:** 1883.

41. AFONSO, L. C., T. M. SCHARTON, L. Q. VIEIRA, M. WYSOCKA, G. TRINCHIERI & P. SCOTT. 1994. The adjuvant effect of interleukin-12 in a vaccine against *Leishmania major.* Science **263:** 235.

42. NORTH, R. J. 1973. Cellular mediators of anti-*Listeria* immunity as an enlarged population of short-lived replicating T cells. J. Exp. Med. **138:** 342.

43. BARZA, M. 1985. Listeriosis in milk. N. Engl. J. Med. **312:** 438.

44. GRAY, M. L. & A. H. KILLINGER. 1966. *Listeria monocytogenes* and listeric infections. Bacteriol. Rev. **30:** 309.

45. SEELIGER, H. P. R. 1961. Listeriosis. Hafner. New York.

46. JURADO, R. L., M. M. FARLEY, E. PEREIRA, R. C. HARVEY, A. SCHUCHAT, J. D. WENGER & D. S. STEPHENS. 1993. Increased risk of *Listeria monocytogenes* meningitis and bacteremia in patients with human immunodeficiency virus infection. Clin Infect. Dis. **17:** 224.

47. ZIEGLER, H. K. & E. R. UNANUE. 1981. Identification of a macrophage antigen-processing event required for I-region-restricted antigen presentation to T lymphocytes. J. Immunol. **127:** 1869.

48. MACKANESS, G. B. 1962. Cellular resistance to infection. J. Exp. Med. **116:** 381.

49. ROTHE, J., W. LESSLAUER, H. LOTSCHER, Y. LANG, P. KOEBEL, F. KONTGEN, A. ALTHAGE, R. ZINKERNAGEL, M. STEINMETZ & H. BLUETHMANN. 1993. Mice lacking the tumor necrosis factor receptor 1 are resistant to TNF-mediated toxicity but highly susceptable to infection by *Listeria monocytogenes.* Nature **364:** 798.

50. HUANG, S., W. HENDRIKS, A. ALTHAGE, S. HEMMI, H. BLUETHMANN, R. KAMIJO, J. VILCEK, R. M. ZINKERNAGEL & M. AQUET. 1993. Immune response in mice that lack the interferon-gamma receptor. Science **259:** 1742.

51. SKEEN, M. J. & H. K. ZIEGLER. 1993. Intercellular interactions and cytokine responsiveness of peritoneal α/β and γ/δ T cells from Listeria-infected mice: Synergistic effects of interleukin-1 and 7 on γ/δ T cells. J. Exp. Med. **178:** 985.

52. SKEEN, M. J. & H. K. ZIEGLER. 1993. Induction of murine peritoneal γ/δ T cells and their role in resistance to bacterial infection. J. Exp. Med. **178:** 971.

53. MOMBAERTS, P. J. ARNOLD, F. RUSS, S. TONEGAWA & S. H. E. KAUFMANN. 1993. Different roles of α/β and γ/δ T cells in immunity against an intracellular bacterial pathogen. Nature **365:** 53.

54. ARMSTRONG, A. S. & C. P. SWORD. 1964. Cellular resistance in listeriosis. J. Infect. Dis. **114:** 258.

55. MACKANESS, G. B. & W. C. HILL. 1969. The effect of anti-lymphocyte globulin on cell-mediated resistance to infection. J. Exp. Med. **129:** 993.

56. KAUFMANN, S. H. E., M. M. SHIMON & H. HAHN. 1979. Specific Lyt 123 T cells are involved in protection against *Listeria monocytogenes* and in delayed-type hypersensitivity to listerial antigens. J. Exp. Med. **150:** 1033.

57. BERCHE, P., J. L. GAILLARD & P. J. SANSONETTI. 1987. Intracellular growth of *L. monocytogenes* as a prerequesite for *in vivo* induction of T cell immunity. J. Immunol. **138:** 2266.

58. BUCHMEIER, N. A. & R. D. SCHREIBER. 1985. Requirement of endogenous interferon-γ production for resolution of *Listeria monocytogenes* infection. Proc. Natl. Acad. Sci. USA **82:** 7404.

59. BERCHE, P., J. L. GAILLARD, C. GEOFFROY & J. E. ALOUF. 1987. T cell recognition of listeriolysin O is induced during infection with *Listeria monocytogenes*. J. Immunol. **139:** 3813.

60. MITSUYAMA, M., K. IGARASHI, I. KAWAMURA, T. OHMORI & K. NOMOTO. 1990. Difference in the induction of macrophage interleukin-1 production between viable and killed cells of *Listeria monocytogenes*. Infect. Immun. **58:** 1254.

61. WIRSING VON KOENIG, C. H., H. FINGER & H. HOF. 1982. Failure of killed *Listeria monocytogenes* vaccine to produce protective immunity. Nature (Lond) **297:** 233.

62. MARSHALL, N. E. & H. K. ZIEGLER. 1991. The role of bacterial hemolysin production in induction of macrophage Ia expression during infection with *Listeria monocytogenes*. J. Immunol. **147:** 2324.

63. SAFLEY, A. S., C. W. CLUFF, N. E. MARSHALL & H. K. ZIEGLER. 1991. Role of listeriolysin-O (LLO) in the T lymphocyte response to infection with *Listeria monocytogenes:* Identification of T cell epitopes of LLO. J. Immunol. **146:** 3604.

64. WENTWORTH, P. A. & H. K. ZIEGLER. 1987. The antigenic and mitogenic response of murine B and T lymphocytes to soluble listerial proteins fractionated by preparative SDS-PAGE. J. Immunol. **138:** 2671.

65. MARSHALL, N. E. & H. K. ZIEGLER. 1991. Lipopolysaccharide responsiveness is an important factor in the generation of antigen-specific T cell responses during infection with gram-negative bacteria. J. Immunol. **147:** 2333.

66. MILLER, M. A., M. J. SKEEN & H. K. ZIEGLER. 1995. Non-viable bacterial antigens administered with IL-12 generate antigen-specific T cell responses and protective immunity against *Listeria monocytogenes*. J. Immunol. **155:** 4817.

67. GREGORY, S. H., L. K. BARCZYNSKI & E. J. WING. 1992. Effector function of hepatocytes and Kupffer cells in the resolution of systemic bacterial infections. J. Leukocyte Biol. **51:** 421.

68. VAN DIJK, H., F. M. HOFHUIS, E. M. BERNS, C. VAN DER MEER & J. M. WILLERS. 1980. Killed *Listeria monocytogenes* vaccine is protective in C3H/HeJ mice without addition of adjuvants. Nature **286:** 713.

69. VAN DER MEER, C., F. M. HOFHUIS & J. M. WILLERS. 1977. Killed *Listeria monocytogenes* vaccine becomes protective on addition of polyanions. Nature **269:** 594.

70. HASENCLEVER, H. F. & W. W. KARAKAWA. 1957. Immunization of mice against *Listeria monocytogenes*. J. Bacteriol. **74:** 584.

71. NÄHER, H., U. SPERLING & H. HAHN. 1985. H-2K-restricted granuloma formation by Ly-2$^+$ cells in antibacterial protection to facultative intracellular bacteria. J. Immunol. **134:** 569.

72. SKEEN, M. J., M. A. MILLER, T. M. SHINNICK & H. K. ZIEGLER. 1996. Regulation of murine macrophage IL-12 production: activation of macrophages *in vivo*, restimulation *in vitro*, and modulation by other cytokines. J. Immunol. **156:** 1196–1206.

Endogenous Vertebrate Antibiotics

Defensins, Protegrins, and Other Cysteine-Rich Antimicrobial Peptides[a]

ROBERT I. LEHRER[b] AND TOMAS GANZ

Department of Medicine
UCLA-Center for the Health Sciences
Los Angeles, California 90095

Animals and plants came late to a world that was already populated by microorganisms. Consequently, the development of potent and broadly effective host defense mechanisms was essential to their survival. Leukocytes and many epithelial tissues of humans and other mammals produce endogenous, cysteine-rich, β-sheet peptide antibiotics. Remarkably high concentrations of such antimicrobial molecules are present in the cytoplasmic granules of most mammalian neutrophils, and analogous peptides are synthesized by cells of the respiratory, gastrointestinal, and urogenital tracts. As similar antimicrobial peptides have been found in amebae, dragonflies, and horseshoe crabs, innate host defense mediated by such peptides is evidently an ancestral feature of the animal immune system. This report centers on two classes of mammalian peptide antibiotics, defensins and protegrins. In addition, several structurally (or at least etymologically) related peptide families found in invertebrates or plants are considered.

The terms "defensins" was devised about a decade ago to describe a family of antimicrobial peptides found in rabbit and human neutrophils.[1,2] More recently three additional peptide families have been designated as defensins: β-defensins, which are present in humans, bovidae, and fowl; insect defensins and plant defensins. In deference to the pressures of linguistic logic and the laws of nominate symmetry, we have used the term "α-defensins" in this study to describe defensins homologous to those found in human and rabbit neutrophils. This designation allows the term "defensins" to be applied unambiguously to a constellation of host defense peptide families, all of which have considerable β-sheet structure, as well as six (α, β, and insect-defensins) or eight (plant defensins) invariant cysteine residues that form intramolecular cystine disulfide bonds. As will be discussed, each defensin family (α, β, insect, and plant) manifests a unique motif, which includes its invariant cysteines plus several other highly conserved residues.

α-DEFENSINS

Six human α-defensins are presently known. Four of them (defensins HNP-1, 2, 3, and 4) are produced by neutrophils, and two (HD5 and HD6) are produced by

[a]Our work in this area is supported by grants from the National Institutes of Health, currently AI 22839 and AI-39745 to RIL, and HL-35640 and AI 38567 to T.G. We thank the Will Rogers Research Institute for their continued support.

[b]Address for correspondence: Robert I. Lehrer, MD, Department of Medicine, CHS 37-062, 10833 LeConte Avenue, Los Angeles, CA 90095–1690 (tel: 310 825-5340; fax: 310 206-8766; e-mail: rlehrer@medicine.medsch.ucla.edu).

Paneth cells, which are specialized secretory cells found at the base of the small intestinal crypts. FIGURE 1 shows the primary amino acid sequences of 20 α-defensins. The six invariant cysteine residues plus the single conserved glycine, glutamic acid, and arginine residues are shown within boxes. Under physiologic conditions, α-defensins are polycationic (positively charged) molecules due principally to their high content of arginine residues. These cysteine residues, which are numbered from the amino terminus in FIGURE 1, are paired as follows: cys 1 → cys 6; cys 2 → cys 4; cys 3 → cys 5. Detailed information about α-defensins, including primary references for many of the following statements, can be found in two recent reviews.[3,4]

By X-ray crystallography,[5] human defensin HNP-3 is an elongated ellipsoidal molecule, 260 × 150 × 150 nm, that is composed largely of a triple-stranded, cystine-stabilized, antiparallel β-sheet. Its highly conserved Arg[6] and Glu[14] mol-

```
Human
  HNP1   A  C Y  C R  I P A  C I A G  E  R R Y  G  T  C I Y Q G R L W A F  C C
  HNP2      C Y  C R  I P A  C I A G  E  R R Y  G  T  C I Y Q G R L W A F  C C
  HNP3   D  C Y  C R  I P A  C I A G  E  R R Y  G  T  C I Y Q G R L W A F  C C
  HNP4   V  C S  C R  L V F  C R R T  E  L R V  G  N  C L I G G V S F T Y  C C  T R V
Rabbit
  NP1  V V  C A  C R  R A L  C L P R  E  R R A  G  F  C R I R G R I H P L  C C  R R
  NP2  V V  C A  C R  R A L  C L P L  E  R R A  G  F  C R I R G R I H P L  C C  R R
  NP3a G I  C A  C R  R R F  C P N S  E  R F S  G  Y  C R V N G A R Y V R  C C  S R R
  NP3b G R  C V  C R  K QLL  C S Y R  E  R R I  G  D  C K I R G V R F P F  C C  P R
  NP4  V S  C T  C R  R F S  C G F G  E  R A S  G  S  C T V N G V R H T L  C C  R R
  NP5  V F  C T  C R  G F L  C G S G  E  R A S  G  S  C T I N G V R H T L  C C  R R
Rat
  RtNP1 V T C Y  C R  R T R  C G F R  E  R L S  G  A  C G Y R G R I Y R L  C C  R
  RtNP2 V T C Y  C R  S T R  C G F R  E  R L S  G  A  C G Y R G R I Y R L  C C  R
  RtNP3     C S  C R  T S S  C R F G  E  R L S  G  A  C R L N G R I Y R L  C C
  RtNP4 A   C Y  C R  I G A  C V S G  E  R L T  G  A  C G L N G R I Y R L  C C  R

                    INTESTINAL α-DEFENSINS

Mouse
  MuCr1  L R D L V  C Y  C R  T R G  C K R R  E R M N  G T  C R K G H L M Y T L  C C  R
  MuCr2  L R D L V  C Y  C R  A R G  C K G R  E R M N  G T  C R K G H L L Y M L  C C  R
  MuCr1α L R D L V  C Y  C R  K R G  C K R R  E R M N  G T  C R K G H L M Y T L  C C  R
Rabbit
  NP6        G I    C A  C R  R R F  C L N F  E Q F S  G Y  C R V N G A R Y V R  C C  S R R
Human
  HD5    A R A T    C Y  C R  T G R  C A T R  E S L S  G V  C E I S G R L Y R L  C C  R
  HD6    T R A F T  C H  C R  R - S  C Y S T  E Y S Y  G T  C T V M G I N H R F  C C  L

cysteine #         1   2      3                  4              5 6
```

FIGURE 1. Primary sequences of 20 myeloid α-defensins. The invariant and highly conserved residues are *boxed,* and positively charged residues (R, K, and H) are *bolded.* Cystine disulfide pairing is shown at the *bottom.* MuCr signifies murine intestinal (Paneth cell) defensins.[54] Additional murine intestinal defensins were described by Ouellette *et al.,*[55] who use a different numbering schema.

ecules form a salt bridge spanning the only non–β-sheet portion of the molecule, and its invariant glycine[24] occupies position 3 of a Type I′ turn. The structures of several other α-defensins were examined by two-dimensional NMR and conform closely to the structure described for HNP-3.

Individual α-defensins differ considerably in their antimicrobial spectrum and relative potency. The latter generally, but imperfectly, parallels their net positive charge. Collectively, the spectrum of antimicrobial activity by α-defensins encompasses gram-positive and gram-negative bacteria, yeast phase and filamentous fungi, many enveloped viruses, and mycobacterial spp. Curiously, human defensins are substantially less potent than animal α-defensins against many human pathogens,

EPITHELIAL β-DEFENSINS

Species	Name				1										4	56	
Human	hβD-1		DHYN	C	VSSG	G	Q	C	LYSA	CP	IFTKIQ	G	T	C	YRGKAK	CC	K
Bovine	TAP		NPVS	C	VRNK	G	I	C	VPIR	CP	GSMKQI	G	T	C	VGRAVK	CC	RKK
	LAP	QGV	RNSQS	C	RRNK	G	I	C	VPIR	CP	GSMRQI	G	T	C	LGAQVK	CC	RRK

MYELOID β-DEFENSINS

Species	Name				1										4	56	
Bovine	BNBD1		DFAS	C	HTNG	G	I	C	LPNR	CP	GHMIQI	G	I	C	FRPRVK	CC	RSW
	BNBD2	V	RNHVT	C	RINR	G	F	C	VPIR	CP	GRTRQI	G	T	C	FGPRIK	CC	RSW
	BNBD5	pEVV	RNPQS	C	RWNM	G	V	C	IPIS	CP	GNMRQI	G	T	C	FGPRIK	CC	RSW
	BNBD10	pEGV	RSYLS	C	WGNR	G	I	C	LLNR	CP	GRNRQI	G	T	C	LAPRVK	CC	R
	BNBD11		GPLS	C	RRNG	G	V	C	IPIR	CP	GPNRQI	G	T	C	FGRPVK	CC	RSW
Avian	Gal 1α		GRKSD	C	FRKN	G	F	C	AFLK	CP	YLTLIS	G	K	C	SRFHL-	CC	KRIW
	Gal 1		GRKSD	C	FRKS	G	F	C	AFLK	CP	SLTLIS	G	K	C	SRFYL-	CC	KRIW
	THP-1		GRKEK	C	LRRN	G	F	C	AFLK	CP	TLSVIS	G	T	C	SRFQV-	CC	
	Gal 2		LF	C	--KG	G	S	C	HFGG	CP	SHLIKV	G	S	C	FGFRS-	CC	KWPWNA

1   2   3   4   56

FIGURE 2. Primary sequences of 12 β-defensins. Invariant residues are *boxed* and cysteine residues are numbered in order of their proximity to the amino terminus. The cysteine connectivity of BNBD-12 (not shown) was determined to be (cys 1 → cys 5; cys 2 → cys 4; cys 3 → cys 6).[14]

suggesting that relative resistance to autogenous defensins may be a species-specific virulence factor.

The amphiphilic nature of α-defensins and their ability to form voltage-gated pores in phospholipid bilayers allow them to perturb the membranes of susceptible microbial targets. The cytotoxic potential of defensins for the host is mitigated by the presence of defensin-binding proteins (including α_2-macroglobulin) in the serum, by the ability of host cells to repair early defensin-mediated cytotoxicity, and by the relatively low concentrations of free defensins found in the plasma.

Myeloid α-defensins are produced in remarkably large amounts (5–10 mg/kg body weight/day) by human bone marrow during neutrophil maturation. They are synthesized as ≈ 10-kD prepro-peptides which are stored in the neutrophil's "azurophil" cytoplasmic granules after stepwise proteolytic processing. Delivery of these granules to nascent phagocytic vacuoles bathes ingested microbes in a formidable brew that contains milligram/milliliter concentrations of defensins, liberally spiced with neutrophil-derived toxic oxidants and other antimicrobial proteins.

β-DEFENSINS

Members of this peptide family were initially discovered in tracheal epithelial cells[6,7] and bovine tongue.[11] The first human β-defensin (hβD-1) was described recently and is produced by vaginal and renal tissues.[12] The primary sequences of several representative β-defensins, including hβD-1, are shown in FIGURE 2. All β-defensins share nine invariant amino acids, including six cysteines, two glycines, and a proline.

Tracheal antimicrobial peptide (TAP), a β-defensin from bovine tracheal mucosa,[6] contains 38 amino acids. It is synthesized as a 64 amino acid prepro-peptide with a 20 amino acid signal sequence and a short (FTQGVG) pro-sequence. Mature TAP killed *Staphylococcus aureus, Escherichia coli, Klebsiella pneumoniae,* and *Candida albicans in vitro.* The antimicrobial activity of the 44 amino acid TAP proβ-defensin has not been reported. *In situ* hybridization studies detected TAP mRNA in periluminal columnar respiratory epithelial cells, but not in basal epithelial cells, bovine alveolar macrophages, or submucosal glands.[7] The TAP gene contains two exons, an intron and an upstream NF-κB sequence. Exon 1 encodes its signal sequence and Exon 2 encodes the short propiece and the mature peptide. Expression of TAP mRNA by bovine tracheal cells in tissue culture was increased by adding lipopolysaccharide (LPS).[13]

Lingual anitmicrobial peptide (LAP), a 42 residue peptide isolated from bovine tongue,[11] manifested antimicrobial activity against *S. aureus, E. coli, Pseudomonas aeruginosa,* and *Candida* spp *in vitro. In situ* hybridization studies revealed LAP mRNA in lingual epithelial cells and demonstrated markedly increased levels in areas of injury.[11] cDNA cloning indicated that LAP was synthesized as a 64 amino acid prepro-peptide, with a 20 residue signal sequence and a two residue (phe-thr) pro-region. LAP mRNA or closely related transcripts were also detected in other epithelial surfaces, including the bronchi, conjunctivae, colon, and urinary tract.

Selsted *et al.*[8] reported the primary sequences of 13 bovine neutrophil β-defensins (BNBDs). These ≈ 5k-Da peptides contained 38-42 residues and were highly cationic. Half of the BNBDs had blocked NH_2-termini that resulted from cyclization of an amino-terminal glutamine residue. Most of the peptides killed *E. coli* ML-35 and *S. aureus* 502A with MICs of approximately 10 μg/ml. The disulfide connectivity of BNBD-12 (cys 1 → cys 5, cys 2 → cys 4; cys 3 → cys 6) differs from that seen in α-defensins.[14]

Three β-defensins (gallinacins) were purified from leukocytes of *Gallus gallus,* the domestic chicken.[9] The peptides contained 36–39 amino acid residues, including numerous arginines and lysines, and were active *in vitro* against *E. coli, Listeria monocytogenes,* and *C. albicans.* Very similar β-defensins have also been purified from turkey polymorphonuclear neutrophils.[10] The existence of β-defensins in and mammals implies that this family of peptides originated before the avian and mammalian lineages diverged, > 150 million years ago.

"BIG DEFENSIN"

An interesting 79 amino acid antimicrobial molecule, recently purified from the cytoplasmic granules of horseshoe crab (*Tachypleus tridentatus*) hemocytes,[15] was named "big defensin" because its carboxy terminal 37 residues showed homology to α-defensins (FIG. 3), whereas its disulfide connectivity (cys 1 → cys 5; cys 2 → cys 4; cys 3 → cys 6) matched that of β-defensins. The 79 a.a. holopeptide was active against gram-positive and gram-negative bacteria and *C. albicans.* After cleavage by trypsin into a 37 residue amino-terminal domain and a 42 residue defensin-like peptide, the former portion was highly active against *S. aureus* but not *Salmonella typhimurium* LT2, whereas the defensin-like segment showed the opposite activity pattern. The defensin-like COOH-terminal domain is highly cationic, due to the presence of 8 arginine, 1 lysine, and 2 histidine residues. The large size of big defensin relative to conventional α or β-defensins resulted from the presence of a 35

```
LIPAIYIGATVGPSVWAYLVALVGAAAVTAANIRRASSDNHSCAGNRGWCRSKCFRHEYVDTYYSAVCGRYFCCRSR

C-terminal segment        RRASSDNHSCAGNRGWCRS-KC-FRHEYVDTYYS-AVCG-R---YF-CCRSR
NP-2 (rat α-defensin)          VTCY-----CRSTRCGFR-ERL----SGA-CGYRGRIYRLCCR
```

FIGURE 3. "Big defensin" from horseshoe crab. The complete primary structure of big defensin is shown on the *top line.* Below this, its defensin like COOH-terminal domain has been aligned with rat neutrophil α-defensin NP-2. *Dashes* represent gaps introduced for purposes of alignment.

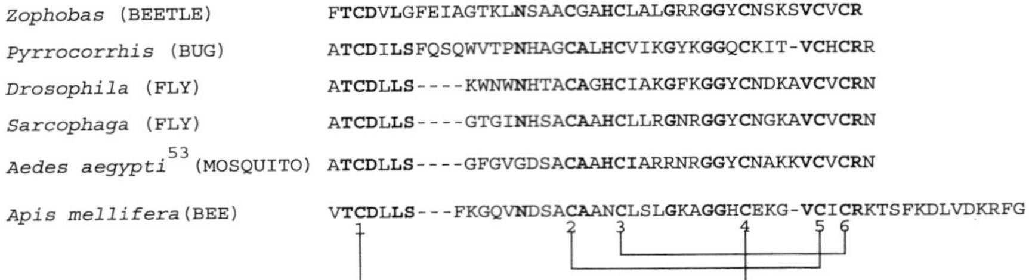

FIGURE 4. Primary sequences of six insect defensins. Invariant and highly conserved residues are *bolded*. *Dashes* represent gaps introduced for purposes of alignment. Cystine disulfide pairing is shown at the *bottom*.

a.a. hydrophobic domain located NH_2-terminal to the cationic, defensin-like COOH-terminus. Perhaps big defensin is an incompletely processed limulid defensin precursor, and the hydrophobic domain is its biologically active pro-piece.

INSECT DEFENSINS

Although insects lack many accoutrements of the vertebrate immune system, including immunoglobulins and complement, they can mount a potent systemic humoral response to microbial challenges by producing multiple, structurally diverse antimicrobial peptides (reviewed in ref. 16), including "insect defensins."

Insect defensins occur in dragonflies,[17] an ancient order of winged insects (*Odonata*) that first appeared during the Carboniferous era, and in *Phormia terranovae,* a fleshfly whose evolutionary forebears appeared 100 million years later. *Drosophila*'s defensin gene is intronless and occurs in a single copy per haploid genome.[18] Analysis of the defensin gene revealed the presence of 5' upstream sequences similar to motifs that regulate acute phase response genes of mammals. Like the α-defensins of mammals, insect defensins are also produced as ≈ 95 amino acid prepro-peptides.

The primary structures of several insect defensins are shown in FIGURE 4. Insect defensins differ from α- and β-defensins in their cysteine disulfide pairing, which is (cys 1 → cys 4, cys 2 → cys 5, cys 3 → cys 6).[19,20] Their molecular conformation includes a β-sheet structure that is linked to an α-helical domain by two disulfide bridges and to a large loop by the third disulfide bridge.[21,22] Bee defensin is 20% longer than typical insect defensins because of the presence of an amphipathic, 10 amino acid COOH-terminal extension.[23] Recombinant insect defensin disrupted the permeability barrier of *Micrococcus luteus,* causing massive loss of intracellular potassium, decreased cellular ATP, partial depolarization, and total respiratory inhibition. Patch clamp studies with giant liposomes suggested that these effects could result from formation of voltage-dependent membrane channels[24] analogous to those formed by α-defensins.[25]

Royalisin, a 5.5-kD insect defensin found in honeybee royal jelly,[19] showed potent antibacterial activity against gram-positive bacteria at ≈ 1 μM, but it was relatively ineffective against gram-negative bacteria. The *Aeschna* (dragonfly) peptide was highly active against gram-positive bacteria and killed at least one gram-negative organism. Insect defensins are induced promptly after the insects are infected or eat microbe-laden food, possibly by a signal transduction system homologous to the NF-κB-IκB regulatory system of mammalian lymphocytes.

PLANT DEFENSINS

Although most experts consider "couch potatoes" to be animals rather than plants, it is noteworthy (in a couch-potatoey way) that plants also respond to injury or infection by producing low molecular weight substances with antimicrobial properties. Among these are plant defensins (FIG. 5) extremely potent antimicrobial 5-kD molecules that contain 49–54 amino acids including *eight* conserved cysteine residues.[26–29] The other invariant residues include 2 glycines, a serine and a glutamic acid. Plant defensins are especially active against filamentous fungi and show homology to the γ-thionins of other wheat and barley, which are induced in response to fungal attack. The γ1 thionin of barley contains 47 amino acids, including its 8 conserved cysteines plus 8 arginines and 3 lysines. Two-dimensional nonmagnetic resonance imaging solution structures of barley and wheat γ-type thionin molecules revealed a small, well defined triple-stranded antiparallel β sheet that was formed by residues 1–6, 31–34, and 39–47 and an α-helical element (residues 16–28) aligned parallel to the β-sheet and connected to it by two cystine disulfide bonds.[30] The overall structure shows considerably resemblance to that of insect defensins.

Plant defensins are found in the outer cell layers of normal radish seeds, and their release during germination suppresses fungal growth around the growing rootlets. Whereas plant defensins are barely detectable in the leaves of uninfected radish plants, they accumulate systemically at high levels after localized fungal infection. Transgenic tobacco plants expressing these antifungal radish peptides show enhanced resistance to *Alternaria,* a fungal leaf pathogen.[28]

AMEBAPORE

The cytoplasmic granules of *Entamoeba histolytica* contain a pore-forming and potently cytotoxic peptide that resembles big defensin in size (77 amino acid residues), in overall cationcity (8 lysines and 1 histidine), and in possessing six conserved cysteines.[31] Amebapore kills gram-positive bacteria by permeabilizing their cytoplasmic membranes.[32] The amebapore molecule is composed entirely of cystine-stabilized α-helices and lacks any β-sheet elements.[33] Despite its 6-cysteine array, its α-helical structure indicates that amebapore is not a defensin. Rather, it

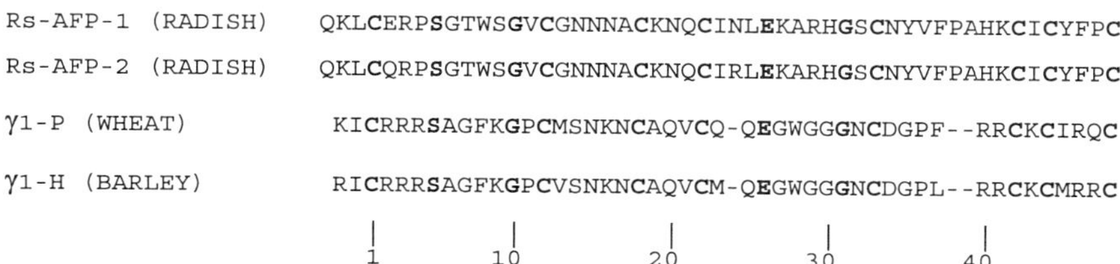

FIGURE 5. Primary sequences of four plant defensins. The eight invariant cysteines and several additional conserved residues have been *bolded.* Residues are numbered according to the radish defensins.

Protegrins

PG-1	RGG	R	LCYCR	RRF	C	V	CV	GR*
PG-2	RGG	R	LCYCR	RRF	C	I	CV	--*
PG-3	RGG	G	LCYCR	RRF	C	V	CV	GR*
PG-4	RGG	R	LCYCR	GWI	C	F	CV	GR*
PG-5	RGG	R	LCYCR	PRF	C	V	CV	GR*

Tachyplesins

TP-1	-K	WCFRVCY	R	G	I	CYR	R	CR*
TP-2	-R	WCFRVCY	R	G	I	CYR	K	CR*
PP-1	RR	WCFRVCY	R	G	F	CYR	K	CR*
PP-2	RR	WCFRVCY	K	G	F	CYR	K	CR*

FIGURE 6. Primary sequences of porcine protegrins and horseshoe crab tachyplesins/polyphemusins. The cysteines are *bolded* and invariant residues are within *shaded boxes. Asterisk* denotes COOH-terminal amidation.

may be related to the saposin peptide family, whose other members include saposins A-D, NK-lysin, domains of acid sphingomyelinase, and acyloxyacylhydrolase.[34]

PROTEGRINS

Protegrins (PGs) constitute a family of antimicrobial peptides (FIG. 6) whose index members, PG-1, 2 and 3, were purified from porcine leukocytes.[35] Protegrins PG 4 and PG-5 were delineated from cDNA and gene-cloning studies[36,37] and have been prepared synthetically. Like invertebrate tachyplesins (FIG. 6), protegrins contain 16–18 amino acid residues, possess 4 conserved cysteines that form intramolecular disulfide bonds, and have amidated COOH-terminal arginine residues. Although protegrins show noteworthy primary sequence homology to rabbit α-defensins NP-3A and NP-6, protegrins (but not defensins) are synthesized at the COOH-terminus of a cathelin-containing peptide precursor.[36] Human protegrins have not yet been described.

Protegrin genes contain 4 exons and 3 introns. Exon I encodes the signal sequence and the first 37 amino acids of the conserved cathelin domain cathelin, Exons II and III encode 36 and 24 additional cathelin residues, respectively, and Exon IV contains the final two cathelin residues followed by the mature protegrin peptide sequence, an amidation consensus sequence, a 3' untranslated region, and the polyadenylation site. The three introns range in size from 152–596 bp. An identical quadripartite gene structure was recently reported[38] for another cathelin-associated porcine antimicrobial peptide, PR-39.

Protegrins kill many gram-negative bacteria *in vitro* including *E. coli, P. aeruginosa, K. pneumoniae,* and *S. typhimurium,* at concentrations of 1–5 μg/ml. Unlike defensins, protegrins display excellent activity in physiologic salt solutions and are active in the presence of serum.[39] The ability of protegrins to bind the lipid A portion of lipopolysaccharide (LPS) may contribute to their potent activity against gram-negative bacteria and their ability to inhibit LPS-stimulated tumor necrosis factor-alpha (TNF-α) production by human leukocytes. Protegrins cause formation of voltage-gated pores in artificial lipid bilayers, especially when these contain LPS.[39]

Protegrin-treated *E. coli* develop a rapid and simultaneous performation of their outer and inner membranes and display scores of small, doughnut-shaped lesions on their outer membrane. These lesions resemble those generated by poly C9 or the membrane attack complex of complement.[39] Transmission EMS showed the presence of ≈ 100-nm diameter holes that traversed the outer and inner membranes and permitted gross leakage of cytoplasmic contents. The outer membrane of protegrin-treated *E. coli* also showed outer membrane ruffling and microvillus formation which resembled the effects induced by polymyxin, an LPS-binding peptide antibiotic produced by *Bacillus polymyxa.*

Circular dichoism spectra of protegrins indicated a predominantly antiparallel β-sheet secondary structure. ATR-FTIR spectra suggested that the β-sheet molecular axis of protegrins was oriented parallel to phospholipid or SDS film surfaces, presaging its hydrophobic insertion into lipid bilayers.[40] Ongoing studies with synthetic protegrin congeners revealed that the successive elimination of the intramolecular disulfide bonds led to parallel loss of β-sheet structure and broad-spectrum microbicidal activity in physiologic salt concentrations.[41,42] The interaction of protegrins with lipid bilayers may underlie their potent ability to inactivate HIV-1.[43]

TACHYPLESINS

Tachyplesins (polyphemusins) are ≈ 2-kD antimicrobial peptides found in horseshoe crab amebocytes (hemocytes).[44,45] The peptides are extremely stable to heat and acidity, retaining their antimicrobial activity after boiling for 30 minutes or exposure to 0.1% trifluoroacetic acid. Tachyplesin-1 has 17 amino acid residues, including 4 arginines and 2 lysines which make it strongly cationic. Its 4 cysteine residues form two intramolecular disulfide bonds and its carboxy-terminal arginine residue is amidated, increasing its net cationicity and conferring resistance to carboxypeptidases. Tachyplesins I and II (TP1 and TP2) and polyphemusins I and II (PP1 and PP2) from *Limulus polyphemus*[46] are shown in FIGURE 6. In this figure, CONH2 indicates a COOH-terminal amide. Whereas the homology of protegrins and defensins is evident from their primary sequences, the similarity of protegrins and tachyplesins is more apparent from their secondary structures which are also shown diagrammatically in FIGURE 7.

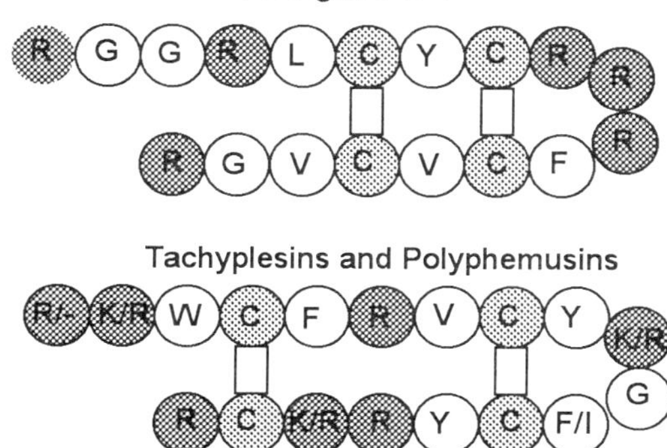

FIGURE 7. Secondary structures of protegrin PG-1 and tachyplesin/polyphemusins. Cationic residues (arg or lys) are *darkly shaded* and cysteins are more *lightly shaded.* The disulfide connectivity is shown. COOH-terminal arginines are amidated in both peptide families.

By two-dimensional NMR spectroscopy,[47] residues 3–8 and 11–16 of tachyplesin I formed an antiparallel β-sheet, connected by a β turn that involved residues 8–11. Rigidity was imparted by disulfide bridges connecting cysteines 1 and 4 and cysteines 2 and 3. Tachyplesin I interacted strongly with neutral and acidic phospholipids, but not with phosphatidylcholine. Its interaction with amphipathic lipid bilayers induced a conformational change.[48]

Polyphemusin II (PP2) was found to inhibit HIV-1 *in vitro*,[49,50] but it was strongly cytotoxic to Molt-4 cells. Analogs of tachyplesins, including (Tyr[4], Lys[6])-TP2 and Tyr,[5,12] Lys[7])-PP2, showed enhanced activity against HIV-1 in conjunction with reduced cytotoxicity.[49] The modified P-2 antiviral congener inhibited HIV-1 induced cytopathic effects and syncytium formation with half-maximal effective concentrations (EC_{50}) of 0.008 and 0.09 μg/ml, a 50% cytotoxic concentration of 54 μg/ml.

Tachyplesin precursors contain 77 amino acids, including a 23 residue prosequence, and contain a remarkable polyanionic nonapeptide (DEDEDDDEE) COOH-terminal to the tachyplesin sequence[51] that may render the peptide inert until its proteolytic processing is completed. Tachyplesins are present in extraordinarily large amounts in the small cytoplasmic granules of horseshoe crab hemocytes and are likely to play a substantial role in this invertebrate's overall antimicrobial defenses.[52]

SUMMARY

Although newly recognized, endogenous cystine-stabilized β-sheet antimicrobial peptides have ancient origins. These peptides can arm circulating phagocytes and cells of the gastrointestinal, respiratory, and genitourinary tracts to resist invasion by bacteria, mycobacteria, fungi, and enveloped viruses. Defensins and protegrin-like peptides are likely to play a considerable role in innate immunity and may provide molecular templates that can be used to generate novel antibiotics for topical and systemic use.

ACKNOWLEDGMENTS

We thank our laboratory associates for their dedicated and invaluable efforts and our colleagues for making this field of study a vital and lively one. We thank Eli Metchnikoff for showing the way.

REFERENCES

1. GANZ, T., M. E. SELSTED, D. SZKLAREK, S. L. HARWIG, K. DAHER, D. F. BAINTON & R. I. LEHRER. 1985. Defensins: Natural peptide antibiotics of human neutrophils. J. Clin. Invest. **76:** 1427–1435.
2. SELSTED, M. E., S. S. HARWIG, T. GANZ, J. W. SCHILLING & R. I. LEHRER. 1985. Primary structures of three human neutrophil defensins. J. Clin. Invest. **76:** 1436–1439.
3. LEHRER, R. I., A. K. LICHTENSTEIN & T. GANZ. 1993. Defensins: Antimicrobial and cytotoxic peptides of mammalian cells. Ann. Rev. Immunol. **11:** 105–128.
4. GANZ, T. & R. I. LEHRER. 1995. Defensins. Pharmac. Ther. **66:** 191–205.
5. HILL, C. P., J. YEE, M. E. SELSTED & D. EISENBERG. 1991. Crystal structure of defensin HNP-3, an amphiphilic dimer: Mechanisms of membrane permeabilization. Science **251:** 1481–1485.

6. DIAMOND, G., M. ZASLOFF, H. ECK, M. BRASSEUR, W. L. MALOY & C. L. BEVINS. 1991. Tracheal antimicrobial peptide: A cysteine-rich peptide from mammalian tracheal mucosa: Peptide isolation and cloning of a cDNA. Proc. Natl. Acad. Sci. USA **88:** 3952–3956.

7. DIAMOND, G., D. E. JONES & C. L. BEVINS. 1993. Airway epithelial cells are the site of expression of a mammalian antimicrobial peptide gene. Proc. Natl. Acad. Sci. USA **90:** 4596–4600.

8. SELSTED, M. E., Y.-Q. TANG, W. L. MORRIS, P. A. McGUIRE, M. J. NOVOTNY, W. SMITH, A. H. HENSCHEN & J. S. CULLOR. 1993. Purification, primary structures and antibacterial activities of β-defensins, a new family of antimicrobial peptides from bovine neutrophils. J. Biol. Chem. **268:** 6641–6648.

9. HARWIG, S. S. L., K. M. SWIDEREK, V. N. KOKRYAKOV, L. TAN, T. D. LEE, E. A. PANYUTICH, G. M. ALESHINA, O. V. SHAMOVA & R. I. LEHRER. 1994. Gallinacins: Cysteine-rich antimicrobial peptides of chicken leukocytes. FEBS Lett. **342:** 281–285.

10. EVANS, E. W., G. G. BEACH & J. WUNDERLICH. 1994. Isolation of antimicrobial peptides from avian heterophils. J. Leuk. Biol. **56:** 661–665.

11. SCHONWETTER, B. S., E. D. STOLTZENBERG & M. A. ZASLOFF. 1995. Epithelial antibiotics induced at sites of inflammation. Science **267:** 1645–1648.

12. BENSCH, K. W., M. RAIDA, H.-J. MAGERT, P. SCHULTZ-KNAPPE & W.-G. FORSSMANN. 1995. hBD-1: A novel β-defensin from human plasma. FEBS Lett. **368:** 331–335.

13. DIAMOND, G. & C. L. BEVINS. 1994. Endotoxin upregulates expression of an antimicrobial peptide gene in mammalian airway epithelial cells. Chest **105**(3 Suppl.): 51S–52S.

14. TANG, Y.-Q. & M. E. SELSTED. 1993. Characterization of the disulfide motif of BNBD-12, an antimicrobial β-defensin peptide from bovine neutrophil. J. Biol. Chem. **268:** 6649–6653.

15. SAITO, T., S. KAWABATA, T. SHIGENATA, Y. TAKAYENOKI, *et al.* 1995. A novel big defensin identified in horseshoe crab hemocytes—isolation, amino acid sequence and antibacterial activity. J. Biochem. **117:** 1131–1137.

16. BOMAN, H. G. 1995. Peptide antibiotics and their role in innate immunity. Ann. Rev. Immunol. **13:** 61–92.

17. BULET, P., S. COCIANCICH, M. REULAND, F. SAUBER, R. BISCHOFF, G. HEGY, A. VAN DORSSELAR, C. HETRU & J. A. HOFFMANN. 1992. A novel insect defensin mediates the inducible antibacterial activity in larvae of the dragonfly *Aeschna cyanea* (Paleoptera, Odonata). Eur. J. Biochem. **209:** 977–984.

18. DIMARCO, J.-L., D. HOFFMANN, M. MEISTER, P. BULET, R. LANOT, J.-M. REICHART & J. A. HOFFMANN. 1994. Characterization and transcriptional profiles of a *Drosophila* gene encoding an insect defensin. A study in insect immunity. Eur. J. Biochem. **221:** 201–209.

19. FUJIWARA, S., J. IMAI, M. FUJIWARA, T. YAESHIMA, T. KAWASHIMA & K. KOBAYASHI. 1990. A potent antibacterial protein in royal jelly. Purification and primary structure of royalisin. J. Biol. Chem. **265:** 11333–11337.

20. KUZUHARA, T., Y. NAKAJIMA, K. MATSUYAMA & S. NATORI. 1990. Determination of the disulfide array in sapecin, an antibacterial peptide of *Sarcophaga peregrina* (flesh fly). J. Biochem. **107:** 514–518.

21. BONTEMS, F., C. ROUMESTAND, B. GILQUIN, A. MENEZ & F. TOMA. 1991. Refined structure of charybdotoxin: Common motifs in scorpion toxins and insect defensins. Science **254:** 1521–1523.

22. BONMATIN, J.-M., J.-L. BONNAT, X. GALLET, F. VOVELLE, M. PTAK, J.-M. REICHART, J. A. HOFFMANN, E. KEPPI, M. LEGRAIN & T. ACHSTETTER. 1992. Two-dimensional ^{1}H NMR study of recombinant insect defensin A in water: Resonance assignments, secondary structure and global folding. J. Biomol. NMR **2:** 235–256.

23. CASTEELS-JOSSON, K., W. ZHANG, T. CAPACI, P. CASTEELS & P. TEMPST. 1994. Acute transcriptional response of the honeydee peptide-antibiotics gene repertoire and required posttranslational conversion of the precursors structures. J. Biol. Chem. **269:** 28569–28575.

24. COCIANCICH, S., A. GHAZI, C. HETRU, J. A. HOFFMAN & L. LETELLIER. 1993. Insect defensin, an inducible antibacterial peptide, forms of voltage-dependent channels in *Micrococcus luteus.* J. Biol. Chem. **268:** 19239–19245.

25. KAGAN, B. L., M. E. SELSTED, T. GANZ & R. I. LEHRER. 1990. Neutrophil antimicrobial peptides (defensins) form voltage-dependent ionic channels in planar lipid bilayer membranes. Proc. Natl. Acad. Sci. USA **87:** 210–214.

26. TERRAS, F. R. G., H. M. E. SCHOOFS, M. F. C. DEBOLLE, F. VAN LEUVEN, S. B. REES, J. VANDERLEYDEN, B. P. A. CAMMUE & W. F. BROEKAERT. 1992. Analysis of two novel classes of antifungal proteins from radish (Raphanus sativus) seeds. J. Biol. Chem. **267:** 15301–15309.

27. TERRAS, F. R. G., S. TORREKENS, F. VAN LEUVEN, R. W. OSBORN, J. VANDERLEYDEN, B. P. A. CAMMUE & W. F. BROEKAERT. 1993. A new family of basic cysteine-rich antifungal proteins from brassicaceae species. FEBS Lett. **316:** 233–240.

28. TERRAS, FF. R. G., K. EGGERMONT, V. KOVALEVA, N. V. RAIKHEL, R. W. OSBORNE, A. KESTER, S. B. REES, S. TORREKENS, F. VAN LEUVEN, J. VANDERLEYDEN, B. P. A. CAMMUE & W. F. BROEKAERT. 1995. Small cysteine-rich antifungal proteins from radish: Their role in host defense. Plant Cell **7:** 573–588.

29. OSBORNE, R. W., G. W. DE SAMBLANX, K. THEVISSEN, I. GODERIS, S. TORREKENS, F. VAN LEUVEN, S. ATTENBOROUGH, S. B. REES & W. F. BROEKAERT. 1995. Isolation and characterization of plant defensins from seeds of *Asteraceae, Fabaceae, Hippocastanaceae* and *Saxifragaceae.* FEBS Lett. **368:** 257–262.

30. BRUIX, M., M. A. JIMENEZ, J. SANTORO, C. GONZALEZ, F. J. COLILLA, E. MENDEZ & M. RICO. 1993. Solution structure of γ1-H and γ1-P thionins from barley and wheat endosperm determined by ^{1}H-NMR: A structural motif. Biochemistry **32:** 715–724.

31. LEIPPE, M., S. EBEL, O. L. SCHOENBERGER, R. D. HORSTMANN & H. J. MULLER-EBERHARD. 1991. Pore-forming peptide of pathogenic *Entamoeba histolytica.* Proc. Natl. Acad. Sci. USA **88:** 7659–7663.

32. LEIPPE, M., J. ANDRA & H. J. MULLER-EBERHARD. 1994. Cytolytic and antibacterial activity of synthetic peptides derived from amoebapore, the pore-forming peptide of *Entamoeba histolytica.* Proc. Natl. Acad. Sci. USA **91:** 2602–2606.

33. LEIPPE, M. & H. J. MULLER-EBERHARD. 1994. The pore-forming peptide of *Entamoeba histolytica,* the protozoan parasite causing human amoebiasis. Toxicology **87:** 5–18.

34. ANDERSSON, M., T. CURSTEDT, H. JORNVALL & J. JOHANSSON. 1995. An amphipathic helical motif common to tumourolytic polypeptide NK-lysin and pulmomary surfactant protein SP-B. FEBS Lett. **362:** 328–332.

35. KOKRYAKOV, V. N., S. S. L. HARWIG, E. A. PANYUTICH, A. A. SHEVCHENKO, G. M. ALESHINA, O. V. SHAMOVA, H. A. KORNEVA & R. I. LEHRER. 1993. Protegrins: Leukocyte antimicrobial peptides that combine features of corticostatic defensins and tachyplesins. FEBS **327:** 231–236.

36. ZHAO, C., L. LIU & R. I. LEHRER. 1994. Identification of a new member of the protegrin family by cDNA cloning. FEBS Lett. **346:** 285–288.

37. ZHAO, C., T. GANZ & R. I. LEHRER. 1995. The structure of porcine protegrin genes. FEBS Lett. **368:** 197–202.

38. GUDMUNDSSON, G. H., K. P. MAGNUSSON, B. P. CHOWDHARY, M. JOHANSSON, L. ANDERSSON & H. G. BOMAN. 1995. Structure of the gene from porcine peptide antibiotic PR-39, a cathelin gene family member: Comparative mapping of the locus for the human peptide antibiotic FALL-39. Proc. Natl. Acad. Sci. USA **92:** 7085–7089.

39. LEHRER, R. I., E. PANYUTICH, A. OREN, Y. SOKOLOV, Y. CHO, S. S. L. HARWIG & B. KAGAN. 1995. Protegrins: Mechanisms of bactericidal activity against Gram-negative bacteria. J. Invest. Med. **43**(Suppl. 2): 288A.

40. WARING, A., S. S. L. HARWIG & R. I. LEHRER. 1995. Conformation and orientation of protegrin-1 in membrane-mimetic environments. Protein Sci. **4**(Suppl 2): 117 (Abstr. 311T).

41. HARWIG, S. S. L., K. M. SWIDEREK, T. D. LEE & R. I. LEHRER. 1995. Determination of disulfide bridges in PG-2, an antimicrobial peptide from porcine leukocytes. J. Peptide Sci. **3:** 207–215.

42. HARWIG, S. S. L., A WARING, H. J. YANG, Y. CHO, L. TAN & R. I. LEHRER. 1995. Studies with synthetic protegrin congeners: Importance of disulfide structures. Protein Sci. **4**(Suppl. 2): 118 (Abstr. 312-T).

43. TAMAMURA, H., T. MURAKAMI, S. HORIUCHI, K. SIGIHARA, A. OTAKA, W. TAKADA, T.

IBUKA, M. WAKI, N. YAMAMOTO & N. FUJI. 1995. Synthesis of protegrins-related peptides and their antibacterial and anti-human immunodeficiency virus activity. Chem. Pharm. Bull. **43:** 853–858.

44. NAKAMURA, T., H. FURUNAKA, T. MIYATA, F. TOKUNAGA, T. MUTA, S. IWANAGA, M. NIWA, T. TAKAO & Y. SHIMONISHI. 1988. Tachyplesin, a class of antimicrobial peptide from the hemocytes of the horseshoe crab (*Tachypleus tridentatus*). Isolation and chemical structure. J. Biol. Chem. **263:** 16709–16713.

45. MUTA, T., T. FUJIMOTO, H. NAKAJIMA & S. IWANAGA. 1990. Tachyplesins isolated from hemocytes of Southeast Asian horseshoe crabs (*Carcinoscorpius rotundicauda* and *Tachypleus gigas*): Identification of a new tachyplesin, tachyplesin III, and a processing intermediate of its precursor. J. Biochem. **108:** 261–266.

46. MIYATA, T., F. TOKUNAGA, T. YONEYA, K. YOSHIKAWA, S. IWANAGA, M. NIWA, T. TAKAO & Y. SHIMONISHI. 1989. Antimicrobial peptides, isolated from horseshoe crab hemocytes, tachyplesin II, and polyphemusins I and II: Chemical structures and biological activity. J. Biochem. **106:** 663–668.

47. KAWANO, K., T. YONEYA, T. MIYATA, K. YOSHIKAWA, F. TOKUNAGA, Y. TERADA & S. IWANAGA. 1990. Antimicrobial peptide, tachyplesin I, isolated from hemocytes of the horseshoe crab (*Tachypleus tridentatus*). NMR determination of the beta-sheet structure. J. Biol. Chem. **265:** 15365–15367.

48. PARK, N. G., S. LEE, O. OISHI, H. AOYAGI, S. IWANAGA, S. YAMASHITA & M. OHNO. 1992. Conformation of tachyplesin I from *Tachypleus tridentatus* when interacting with lipid matrices. Biochemistry **31:** 12241–12247.

49. MASUDA, M., H. NAKASHIMA, T. UEDA, H. NABA, R. IKOMA, A. OTAKA, Y. TERAKAWA, H. TAMAMURA, T. IBUKA, T. MURAKAMI *et al.* 1992. A novel anti-HIV synthetic peptide, T-22 (Tyr^{5,12}, Lys^{7}-polyphemusin II). Biochem. Biophys. Res. Comm. **189:** 845–850.

50. TAMAMURA, H., M. KURODA, M. MASUDA, A. OTAKA, S. FUNAKOSHI, H. NAKASHIMA, N. YAMAMOTO, M. WAKI, A. MATSUMOTO & J. M. LANCELIN. 1993. A comparative study of the solution structures of tachyplesin I and a novel anti-HIV synthetic peptide, T22 (Tyr5, 12, Lys7-polyphemusin II), determined by nuclear magnetic resonance. Biochim. Biophys. Acta. **1163:** 209–216.

51. SHIGENAGA, T., T. MUTA, Y. TOH, F. TOKUNAGA & S. IWANAGA. 1990. Antimicrobial tachyplesin peptide precursor. cDNA cloning and cellular localization in the horseshoe crab (*Tachypleus tridentatus*). J. Biol. Chem. **265:** 21350–21354.

52. IWANAGA, S., T. MUTA, T. SHIGENAGA, Y. MIURA, N. SEKI, T. SAITO & S. KAWABATA. 1994. Role of hemocyte-derived granular components in invertebrate defense. Ann. NY Acad. Sci. **712:** 102–116.

53. CHALK, R., C. M. R. ALBUQUERQUE, P. J. HAM & H. TOWNSON. 1995. Full sequence and characterization of two insect defensins from the mosquito *Aedes aegypti*. Proc. R. Soc. Lond. B. **261:** 217–221.

54. HARWIG, S. S. L., P. B. EISENHAUER, N. P. CHEN & R. I. LEHRER. 1995. Cryptdins: Endogenous antibiotic peptides of small intestinal Paneth cells. *In* Advances in Mucosal Immunology. J. Mestecky *et al.*, Eds.: 251–255. Plenum Press. New York.

55. OUELLETTE, A. J., M. M. HSIEH, M. T. NOSEK, D. F. CANP-GAUCI, K. M. HUTTNER, R. N. BUICK & M. E. SELSTED. 1994. Mouse Panethy cell defensins: Primary structures and antibacterial activities of numerous cryptdin isoforms. Infect. Immun. **62:** 5040–5047.

Identification of Export Proteins from *Mycobacterium tuberculosis* That Interact with SecA

M. U. OWENS,[a] M. G. SCHMIDT,[b] C. H. KING,[a]
AND F. D. QUINN[a]

[a]*Division of AIDS, STD, and TB Laboratory Research
National Center for Infectious Diseases
Centers for Disease Control and Prevention
Atlanta, Georgia 30333*

[b]*Department of Microbiology and Immunology
Medical University of South Carolina
Charleston, South Carolina 29425*

Several recent studies indicate that soluble and membrane-bound proteins may play important roles in the virulence of intracellular pathogens including *Mycobacterium tuberculosis* (MTB).[1,2] Our goal is to understand the protein secretion process of MTB and to identify factors that are secreted by the bacterium, thereby providing important information on the molecular pathogenesis of MTB as well as the immune response generated during infection.

With the use of degenerate primers based on a conserved *Escherichia coli* SecA sequence and biased towards the G + C content of *Mycobacterium,* a 750-base pair (bp) *secA* fragment was amplified from *M. tuberculosis* H37Rv chromosomal DNA. The sequence of this fragment was used to develop specific primers which were used in a single specific primer polymerase chain reaction (SSP-PCR).[3]

Using SSP-PCR, we identified two overlapping fragments of the *secA* gene from MTB and found them to be homologous to the *secA* genes of other prokaryotic and eukaryotic species. The nucleotide sequence obtained displays 59% identity with the *secA* gene from *Caulobacter crescentus* in a 1107-bp overlap and 60.2% identity with the *E. coli secA* gene in a 636-bp overlap. Homology is more extensive in the amino acid sequence comparisons, particularly in regions involved in adenosine triphosphate (ATP) binding where the protein sequences are almost completely conserved (FIG. 1).

SecA plays an indispensible role in the protein export process in *E. coli* and *Bacillus subtilis,* and a similar role is suspected in MTB.[4,5] Isolation of this gene may provide opportunities to identify proteins that are secreted from the myobacteria.

Currently, we are creating a gene fusion of the MTB *secA* gene fragment and GAL4 DNA binding domain in a plasmid vector (pGBT9) that can be used in a yeast two-hybrid system (Clontech Matchmaker Two-Hybrid System).[6] Using this method, we will identify export proteins that specifically interact with the SecA protein. Genes for these proteins can then be further evaluated as to their importance in the virulence and pathogenesis of MTB.

MRT	G	EG	K	T	L
MRT	G	EG	K	T	L
MKT	G	EG	K	T	L
MKT	G	EG	K	T	L
MRT	G	EG	K	T	L

E. coli
M. tuberculosis
B. subtilis
P. lutherii
C. crescentus

A.

EAF	AVVREAS	KR	V
EAF	TVARPA–	CR	V
EAF	AVVREAS	RR	V
EAF	GLVWEAS	LR	V
EAF	AVVREAS	KR	V

E. coli
M. tuberculosis
B. subtilis
P. lutherii
C. crescentus

B.

FLGLTVG	INLPGMPA
FLGLQVG	VILATMTP
FLGLTVG	LNLNSMSK
FLGLSVG	LILADMNR
FLGLSYG	VIVNGLSQ

E. coli
M. tuberculosis
B. subtilis
P. lutherii
C. crescentus

C.

FIGURE 1. Amino acid comparisons and conservation of three putative ATP binding sites in SecA. (A) ATP catalytic site spanning residues 102–110 of *E. coli* SecA. The lysine residue is required for protein function in *B. subtilis*. (B) ATP binding site and adjacent conserved residues; region spans amino acids 66–78 in *E. coli*. (C) ATP binding site covering residues 149–163 in *E. coli*.

REFERENCES

1. BIELECKI, J., P. YOUNGMAN, P. CONNELLY & D. A. PORTNOY. 1990. *Bacillus subtilis* expressing a haemolysin gene from *Listeria monocytogenes* can grow in mammalian cells. Nature **345:** 175–176.
2. SANSONETTI, P. J. 1991. Genetic and molecular basis of epithelial cell invasion by Shigella species. Rev. Infect. Dis. **13:** 92.
3. SHYAMALA, V. & G. F. AMES. 1989. Genome walking by single-specific-primer polymerase chain reaction: SSP-PCR. Gene **84:** 1–8.
4. OLIVER, D. B. 1993. SecA protein: Autoregulated ATPase catalysing preprotein insertion and translocation across the *Escherichia coli* inner membrane. Mol. Microbiol. **7:** 159–165.
5. PUGSLEY, A. P. 1993. The complete general secretory pathway in gram-negative bacteria. Microbiol. Rev. **57:** 50–108.
6. FIELDS, S. & O. SONG. 1989. A novel genetic system to detect protein-protein interactions. Nature **340:** 245–246.

Fab′ Fragments of a mAb to a Member of Family 2 of Trans-sialidases of *Trypanosoma cruzi* Block Trypanosome Invasion of Host Cells and Neutralize Infection by Passive Immunization[a]

FERNANDO VILLALTA,[b,c] CASSANDRA M. SMITH,[d]
JAMES M. BURNS, JR.,[d] GAUTAM CHAUDHURI,[b]
AND MARIA F. LIMA[d]

[b]Division of Biomedical Sciences and
[d]Department of Microbiology
Meharry Medical College
Nashville, Tennessee 37208

Trypanosoma cruzi, the protozoan that causes Chagas' disease and affects millions of people in South and Central America, must attach to mammalian cells before it can invade them. Trypanosome determinants that bind to host cell receptors[1] during invasion may be of interest for developing vaccines and receptor-blocking therapies. It was recently shown that *T. cruzi* trans-sialidase activity is seen in a few members of a large multigene family that encodes an array of trans-sialidase–related surface proteins ranging from 80–220 kD classified in four families (reviewed in refs. 2, 3, and 4). Several possible functions have been attributed to the surface trans-sialidase families of *T. cruzi*, including cellular adhesion and invasion, parasite survival, immune evasion, autoimmunity, and virulence or pathogenicity. However, the precise biologic function of these molecules in *T. cruzi*–host cell interactions is unknown. In the present study we examine the ability of a monoclonal antibody (mAb) or its Fab′ fragments to a member of family 2 of trans-sialidases to inhibit trypanosome binding and invasion of host cells and to neutralize *T. cruzi* infection in BALB/c mice by passive immunization.

MATERIAL AND METHODS

The highly invasive trypomastigote clone MMC 20A of the Tulahuen strain of *T. cruzi*[5] was used in this work. Monoclonal antibodies were produced as previously described[6] and purified using a Mannan binding column (Pierce) followed by

[a]This work was supported in part by grants AI-25637, HL03149, G12RR03032, and 2SO6GM08037 from the National Institutes of Health, HRD 9255157 from the National Science Foundation, and PCE-5053-G-00-3051-00 from the United States Agency for International Development. C.M.S. is a recipient of a Patricia Roberts Harris fellowship from the Department of Education.
[c]To whom all correspondence should be addressed.

Superose gel filtration using FPLC. Monovalent Fab fragments (Fab′) were purified using a Pierce purification kit followed by Superose gel filtration using FPLC. Trypomastigote binding and entry into rat heart myoblasts, Vero cells, and unelicited mouse peritoneal macrophages were performed as previously described.[5,7] Passive

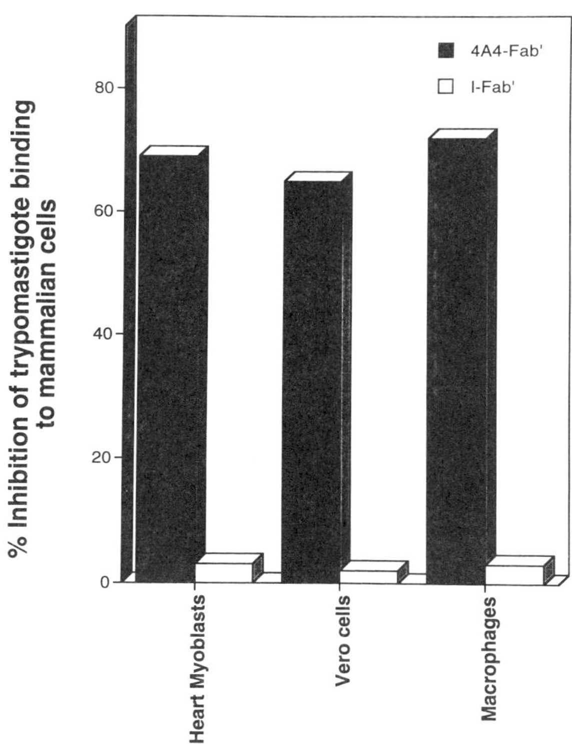

FIGURE 1. Monovalent Fab fragments of mAb 4A4 inhibit the binding of *T. cruzi* trypomastigotes to heart myoblasts, fibroblasts, and unelicited CBA mouse peritoneal macrophages. 1×10^7 trypomastigotes resuspended in DMEM-BSA were incubated with 4A4-Fab′ or I-Fab′ at a concentration of 1 μg/ml or DMEM-BSA for 1 hour at 4°C and added to cell micromonolayers in triplicate and incubated as described.[5,7] Inhibition of trypomastigote binding to mammalian cells was determined by the following formula: % inhibition = $(1 - X/Y)\ 100$, where X is the number of bound parasites per 200 cells in the presence of 4A4-Fab′ or I-Fab′ and Y is the number of parasites bound per 200 cells in the presence of DMEM-BSA. This is a representative experiment of three that were independently performed.

immunization of 4-week-old BALB/c mice with monoclonal antibodies was performed as indicated in the legend to FIGURE 2.

RESULTS AND DISCUSSION

In early previous studies, our group identified the surface gp83 of *T. cruzi* trypomastigotes as a mammalian host cell binding molecule involved in trypanosome attachment and entry into mammalian cells.[5] The addition of either purified gp83 or a monoclonal antibody (4A4) against gp83 to heart myoblast monolayers strongly competed with trypanosome binding and entry into heart myoblasts.[6,8] This trypanosome glycoprotein is expressed more on the surface of highly than weakly infective trypomastigote clones.[5] Because expression of this molecule correlates with infectivity of trypomastigote clones, we hypothesized that it modulates trypanosome invasiveness. We cloned and sequenced the gene coding for this cell adhesion molecule and

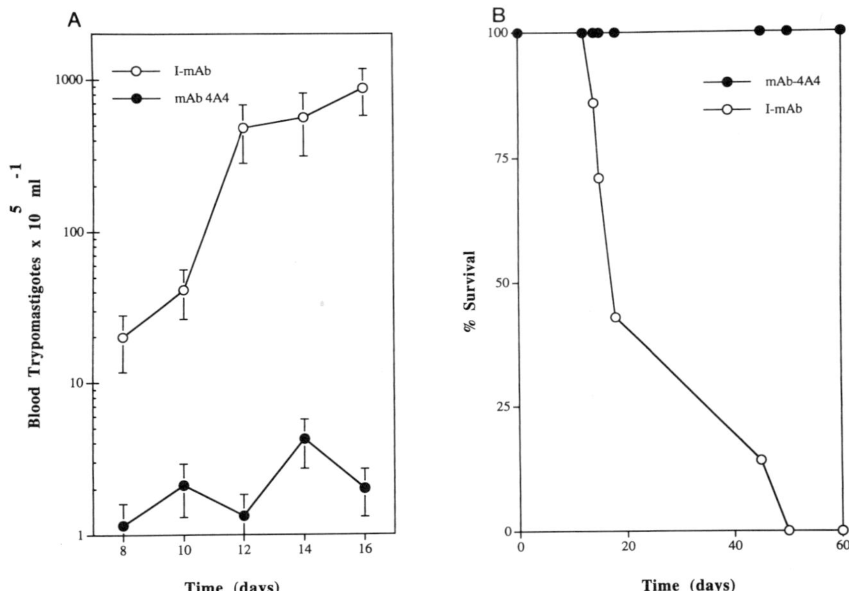

FIGURE 2. Passive immunization of BALB/c mice with mAb 4A4 confers strong protection against lethal challenge with *T. cruzi*. Parasitemia (**A**) and mortality (**B**) of BALB/c mice after passive transfer of mAb 4A4 or I-mAb. Either mAb 4A4 or I-mAb at a concentration of 20 μg in phosphate-buffered saline solution were administered into 4-week-old BALB/c mice ($n = 10$) 2 hours before iv challenge with 2×10^3 blood trypomastigotes followed by three consecutive ip injections of either mAb 4A4 or I-mAb at the same concentration for the next 3 consecutive days. Parasitemia (**A**) was monitored from 5 μl of tail blood. Each point represents the mean of parasitemia at the indicated day of infection with 1 SD. Differences in parasitemia between mice treated with mAb 4A4 and I-mAb at all points were statistically significant ($p \leq 0.01$) as determined by Student's *t* test. This is a representative experiment of three that were independently performed.

found that it belongs to family 2 of trans-sialidases. Furthermore, we found that the native gp83 or recombinant protein expressed in *Escherichia coli* presents both sialidase and trans-sialidase activities. We reasoned that if *T. cruzi* trypomastigotes bind mammalian cells through gp83 trans-sialidase to penetrate these cells, then monovalent Fab fragments of mAb 4A4 (4A4-Fab′) that block the binding of this molecule to heart myoblasts should inhibit the attachment of trypomastigotes to heart myoblasts and prevent trypanosome internalization into these cells. Results from these experiments show that 4A4-Fab' effectively blocked the attachment of trypomastigotes to heart myoblasts, Vero cells and unelicited CBA mouse peritoneal macrophages (FIG. 1), and prevented trypanosome internalization into these cells. An irrelevant mAb of the same class (I-Fab') failed to inhibit *T. cruzi* trypomastigote binding (FIG. 1) and internalization into these cells. These results strongly suggest that *T. cruzi* trypomastigotes attach to phagocytic and nonphagocytic cells through the gp83 trans-sialidase to invade these cells and that the mAb 4A4 recognizes an epitope on the gp83 trans-sialidase that is required for *T. cruzi* binding to promote entry into mammalian cells.

We tested whether the administration of mAb 4A4 into BALB/c mice could neutralize the infectivity of *T. cruzi* trypomastigotes. Results presented in FIGURE 2 show that iv administration of mAb 4A4 into BALB/c mice 2 hours before iv lethal challenge with *T. cruzi* blood trypomastigotes followed by three ip doses of mAb 4A4 resulted in a dramatic reduction in the levels of parasitemia (FIG. 2A). After 50 days, the mortality of mice receiving the irrelevant mAb of the same class (I-mAb) was 100%, whereas mortality was 0% in the group of mice receiving mAb 4A4 (FIG. 2B). Similar results were observed in our laboratory when 4A4-Fab' was used. Given the remarkable neutralization effect on *T. cruzi* infection by passive immunization of BALB/c mice with mAb 4A4, we conclude that the epitope recognized on the gp83 trans-sialidase of *T. cruzi* trypomastigotes by mAb 4A4 is a candidate for vaccine development. To identify the epitope required for parasite binding on gp83 trans-sialidase recognized by mAb 4A4, a series of carboxyl terminally truncated recombinant peptides was produced. Synthesis of the synthetic epitope recognized by mAb 4A4 for vaccine development is in progress in our laboratory. These results indicate that the epitope on gp83 trans-sialidase recognized by mAb 4A4 and required for trypanosome binding to mammalian cells to promote trypanosome entry is an attractive candidate for immunologic intervention in *T. cruzi* infection.

REFERENCES

1. VILLALTA, F., A. RUIZ-RUANO, A. A. VALENTINE & M. F. LIMA. 1993. Mol. Biochem. Parasitol. **61**: 217–230.
2. CROSS, G. A. M. & G. B. TAKLE. 1993. Annu. Rev. Microbiol. **47**: 385–411.
3. COLLI, W. 1993. FASEB J. **7**: 1257–1264.
4. SCHENKMAN, S., D. EICHINGER, M. E. A. PEREIRA & V. NUSSENZWEIG. 1994. Annu. Rev. Microbiol. **48**: 499–523.
5. LIMA, M. F. & F. VILLALTA. 1989. Mol. Biochem. Parasitol. **33**: 159–170.
6. VILLALTA, F., M. F. LIMA, A. RUIZ-RUANO & L. ZHOU. 1992. Biochem. Biophys. Res. Commun. **182**: 6–13.
7. VILLALTA, F. & F. KIERSZENBAUM. 1984. J. Immunol. **133**: 3338–3343.
8. VILLALTA, F., M. F. LIMA & L. ZHOU. 1990. Biochem. Biophys. Res. Commun. **172**:925–931.

Nitric Oxide Production by Human Alveolar Macrophages in Pulmonary Disease

PHILLIP STEINER,[a] LINDA EFFEREN,[b]
HELEN G. DURKIN,[c] GEORGE K. JOSEPH,[c]
AND MAJA NOWAKOWSKI[c,d]

Departments of Pediatrics,[a] Medicine,[b] and Pathology[c]
SUNY Health Science Center at Brooklyn
450 Clarkson Ave., Box 25
Brooklyn, New York 11203–2098

Nitric oxide (NO), a product of nitric oxide synthase (iNOS), is a physiologic messenger with a multitude of activities in the immune, nervous, and cardiovascular systems.[1–3] Although the role of NO in inflammation and bactericidal and tumoricidal macrophage activity is well established, demonstration of iNOS-like activity in human macrophages has proven remarkably difficult.

The present studies focused on detecting and characterizing NO production by human alveolar macrophages (hAM) from children with primary tuberculosis ($n = 5$, age range 8 months to 4.5 years) and adults with sarcoidosis ($n = 4$), adenocarcinoma ($n = 2$), and other pulmonary diseases ($n = 6$). Bronchoalveolar lavage fluid (BALF) was obtained during bronchoscopy with lavage for diagnostic purposes. Cells were isolated from BALF, as previously described,[4] and divided into aliquots for differential staining (DiffQuik) of Cytospin preparations, analysis of surface markers by flow cytometry (FACSCAN), and culture with or without recombinant human interferon gamma (IFN-γ). The amount of NO released into culture supernatants was assessed at 2–5 days by measuring the stable and product of NO, NO_2^-, using the Griess reaction as described.[5]

TABLE 1 summarizes the clinical and laboratory characteristics of the patients and their BALF cells. Pediatric patients acquired primary pulmonary tuberculosis (TB) from adults with active TB, usually family members, and responded favorably to antituberculosis treatment. All had total BALF cell and differential counts within the normal range. Two of the children with primary TB had highly elevated BALF CD4/CD8 ratios, whereas three had inverted CD4/CD8 ratios. By contrast, peripheral blood surface marker profiles were close to normal (data not shown). This finding is in agreement with our earlier studies of BALF lymphocyte surface marker expression in pediatric primary TB.[6] Two adult patients with clinical sarcoidosis

---

[d]To whom correspondence should be addressed.

had elevated BALF lymphocytes, and three had elevated CD4/CD8 ratios, as expected.

Alveolar macrophages from two of five children with TB produced NO spontaneously (2.4 and 1.6 nmol/ml, respectively), and the amounts were increased two to threefold on stimulation with IFN-γ; hAM from two others showed no spontaneous NO production, but it was induced by IFN-γ; hAM from one child were negative with or without stimulation (FIG. 1A).

Alveolar macrophages from adult patients with a variety of pulmonary diseases produced much more NO (1.6–39.6 nmol/ml), but did not respond to IFN-γ stimulation, and the level of NO production was characteristic of each individual (FIG. 1B).

TABLE 1. Clinical and Laboratory Parameters of Study Subjects

Age Group	Sex	Clinical Diagnosis	BALF Cell Recovery ×10⁶/ml	Differential AM	L	PMN	Lumphocyte Surface Markers CD3	CD4	CD8	CD19
				% Total			% Total			
Pediatric	M	Primary TB	0.15	98	1	1	74.2	11.3	32.3	14.7
	M	Primary TB	0.25	80	17	3	80.7	63.8	17.2	5.4
	M	Primary TB	0.48	99	1	0	35.5	10.9	17.9	11.7
	F	Primary TB	0.60	88	12	0	96.7	74.7	19.6	3.0
	F	Primary TB	0.13	89	8	3	74.1	25.0	49.9	22.9
Adult	F	Sarcoidosis	0.22	76	22	2				
	F	Sarcoidosis	0.33	93	4	3	68.0	41.4	26.2	0.2
	F	Sarcoidosis	0.20	48	50	2	83.0	58.6	24.1	0.3
	F	Sarcoidosis	0.36	95	4	1	87.2	64.3	22.9	1.0
	F	Adenocarcinoma	0.17	98	2	0				
	M	Adenocarcinoma	0.17							
	F	Int. pneumonia	0.45	69	29	2	88.5	23.2	68.2	1.1
	F	PCP	0.90	54	10	36	56.1	0.8	38.5	1.3
	M	PCP	0.10	78	16	6				
	M	? (HIV+)	0.52							
	F	? (HIV+)	0.60	56	36	8				
	M	?	0.70	76	19	5	97.6	45.1	55.8	0.3

Abbreviations: AM = alveolar macrophages; BALF = bronchoalveolar lavage fluid; L = lumphocytes; PMN = polymorphonuclear lymphocytes.

Taken together, these studies demonstrate that hAM from patients with pulmonary diseases are capable of producing significant amounts of NO and in certain situations (children with primary TB) respond to IFN-γ stimulation. The regulation and the nature of signals triggering NO production by hAM remain to be elucidated. It is of interest that a recent study reported induction of NO generation by human PBMC in the presence interleukin-4, implying that NO may be involved in regulation of IgE production.[6] Understanding the regulatory pathways controlling NO production by terminally differentiated human macrophages such as hAM and other tissue mononuclear phagocytes is of central importance in delineating the role of NO in the immune response and inflammation.

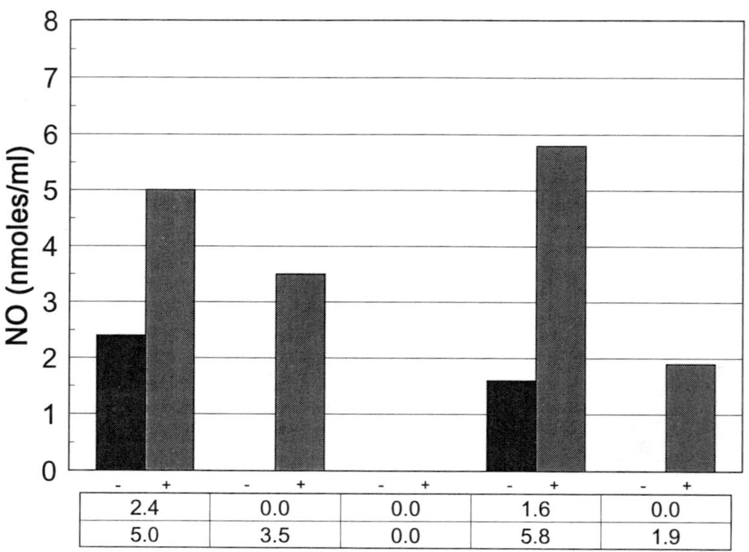

-	+	-	+	-	+	-	+	-	+
2.4		0.0		0.0		1.6		0.0	
5.0		3.5		0.0		5.8		1.9	

Children with Primary TB

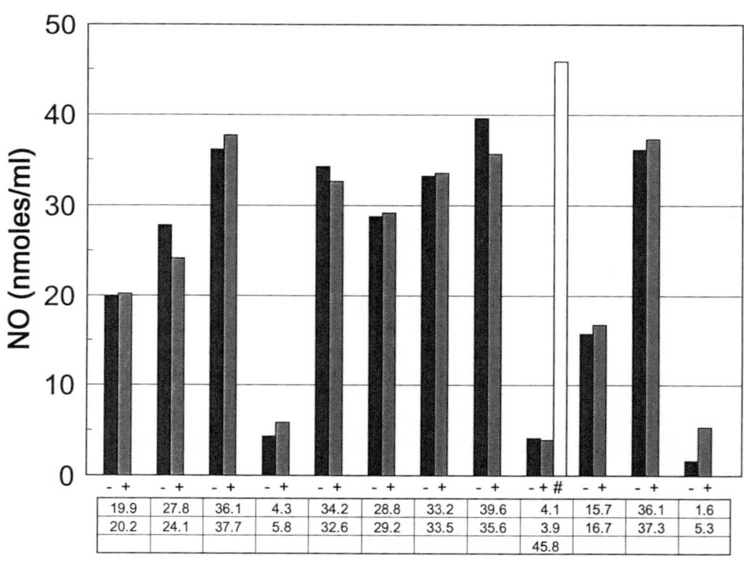

-	+	-	+	-	+	-	+	-	+	-	+	-	+	-	+	-	+	#	-	+	-	+	-	+
19.9		27.8		36.1		4.3		34.2		28.8		33.2		39.6		4.1			15.7		36.1		1.6	
20.2		24.1		37.7		5.8		32.6		29.2		33.5		35.6		3.9			16.7		37.3		5.3	
																45.8								

Adults with pulmonary disease

FIGURE 1. NO production by hAM from children with primary tuberculosis (TB) (**top**) and adults with pulmonary diseases (**bottom**). Amounts of nitric oxide (NO_2^-) in culture supernatants were determined at 2–5 days. Symbols: − = control; + = recombinant human IFN-γ, 500 U/ml; # = IFN-γ, 500 U/ml; lipopolysaccharide, 1 μg/ml. The order of patients (*left to right*) corresponds to the order in TABLE 1.

REFERENCES

1. VALLANCE, P. & S. MONCADA. 1994. Nitric oxide—from mediator to medicines. J. Roy. Coll. Physicians Lond. **28**: 209–219.
2. NATHAN, C. & Q. XIE. 1994. Nitric oxide synthases: Roles, tolls, and controls. Cell **78**: 915–918.
3. SCHMIDT, H. H. H. & U. WALTER. 1994. NO at work. Cell **78**: 919–925.
4. NOWAKOWSKI, M., L. CLARKE, R. AMARO, M. G. PELLEGRINO, M. F. SIERRA & P. STEINER. 1992. Characterization of cells, immunoglobulins, and immune complexes present in the bronchoalveolar lavage of pediatric AIDS patients. Regional Immunol. **4**: 34–40.
5. GREEN, L. C., D. A. WAGNER, J. GLOGOWSKI, P. L. SKIPPER, S. WISHNOK & S. R. TANNENBAUM. 1982. Analysis of nitrate and nitrate and (^{15}N) nitrate in biological fluids. Ann. Biochem. **126**: 131–139.
6. NOWAKOWSKI, M., S.-P. CHAN, P. STEINER, S. CHICE & H. G. DURKIN. 1992. Different distributions of lung and blood lymphocyte subsets in pediatric AIDS or tuberculosis. Ann. Clin. Lab. Sci. **22**: 377–384.

Potent Bactericidal Activity Towards Gram-Positive Bacteria of Mammalian Group II Phospholipase A2 Mobilized in Inflammatory Fluids

LISA M. MADSEN, YVETTE WEINRAUCH,
AND JERROLD WEISS[a]

Department of Microbiology
New York University School of Medicine
New York, New York 10016

The role of the complement system in humoral defense against gram-negative bacteria has long been recognized. Extracellular antimicrobial activity against gram-positive bacteria has also been identified in serum and inflammatory fluids, but the molecular determinants of this activity are undefined.[1,2] We recently demonstrated that the extracellular fluid of (acute) rabbit peritoneal inflammatory exudates contains potent antimicrobial activity that is not present in plasma either before or during the induction of this localized inflammatory response.[3] The antimicrobial spectrum of the inflammatory (ascitic) fluid includes a wide range of gram-negative and gram-positive bacteria[3] and at least certain fungi (e.g., *Candida albicans*) (Weinrauch and Foreman, unpublished observations). Activity toward encapsulated, complement-resistant *Escherichia coli* is due to the synergistic action of the bactericidal/permeability-increasing protein (BPI) and p15s that are likely secreted from polymorphonuclear leukocytes during the inflammatory response (FIG. 1).[3]

Purification of antibacterial activity in ascitic fluid towards *Staphylococcus aureus* has revealed that its activity is due to a 14-kD (Group II) phospholipase A2 (PLA2) (FIG. 1).[4] The potency and concentration (~ 200 ng/ml) of this enzyme in ascitic fluid can fully account for the antistaphylococcal activity of ascitic fluid. More than 99% of 10^7 *S. aureus* are killed per milliliter of ascitic fluid. Neutralizing antibodies to this rabbit PLA2 fully inhibit the bactericidal activity of ascitic fluid towards *S. aureus,* and the addition of a functionally similar but antigenically distinct recombinant human Group II PLA2 fully restores the antistaphylococcal activity of ascitic fluid pretreated with anti-PLA2 serum.[4]

The potency of rabbit and human Group II PLA2 towards *S. aureus* is remarkable (LD_{90} vs 10^6 bacteria/ml is about 10–50 ng/ml [1–3 nM PLA2]). Unlike the antimicrobial activity of many host peptides and proteins that have been described,[5] the bactericidal activity of PLA2 is fully manifest within natural biologic fluids. The absence of bactericidal activity towards *S. aureus* in plasma reflects low levels of this PLA2; the addition to plasma of purified PLA2 to levels reached during systemic inflammatory response confers potent cytotoxic activity towards *S. aureus* and several other species of gram-positive bacteria including *S. epidermidis, S. saprophyticus,* nonencapsulated *Streptococcus pneumoniae, S. salivarius, S. pyogenes,* and *Enterococcus faecalis.*[4] Bactericidal activity is a Ca^{2+} dependent, dependent on catalytically active enzyme and accompanied by virtually quantitative degradation of bacterial envelope phospholipids.[4]

---

[a] Address for correspondence: Department of Microbiology, New York University School of Medicine, 550 First Avenue, Medical Science Building 223, New York, NY 10016 (tel: 212/263-5118; fax: 212/263-8276).

The potent activity of these enzymes towards gram-positive bacteria contrasts sharply with their inability to act alone, at physiologically relevant doses, against gram-negative bacteria (TABLE 1). However, in concert with other host defense systems such as BPI and complement, both rabbit and human Group II PLA2 (e.g., PLA2 present in PMN and inflammatory fluids) displays potent degradative activity and contributes to the

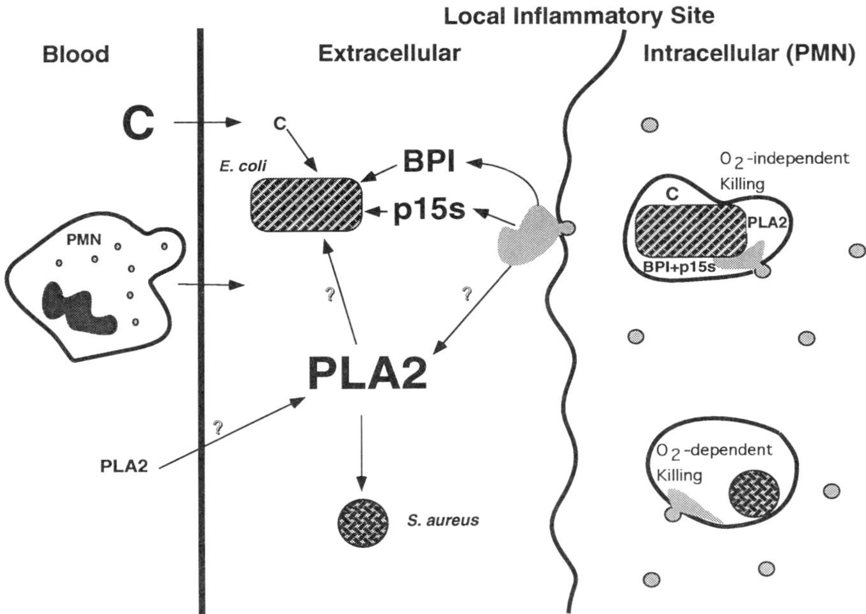

FIGURE 1. Mobilization of host defenses at local inflammatory sites. Possible roles for PLA2. Acute host responses to bacterial invasion include emigration of PMN and transudation of plasma proteins (including complement [C] components and possibly PLA2 secreted from stimulated hepatocytes and/or platelets) across endothelium to the site of infection. In contrast to C, extracellular levels of PLA2, BPI, and p15s at (local) sites of inflammation greatly exceed resting plasma levels. BPI and p15s in the inflammatory fluid likely reflect release from granule stores in PMN. Inflammatory fluid PLA2 may originate from other stimulated cells in the local environment. Intracellular killing of *E. coli* ingested by PMN appears to reflect the combined action of granule-associated BPI, p15s, and PLA2 and extracellular C and PLA2 that coat bacteria before phagocytosis. By contrast, intracellular killing of *S. aureus* by PMN is more greatly dependent on oxidative mechanisms.

destruction of gram-negative bacteria by the host (TABLE 1).[6–8] BPI-dependent PLA2 activity depends on both the enzyme's catalytic machinery, highly conserved in all 14-kD PLA2, and a discrete surface region near the NH_2-terminus rich in basic residues that mediates PLA2 binding to injured bacteria.[7] The latter property is expressed by only a subset of the 14-kD PLA2s (TABLE 1).[7] Similarly, the potent antistaphylococcal activity of mammalian Group II PLA2 is not expressed by many other 14-kD PLA2 (TABLE 1).[4] A basic isozyme in snake (*Naja mossambica mossambica*) venom expresses potent BPI-dependent activity toward *E. coli* but no cytotoxicity towards *S. aureus,* indicating that the structural determinants of PLA2 activity towards gram-positive bacteria and against BPI-treated gram-negative bacteria are distinct.

The dependence of the potent antibacterial activities of mammalian Group II PLA2 on structural properties shared by these enzymes but not by many other closely related members of this enzyme family is consistent with the belief that this is an evolved physiologic function of this enzyme and that its mobilization during inflammation is an integral element of the host's response to microbial invasion. Group II PLA2 is also prominent in several other body fluids (e.g., secretions of lacrimal glands [tears], Paneth cells [intestinal epithelium], and seminal fluid) where innate defenses to invading bacteria are likely to be essential.[9–11] Future studies will further address the contribution of this PLA2 to host defenses.

TABLE 1. Comparison of Activities of Various 14-kD PLA2s

PLA2	*S. aureus* LD$_{90}$ (ng/ml)	Untreated *E. coli* (ng/10^7 bacteria)[a]	BPI-Treated *E. coli* (ng/10^7 bacteria)[a]
Rabbit ascitic fluid (II)[b]	10	Not active (1,000)	2
Human secretory (II)	50	Not active (1,000)	2
Pig pancreas (I)	Not active (20,000)[c]	Not active (1,000)	Not active (1,000)
Naja mossambica mossambica (I)			
CMI (acidic)	Not active (80,000)	Not active (1,000)	Not active (1,000)
CMIII (basic)	Not active (100,000)	Not active (1,000)	2

[a]PLA2 dose required to produce degradation of $\geq 10\%$ of phospholipids of BPI-treated *E. coli.*
[b]Number in parentheses refers to group of 14-kD PLA2s.
[c]Highest dose tested.

REFERENCES

1. DONALDSON, D. M. & J. G. TEW. 1977. Beta-Lysin of platelet origin. Bacteriol. Rev. **41:** 501–513.
2. MYRVIK, Q. N. 1956. Serum bactericidins active against gram positive bacteria. Ann. N.Y. Acad. Sci. **66:** 391–400.
3. WEINRAUCH, Y., A. FORMAN, C. SHU, K. ZAREMBER, O. LEVY, P. ELSBACH & J. WEISS. 1995. Extracellular accumulation of potently microbicidal bactericidal/permeability-increasing protein and p15s in an evolving sterile rabbit peritoneal inflammatory exudate. J. Clin. Invest. **95:** 1916–1924.
4. WEINRAUCH, Y., P. ELSBACH, L. M. MADSEN, A. FOREMAN & J. WEISS. 1996. The potent anti-*Staphylococcus aureus* activity of a sterile rabbit inflammatory fluid is due to a 14 kD phospholipase A2. J. Clin. Invest. **97:** 250–257.
5. LEVY, O. 1995. Antibiotic proteins of PMN. Eur. J. Haematol. **56:** 263–277.
6. WRIGHT, G. C., J. WEISS, K. S. KIM, H. VERHEIJ & P. ELSBACH. 1990. Bacterial phospholipid hydrolysis enhances the destruction of *Escherichia coli* ingested by rabbit neutrophils. Role of cellular and extracellular phospholipases. J. Clin. Invest. **85:** 1925–1935.
7. WEISS J., M. INADA, P. ELSBACH & R. M. CROWL. 1994. Structural determinants of the action against *Escherichia coli* of a human inflammatory fluid phospholipase A2 in concert with polymorphonuclear leukocytes. J. Biol. Chem. **269:** 26331–26337.
8. MADSEN, L. M., M. INADA & J. WEISS. 1996. Determinants of activation by complement of Group II phospholipase A2 acting against *Escherichia coli.* Infect. Immun. **64:** 2425–2430.
9. NEVALAINEN, T. J., H. J. AHO & H. PEURAVUORI. 1994. Secretion of group 2 phospholipase A2 by lacrimal glands. Invest. Ophthalmol. & Vis. Sci. **35:** 417–421.
10. HARWIG, S. S., L. TAN, X. D. QU, Y. CHO, P. B. EISENHAUER & R. I. LEHRER. 1995. Bactericidal properties of murine intestinal phospholipase A2. J. Clin. Invest. **95:** 603–610.
11. NEVALAINEN, T. J., K.-M. MERI & M. NEIMI. 1993. Synovial-type (group II) phospholipase As human seminal plasma. Andrologia **25:** 355–358.

Structure-Function Studies with *Neisseria gonorrhoeae* Opa Outer Membrane Proteins Expressed in *Escherichia coli*

D. SIMON,[a] J. T. LIU,[a] M. S. BLAKE,[b] C. R. BLAKE,[b] AND R. F. REST[a]

[a]*Department of Microbiology and Immunology Medical College of Pennsylvania and Hahnemann University Philadelphia, Pennsylvania 19102–1192*

[b]*Department of Biochemistry The University of Iowa Ames, Iowa*

Gonorrhea is a sexually transmitted disease with high morbidity, especially in minorities and females, and represents a tremendous burden to US and other health care systems. No vaccine is available. *Neisseria gonorrhoeae* Opa proteins comprise a family of ~ 25– ~ 30-kD outer membrane proteins that mediate gonococcal adhesion to and invasion of human epithelial cells and association with human neutrophils.[1] Gonococci possess about 11 *opa* genes and can express 0–3 or more Opa proteins at once. Each *opa* is expressed, that is, is turned on or off, independently of other *opas*. Opa phase and antigenic variation occur at a rate of about 10^{-3} per cell per generation. Gonococci also have other phase and antigenically variable surface components that mediate cellular adhesion and invasion, thus complicating studies of Opa structure-function relationships. To better study Opa function, we expressed *opa* genes in *Escherichia coli* and observed that *E. coli (opa)* closely approximate gonococcal adhesion and invasion to epithelial cells,[2] neutrophils,[3] and human fallopian tube organ culture.[4]

Here we report on studies of specific internal and exonuclease III (exoIII) deletions of an *opa* gene, *opaP* from strain F62SF, to gain a better understanding of Opa's structure-function relationships. For these studies we used a β-*lactamase/opa* gene fusion in pGEM3Z expressed in *E. coli* DH5α. We wanted to determined the shortest expressed Opa protein that could mediate association with epithelial cells and neutrophils. The shortest 3′ deletion resulted in a bla-opa protein of 224 amino acids (parent is 244 amino acids), which abolished the ability of Opa to mediate invasion of ME-180 cervical epithelial cells by *E. coli (opa)*; however, the same deletant completely retained its ability to interact with neutrophils. Surprisingly, Opa deletants possessing as few as 113 or 115 amino acids adhered to neutrophils five- to six-fold greater than did other Opa deletants or the complete Opa. When exoIII deletions extended past amino acid 113 into the carboxyl end of the HV1 region, all Opa protein function was lost.

A 6 amino acid stretch immediately downstream of the HV1 region of all Opas shows homology with the carbohydrate-binding domain of human hepatocyte asialoglycoprotein receptors (ASGP-R)s.[5] It was hypothesized that this region is responsible for binding of Opa to human cellular glycoconjugates. To test this hypothesis we made an internal, in-frame deletion of 12 amino acids encompassing the putative carbohydrate-binding domain of ASGP-Rs. *E. coli* expressing the resulting protein of 232 amino acids showed a > 100-fold reduction in invasion of ME-180 epithelial cells compared to the parent. The deletion had little effect on *E. coli (opa)* adhesion to neutrophils or stimulation of the oxidative burst.

Our observations suggest that: (1) Opa-mediated association with human epithelial cells and neutrophils occurs by at least two different mechanisms; it is likely that two different classes of Opa receptors exist on epithelial cells and neutrophils, respectively. (2) At least two regions of Opa proteins affect the ability of Opa to mediate bacterial invasion of epithelial cells: the COOH-terminus (<20 amino acids), based on exoIII studies, and the region containing amino acids homologous to the carbohydrate-binding site of human hepatocyte ASGP-Rs, as determined by deletion studies. (3) Amino terminal fragments of OpaP as small as 113 amino acids mediate bacterial association with human neutrophils, indicating that the carboxyl half of Opa molecules are not involved in interactions with neutrophils.

REFERENCES

1. MEYER, T. F., J. POHLNER & J. P. M. VAN PUTTEN. 1994. Curr. Topics Microbiol. Immunol. **192:** 283–317.
2. SIMON, D. & R. F. REST. 1992. Proc. Natl. Acad. Sci. USA **89:** 5512–5516.
3. BELLAND, P. J., T. CHEN, J. SWANSON & S. H. FISHER. 1992. Mol. Microbiol. **6:** 1729–1737.
4. GORBY, G., D. SIMON & R. F. REST. 1994. Ann. N.Y. Acad. Sci. **730:** 286–289.
5. BLAKE, M. S., C. M. BLAKE, M. A. APICELLA & R. E. MANDRELL. 1995. Infect. Immun. **63:** 1434–1439.

Models for Pathogenesis of
Mycobacterium avium

E. G. LONG,[a,b] K. A. BIRKNESS,[a] G. W. NEWMAN,[a]
F. D. QUINN,[a] E. P. EWING, JR,[a] J. H. BARTLETT,[a]
C. H. KING,[a] M. A. YAKRUS,[a] AND
C. R. HORSBURGH, JR.[c]

*[a]National Center for Infectious Diseases
Centers for Disease Control and Prevention
and
[c]Emory University School of Medicine
Atlanta, Georgia 30333*

We explored the use of tissue monolayers and embryonated hens' eggs as models for the study of the pathogenesis of *Mycobacterium avium*. Cell mololayers from six human transformed and cancerous cell lines revealed that bacteria attached in numbers six times greater to spindle-shaped cells than to rounded cells, but these experiments did not distinguish between patient and environmental strains and the infected cells did not show any pathogenic effects of the bacteria.

When 8-day-old embryonated hens' eggs were infected via the amniotic sac with suspensions containing 1×10^7 colony-forming units (CFU), patient strains caused 40–90% mortality and environmental strains caused 10–30% mortality. These difference were statistically significant ($p = 0.0205$). Strains of *M. avium* isolated from the blood of infected patients were twice as virulent as strains isolated from sputum and bronchoalveolar fluid (BAL). Virulence was defined as the percentage mortality in groups of infected eggs compared to control groups injected with sterile medium. Virulence of most strains decreased with passage through eggs. The mean percentage of eggs killed by two strains of *M. avium* isolated from blood was 44.3% after the first infection. This decreased to 21.4% at the next passage ($p = 0.0152$), to 12.90% at the third passage ($p = 0.0136$), and to 5.0% at the fourth passage ($p = 00.0032$). Mortality in the controls averaged 3.0 (Fig. 1).

The site of infection in the egg was usually the mesodermal layer of the chorioallantoic membrane (CAM). A few small granulomas containing acid-fast bacteria were seen in the liver but not in other organs. Death of chicken embryos may have resulted from destruction of the mesodermal layer of the CAM with consequent respiratory failure. Bacteria could be recovered from all fluids in dead and apparently healthy chicken embryos.

Reports indicate that colonies producing rough and granular colonies (RG) were more virulent than smooth and domed variants (SmD) when inoculated intravenously into chickens.[1] In other reports, beige mice were more susceptible to isolates from AIDS patients that formed smooth transparent colonies.[2] Earlier studies have associated virulence in chicken and mice to strains that produce transparent colonies.[3,4]

---

[b]Address for correspondence: Earl G. Long, PhD, G-11, DASTLR/NCID, Centers for Disease Control, Atlanta, GA 30333.

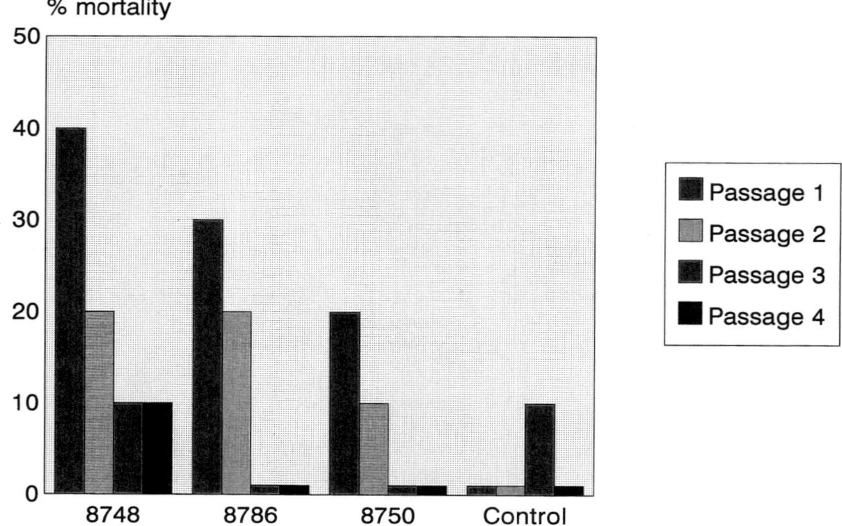

FIGURE 1. Reduction of virulence of *Mycobacterium avium* with passage through eggs.

We did not find any differences in colony morphology between strains that differed in their ability to kill eggs.

REFERENCES

1. MORITA, Y., M. ARAI, O. NOMURA, S, MARUYAMA & Y. KATSUBE. 1994. Avian tuberculosis which occurred in an imported pigeon and pathogenesis of the isolates. J. Vet. Med. Sci. **56:** 585–587.
2. REDDY, V. M., K. PARIKH, J. LUNA-HERRERA, J. O. FALKINGHAM, III, S. BROWN & P. R. J. GANGADHARAM. 1994. Comparison of virulence of *Mycobacterium avium* complex (MAC) strains isolated from AIDS and non-AIDS patients. Microb. Pathog. **16:** 121–130.
3. MOEHRING, J. M. & M. R. SOLOTOROVSKY. 1965. Pathogenicity of transparent, opaque and rough variants of *Mycobacterium avium* in chickens and mice. Am. Rev. Respir. Dis. **92:** 499–506.
4. SCHAEFER, W. B., C. L. DAVIS & M. L. COHN. 1970. Pathogenesis of transparent, opaque, and rough variants of *Mycobacterium avium* in chickens and mice. Am. Rev. Respir. Dis. **102:** 499–506.

The *Bcg* Gene (*Nramp1*) Does Not Determine Resistance of Mice to Virulent *Mycobacterium tuberculosis*

EVA MEDINA AND ROBERT J. NORTH

The Trudeau Institute
Saranac Lake, New York 12983

Some strains of mice are more resistant than others to a range of intracellular pathogens, including the vaccine Bacillus-Calmus-Guérin (BCG) strain of *Mycobacterium bovis,* because they possess the dominant resistance allele of a gene (*Nramp1*) in the *Ity/Lsh/Bcg* locus of chromosome 1 (reviewed in refs. 1 and 2). In BCG infection the superior resistance of mice with the resistance allele (*Bcg^r*) over those with the susceptible allele (*Bcg^s*) of the gene has been measured as decreased bacterial growth in the spleen before the onset of specific immunity. The purpose of our study was to determine if the same applies to infection with a virulent strain of *M. tuberculosis.*

METHODS

Bcg^r DBA/2, *Bcg^s* BALB/c, CD2F1 (DBA/2 × BALB/c), and *Bcg^r* congenic C.D2-N20 mice (BALB/c mice with the *Ity/Lsh/Bcg* locus of DBA/2 mice) were employed. They were infected intravenously with approximately 10^5 colony-forming units (cfu) of the H37Rv strain of *M. tuberculosis* (TMC 102) or 5×10^2 cfu of the same strain by aerosol. Infection was followed against time in the liver, spleen, and lung by plating homogenates of these organs on nutrient agar (7H11) and counting colonies 2–3 weeks later. Survival of additional mice was recorded over time. Histology of the lungs was performed on 5- or 10-μm thick sections stained for acid-fast bacilli with a modified basic fuchsin stain and counterstained with methylene blue.

RESULTS AND DISCUSSION

Contrary to expectation, *Bcg^r* DBA/2 mice were less, rather than more, resistant than *Bcg^s* BALB/c mice to infection with *M. tuberculosis H37Rv* initiated via the intravenous or respiratory route. This was evidenced by an inferior ability of DBA/2 mice to restrict the growth of *M. tuberculosis* in their lungs, but not in their liver and spleen, after the onset of expression of immunity at about day 20 postinoculation. More convincing evidence was seen in the mortality data which showed that DBA/2 mice died much earlier (MST = 84 days) than did BALB/c mice (MST = 290 days). Importantly, the resistance of F1 hybrid mice produced by DBA/2 and BALB/c parents was identical to that of *Bcg^s* BALB/c mice. The absence of a role for the *Bcg^r* allele in immunity to *M. tuberculosis* infection is also convincingly illustrated by the results of an experiment with DBA/2, BALB/c, and congenic C.D2-N20 mice. FIGURE 1 shows that *Bcg^r* BALB/c mice could cause 10 times less growth of *M.*

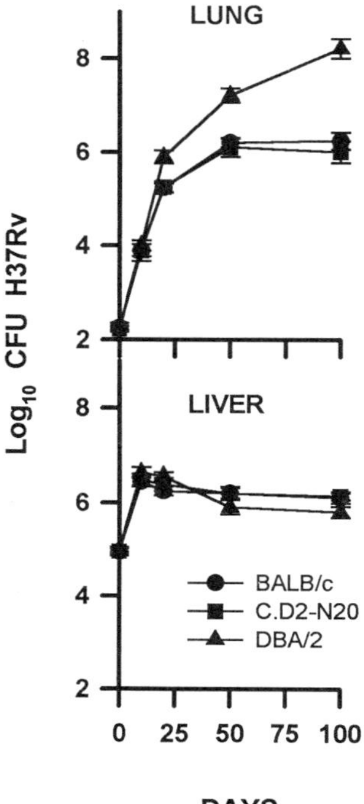

FIGURE 1. *Bcg^s* BALB/c can cause 100 times less growth of *M. tuberculosis* in their lungs than can *Bcg^r* DBA/2 mice.

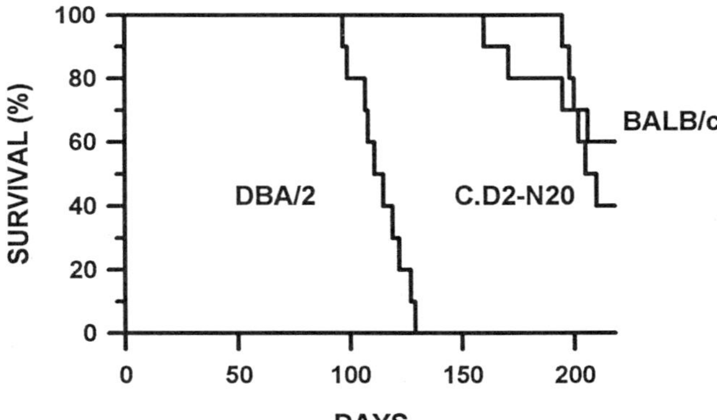

FIGURE 2. Congenic *Bcg^r* mice are similar to BALB/c mice in that they can survive much longer (MST = 200 days) than can DBA/2 mice (MST = 110 days).

tuberculosis in their lungs, but not in other organs, than could *Bcg*^r DBA/2 mice. Congenic *Bcg*^r C.D2-N20 mice were similar to BALB/c mice in this regard. They were also similar (FIG. 2) to BALB/c mice in being able to survive much longer (MST = 200 days) than can DBA/2 mice (MST = 110 days). Therefore, there can be little doubt that the resistant allele of the *Nramp1* gene, although providing mice with superior natural resistance to *Salmonella typhimurium, Leishmania donovani,* and BCG,[3] has no measurable influence on resistance to infection with virulent *M. tuberculosis.* This demonstration that the superior anti-*M. tuberculosis* resistance of BALB/c over DBA/2 mice is expressed only in the lung is important, because of evidence showing that in mice,[4] as in most human,[5] tuberculosis is predominantly a disease of the lung. The *Bcg*^r gene, on the other hand, provides mice with a resistance advantage against BCG (an attenuated organism) only in the spleen, an organ that normally is not susceptible to *M. tuberculosis* infection. Moreover, histologic study of the lungs of *M. tuberculosis*-infected DBA/2 and BALB/c mice revealed that earlier death of the former mice is associated with more extensive lung pathology and with lesions containing much higher numbers of acid-fast bacilli.

CONCLUSION

The resistant allele of the *Nramp1* gene in the *Ity/Lsh/Bcg* locus of mouse chromosome 1 does not determine resistance to infection with virulent *M. tuberculosis.*

REFERENCES

1. VIDAL, S. M., D. MALO, K. VOGAN, E. SKAMENE & P. GROS. 1993. Natural resistance to infection with intracellular parasites: Identification of a candidate gene for *Bcg.* **73:** 469–485.
2. VIDAL, S., M. L. TREMBLAY, G. GOVONI, S. GAUTHIER, G. SEBASTIANI, D. MALO, E. SKAMENE, M. OLIVER, S. JOTHY & P. GROS. 1995. The *Ity/Lsh/Bcg* locus: Natural resistance to infection with intracellular parasites is abrogated by disruption of the *Nramp* gene. J. Exp. Med. **182:**
3. SKAMENE, E., P. GROS, A. GORGET, P. A. L. KONGSHAVN, C. S. CHARLES & B. A. TAYLOR. 1982. Genetic regulation of resistance to intracellular pathogens. Nature **297:** 506–509.
4. DUNN, P. L. & R. J. NORTH. 1995. Virulence ranking of some *Mycobacterium tuberculosis* and *Mycobacterium bovis* strains according to their ability to multiply in the lungs, induce lung pathology, and cause mortality in mice. Infect. Immun. **63:** 3428–3437.
5. HOPEWELL, P. C. 1994. Overview of clinical tuberculosis. *In* Tuberculosis: Pathogenesis, Protection and Control. B. R. Bloom, Eds. 25–46. ASM Press, Washington DC.

Both Epidermal Growth Factor-Like Domains of the Merozoite Surface Protein-1 from *Plasmodium yoelii* Are Required for Protection from Malaria

PAUL A. CALVO, THOMAS M. DALY,
AND CAROLE A. LONG

Department of Microbiology and Immunology
Mail Stop 410
Medical College of Pennsylvania and
Hahnemann University
Broad and Vine Sts.
Philadelphia, Pennsylvania 19102

The erythrocytic stages of parasite development are responsible for the morbidity and mortality associated with malaria. A leading human vaccine candidate antigen directed to these stages is the merozoite surface protein-1 (MSP-1). MSP-1 in the rodent model *Plasmodium yoelii* is a 230-kD polypeptide that is proteolytically processed on the merozoite surface prior to invasion of erythrocytes. Recently, our laboratory demonstrated that a 12-kD carboxyl-terminal region of the MSP-1 could be produced in *Escherichia coli* as a fusion protein with glutathione-*S*-transferase, retaining native configuration. This region contains 10 cysteine residues believed to be arranged as two epidermal growth factor (EGF)-like domains. Immunization of naive mice with this fusion protein elicits a protective host immune response that is predominately mediated by antibodies. We hypothesized that the first EGF-like domain may be sufficient to elicit a protective response because of the identification of monoclonal antibodies (which map to this region) that inhibit erythrocytic infections both *in vitro* and *in vivo*.

To examine the possible role of the individual EGF-like domains in protection, we generated homologous fusion proteins containing either the first or the second EGF-like domains. Although all animals developed some level of antibody in response to the various immunogens, only those animals immunized with both EGF-like domains produced antibodies that could recognize the native MSP-1 molecule. Antibodies generated against the individual EGF-like domains did cross-react with the double EGF-like domain structure, suggesting that the immunogens had retained elements of native configuration. Mice immunized with the first EGF-like domain developed antibody titers specific to that region comparable to those of animals immunized with both domains, whereas mice immunized with the second EGF-like domain developed specific antibody titers that were decreased threefold (FIG. 1). Isotypic analysis of these antibodies did not demonstrate an appreciable difference in the groups immunized with either both or the first EGF-like domain. The parasitemia profiles of mice immunized with the various fusion proteins showed that only those animals receiving both EGF-like domains, which all produced antibodies recognizing native MSP-1, were protected

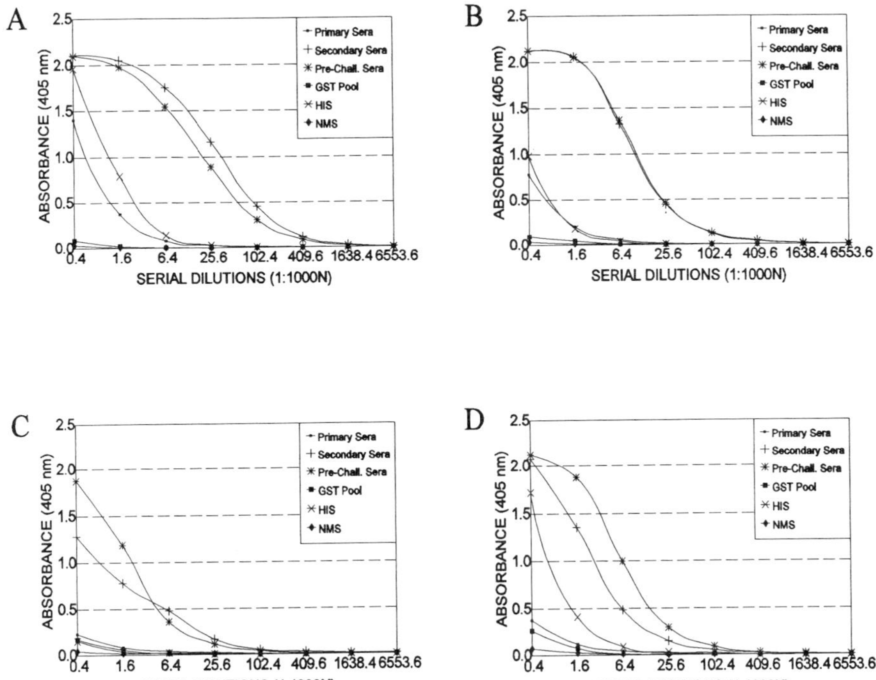

FIGURE 1. Time course of antibody production in response to immunization. Antibody production was followed by direct-binding ELISA using serial dilutions of antisera produced in response to immunization with (**A**) GST-PyC2, (**B**) GST-PyC3, (**C**) GST-PyC4, and (**D**) GST-PyC3 + GST-PyC4 (20 μg of carboxyl-terminal MSP-1 material) following the first, second, and third administration of immunogen. Each point represents the average of five animals. Antigen used in each ELISA was the respective MSP-1 region of the fusion protein cleaved free from GST using thrombin. Abbreviations: GST pool polyclonal anti-GST sera; HIS = *P. y. yoelii* 17X hyperimmune sera; NMS = normal mouse sera.

from a lethal challenge infection (FIG. 2). Mice immunized with either of the individual domain fusion proteins or a mixture of the two fusion proteins showed a slight delay in the onset of parasitemia, but were unable to control their infections with maximal parasitemias in excess of 50%. These observations suggest that determinants unique to the secondary structure generated by the double EGF-like

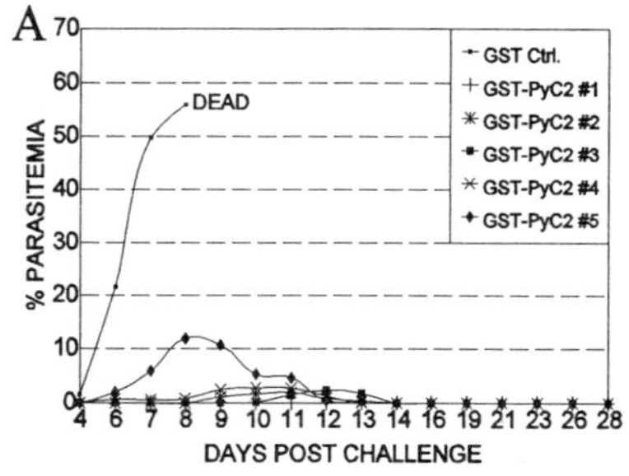
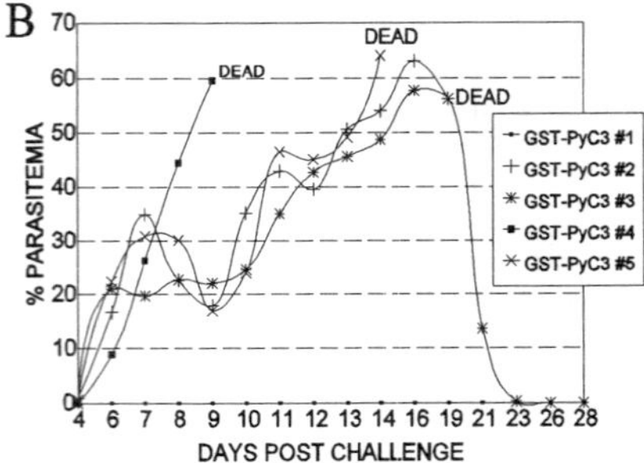
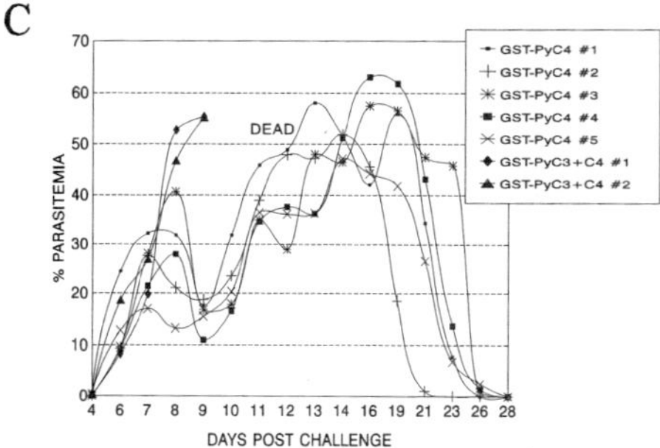

FIGURE 2. Parasitemia profiles of immunized animals challenged with *P. y. yoelii* 17XL. Inbred BALB/c ByJ mice were immunized with GST, or the various fusion proteins, assessed serologically, and then challenged with 1×10^4 *P. y. yoelii* 17XL parasitized erythrocytes 2 weeks after the third immunization. Parasitemia was followed by microscopic analysis of daily blood films from mice immunized with (**A**) GST or GST-PyC2, (**B**) GST-PyC3, and (**C**) GST-PyC4 or GST-PyC3 + GST-PyC4. GST control animals are the average of five mice. Parasitemia is reported as the percentage of infected versus total erythrocytes.

domains may be necessary for the generation of antibodies that can recognize the native configuration of MSP-1 and that these antibodies may play an important role in protection.

Role of Passive Humoral Immunity in Experimental Mycetoma by *Nocardia brasiliensis*

MARIO C. SALINAS-CARMONA

AND ERNESTO TORRES-LÓPEZ

Department of Immunology
Facultad de Medicina y Hospital Universitario
Universidad Autónoma de Nuevo León
Monterrey, N. L., Mexico 64460

Mycetoma is a chronic infectious disease that affects skin and underlying tissues, but in some cases it can extend and destroy bone and adjacent organs. This disease may be produced by fungi (eumycetoma) or bacteria (actinomycetoma).[1] In Mexico, mycetoma is produced frequently by *Nocardia brasiliensis* (86%). We previously showed that sera from patients with actinomycetoma strongly react with p61, p26, and p24 proteins on Western blot assay.[2] The p24 protein was isolated from a defatted *N. brasiliensis* cell extract using simple physicochemical techniques.[3] When used as antigen in a solid phase ELISA, the anti-p24 antibody concentration was directly correlated with the severity of mycetoma lesions.[4] It has been suggested that *N. brasiliensis* proteases may be involved in the pathogenesis of actinomycetoma,[5] but this is not completely clear.

Innate and adoptive immunity may play a role in host resistance to *N. brasiliensis* infection in both murine models and humans. Histopathologic study of a typical mycetoma lesion shows polymorphonuclear cells, usually neutrophils surrounding *N. brasiliensis* microcolonies forming an abscess; large activated macrophages are also present in the outer limits of the abscess. Host resistance to nocardial infection has been extensively studied in mice using *N. asteroides,* and it has been suggested that anti-*N. asteroides* antibodies play no role; perhaps they worsen the lesion.[6] In the present study we inoculated 1×10^7 *N. brasiliensis* colony-forming units (CFU) in the footpad of BALB/C and C57 BL/6 mice. Mycetoma was fully established 28 days after infection in these immunocompetent strains. Spontaneous regression of mycetoma lesions started 150 days after infection, and 100% of infected mice recovered from the foot lesions as summarized in TABLE 1. We demonstrated that p61, p26, and p24 are the immunodominant antigens by Western blot analysis using *N. brasiliensis* defatted antigen. BALB/c mice and New Zealand white rabbits donated the serum for the adoptive transfer experiments; animals were immunized with heat-killed *N. brasiliensis* cells and incomplete Freund's adjuvant. Two additional injections, one subcutaneous and one intramuscular, were given before collecting blood. Serum was heat inactivated, sterilized by millipore filtration, and pooled; an aliquot was analyzed by Western blot, anti-*N. brasiliensis* antibody concentration being determined by ELISA. We injected 0.1 ml of the hyperimmune serum intramuscularly on days 1, 7, 14, and 28 after infection with the *N. brasiliensis* cell. Daily evaluation sought mycetoma signs for each treated mouse.

We also included one group of mice injected with hyperimmune sera that had

TABLE 1. Clinical Evaluation of *N. brasiliensis* Experimental Mycetoma in Immunocompetent Mice[a]

| | Days after Infection | | | | | |
Mouse Strain	7	14	28	90	150	200
BALB/c	+ +	+ + +	+ + + +	+ + + +	+ + +	+ +
C57BL/6	+ +	+ + +	+ + + +	+ + + +	+ + +	+

[a]Inflammation is present on day 7, but the full-blown lesion is seen from day 28 to day 90. Symbols: + = only inflammation, 5 mm; + + = inflammation plus abscess and ulceration; + + + = inflammation, abscess, and granule discharge; + + + + = fully established mycetoma.

recovered after 200 days of infection. This serum was shown to have high titer of anti-*N. brasiliensis* antibodies by ELISA. The results summarized in TABLE 2. demonstrate that only the sera from heat-killed *N. brasiliensis*-immunized mice prevented infection. By contrast, sera from spontaneously recovered mice or rabbits did not confer this protective effect. To further investigate the role of antibodies in healing an established lesion, we injected sera at the same doses and route into BALB/c mice with typical mycetoma lesions on day 90 after infection. An additional series of four injections were given with no effect whatsoever. Therefore, we conclude that the anti-*N. brasiliensis* antibodies present in the sera of hyperimmune mice are responsible for the protection against mycetoma lesions.

TABLE 2. Hyperimmune Sera from BALB/c Mice Prevent the Mycetoma Lesions When Obtained from Heat-Killed *N. brasiliensis*-Immunized Animals

Healthy Male BALB/C Mice Infected on Day 1		Source of Hyperimmune Sera		Effect
	+	Mice immunized with heat-killed *N. brasiliensis*	45 days $\longrightarrow$	PROTECTION (No Mycetoma)
	+	Mice recovered from mycetoma	45 days $\longrightarrow$	Mycetoma + + + +
	+	Rabbit immunized with heat-killed *N. brasiliensis*	45 days $\longrightarrow$	Mycetoma + + + +
	+	Rabbit immunized with *N. brasiliensis* cell extract	45 days $\longrightarrow$	Mycetoma + + + +
	+	Sterile saline solution	45 days $\longrightarrow$	Mycetoma + + + +

$n = 30$

REFERENCES

1. WELSH, O., M. C. SALINAS-CARMONA & M. A. RODRÍGUEZ. 1994. Mycetoma In infectious diseases, 5th Ed. P. D. Hoeprich, M. C. Jordan & A. R. Ronald, Eds. Chapt. 174: 1402–1406. J.B. Lippincott Co. Philadelphia, PA.
2. SALINAS-CARMONA, M. C., L. VERA, O. WELSH & M. A. RODRÍGUEZ. 1992. Antibody response to *Nocardia brasiliensis* antigens in man. Zentralbl. Bakteriol. **276:** 290–397.
3. VERA-CABRERA, L., M. C. SALINAS-CARMONA, O. WELSH & M. A. RODRÍGUEZ. 1992. Isolation and purification of two immunodominant antigens from *Nocardia brasiliensis*. J. Clin. Microbiol. **30:** 1183–1188.
4. SALINAS-CARMONA, M. C., O. WELSH & S. M. CASILLAS. 1993. Enzyme-linked immunosorbent assay for serological diagnosis for *Nocardia brasiliensis* and clinical correlation with mycetoma infections. J. Clin. Microbiol. **31:** 2901–2906.
5. SALINAS-CARMONA, M. C., L. PEREZ, O. WELSH & M. G. RINALDI. 1992. Identification of intracellular proteases from *Nocardia brasiliensis*. J. Mycol. Méd. **2:** 183–188.
6. BEAMAN, B. L., M. E. GERSHWIN, A. AHMED, S. M. SCATES & R. DEEM. 1982. Response of CBA/N × DBA2/F mice to *Nocardia asteroides*. Infect. Immun. **35:** 111–116.

A Nontoxic Chimeric Cholera Toxin Analog[a]

M. BOESMAN-FINKELSTEIN,[b] J. W. PETERSON,[c]
L. S. THAI,[b] AND R. A. FINKELSTEIN[b,d]

[b]*Department of Molecular Microbiology and Immunology*
University of Missouri School of Medicine
Columbia, Missouri 65212

[c]*Department of Microbiology and Immunology*
School of Medicine
University of Texas Medical Branch
Galveston, Texas 77555-1019

Cholera enterotoxin (CT) has two major epitypes, CT-1 and CT-2, defined by immunologic differences in their B subunits. The prototype CT, CT-1, is produced by classic biotype Inaba serotype *Vibrio cholerae* strain 569B, by other classic biotype strains, and by the "Gulf Coast" El Tor biotype. CT-2 is produced by El Tor biotype Ogawa serotype strain 3083, by other El Tor strains, and by the new serogroup O139 (syn, Bengal). The epitypes are easily differentiated by monoclonal antibodies. Quantitative cross-neutralization studies revealing the superior neutralizing activity of homologous antisera imply that the differences may be significant in antitoxic immunity. Although the B subunits of CT are immunodominant, evidence suggests that CT or CT analogs and derivatives are more effective antigens and adjuvants than is the B subunit protein by itself.[1]

We previously[2] introduced substitutions, Arg-7 → Lys and Glu-112 → Gln, in the A subunit of CT, thus eliminating its enzymatic/toxic activity. The gene encoding a nontoxic analog, CT-2* (carrying the B-2 subunit), was introduced into *V. cholerae* strains including CVD103, an attenuated classic biotype mutant candidate vaccine strain that produces the B subunit (but not the A subunit) of CT-1. The present work shows that the recombinant strain now produces a chimeric nontoxic analog holotoxin protein containing both CT-B-1 and CT-B-2 subunits.

The protein was purified to homogeneity (FIG. 1) from syncase medium fermentor cultures of CVD103/CT-2*. The recombinant protein reacts, in checkerboard immunoblots,[3] with specific mouse monoclonal antibodies against the A* subunit and both CT-B-1 and CT-B-2 (FIG. 2). This suggests that the protein may be chimeric, but it is also consistent with the existence of two kinds of CT*, one consisting of CT-A*-B-1 and one of CT-A*-B-2. This question was resolved by enzyme-linked immunosorbent assays (ELISA) of toxin analog eluted from an affinity column containing immobilized monoclonal antibodies specific for CT-B-1. The eluted antigen reacted equally well with monoclonal antibodies specific for both CT-B-1 and CT-B-2. Because only molecules containing CT-B-1 antigen were trapped on the affinity column and the eluted protein contained both epitypes, we

[a]This work was supported in part by Public Health Service National Institutes of Health grants AI17312 and AI21463 to R.A.F. and J.W.P., respectively.

[d]Corresponding author.

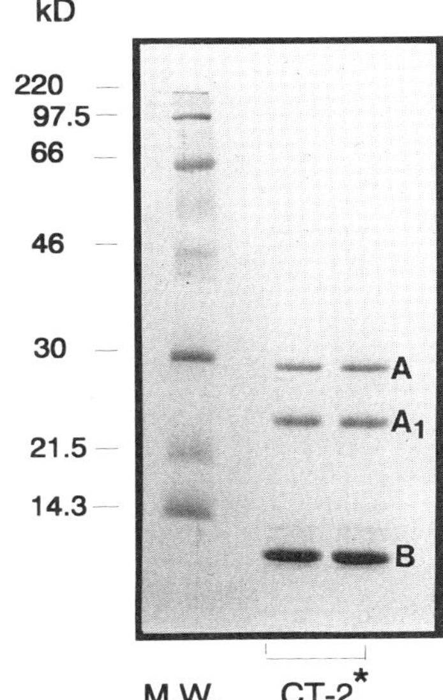

FIGURE 1. SDS-PAGE of purified CT holotoxin analog protein, CT-2*, produced by CVD103/CT-2*.

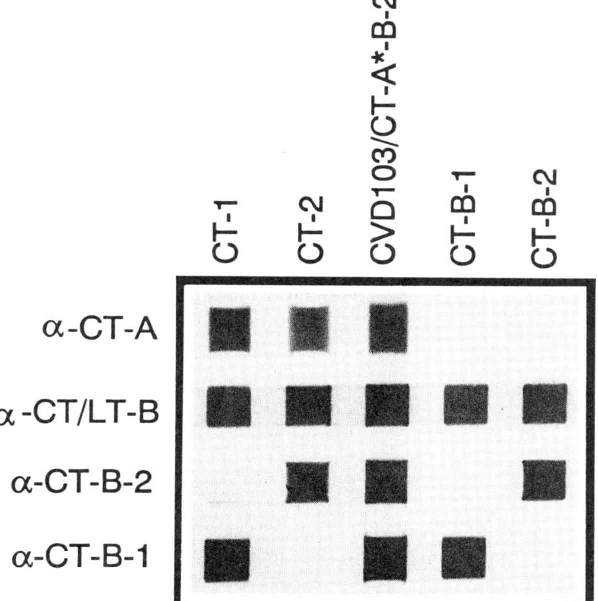

FIGURE 2. Checkerboard immunoblot of reactions of (*left side, top to bottom*) monoclonal mouse anti-CT-A, promiscuous monoclonal mouse anti-CT-B/LT-B, specific mouse monoclonal anti-CT-B-2, specific mouse monoclonal anti-CT-B-1 vs (*top, left to right*) CT-1, CT-2, CVD 103/CT-2*, CT-B-1, and CT-B-2.

conclude that the recombinant strain produces CT-A* and the two epitypes of CT-B on the same nontoxic holotoxin analog molecule.

The recombinant strain producing the chimera may have advantages over the original construct in induction of immunity against El Tor and O139 strains that produce CT-B-2. The protein may also be useful in conjugate vaccines[4] including those directed against O139.

REFERENCES

1. FINKELSTEIN, R. A. 1995. Why do we not yet have a suitable vaccine against cholera? *In* Advances in Mucosal Immunology. J. Mestecky *et al.,* Eds.: 1633–1640. Plenum Press. New York.
2. HÄSE, C. C., L. S. THAI, M. BOESMAN-FINKELSTEIN, V. L. MAR, W. N. BURNETTE, H. R. KASLOW, L. A. STEVENS, J. MOSS & R. A. FINKELSTEIN. 1994. Construction and characterization of recombinant *Vibrio cholerae* strains producing inactive cholera toxin analogs. Infect. Immun. **62:** 3051–3057.
3. KAZEMI, M. & R. A. FINKELSTEIN. 1990. Study of epitopes of cholera enterotoxin-related enterotoxins using checkerboard immunoblotting. Infect. Immun. **58:** 2352–2360.
4. GUPTA, R. K., S. C. SZU, R. A. FINKELSTEIN & J. B. ROBBINS. 1992. Synthesis, characterization, and some immunologic properties of conjugates composed of the detoxified lipopolysaccharide of *Vibrio cholerae* O1 serotype Inaba bound to cholera toxin. Infect. Immun. **60:** 3201–3208.

Bismuth–Dimercaprol Exposes Surface Components of *Klebsiella pneumoniae* Camouflaged by the Polysaccharide Capsule

P. DOMENICO,[a] J. M. TOMAS,[b] S. MERINO,[b] X. RUBIRES,[b] AND B. A. CUNHA[a]

[a]*Winthrop-University Hospital*
Mineola, New York 11501

[b]*University of Barcelona*
Barcelona, Spain

Encapsulated gram-negative bacteria are among the leading causes of morbidity and mortality in the hospital environment. The pathogenicity of these bacteria is often predicated on the production of capsular polysaccharide (CPS) which envelopes bacteria and shields them from host defenses.[1] Bacteria also release large quantities of CPS, which is complexed with endotoxin[2] and may neutralize antibodies that would otherwise attach to and opsonize bacteria.[3] A vaccine approach to the capsule is usually not practical, because a variety of capsular serotypes are associated with disease. Furthermore, CPS is a poor immunogen.

An alternative therapeutic approach is the suppression of CPS expression. Agents such as salicylate or bismuth limit the expression of CPS.[4] Bismuth–dimercaprol (BisBAL) is a new agent with enhanced antimicrobial activity. BisBAL is bacteriostatic, producing MICs of 10–25 μg/ml for most bacteria. At subMIC concentrations (3–5 μg/ml), BisBAL reduced *Klebsiella pneumoniae* O1:K2 CPS expression by 60–90%, as determined by a chemical assay for uronic acid (Fig. 1). Reduction in CPS expression resulted in exposure of subsurface structures, as measured in biologic assays. Phagocytosis of BisBAL-treated O1:K2 cells by human polymorphonuclear leukocytes increased from <10 to >300 per 100 polymorphonuclear leukocytes (FIG. 1), but phagocytosis still required complement and anti-K2 (diluted 1:40 to minimize agglutination) or anti-O1 antiserum. By contrast, the biocide chlorhexidine had little effect on CPS expression and no effect on phagocytosis at subMIC concentrations (FIG. 1). BisBAL potency is ≥100-fold greater than that of other bismuth compounds.

Reactivity of monoclonal antibodies specific for the O1-antigen lipolysaccharide or the lipopolysaccharide core also increased markedly with BisBAL treatment. Whole cells of *K. pneumoniae* O1:K1 or O1:K2, but not O1:K⁻, grown in the presence of subMIC BisBAL reacted to monoclonal antibodies in a dose-dependent manner in ELISA. Using anti-O1 monoclonal antibodies, absorbance (A_{405}) increased from <0.1 to 0.85 for O1:K1, from 0.72 to 1.49 for O1:K2, but remained in 1.67 for O1:K⁻ cells treated with 5 μg/ml BisBAL.

BisBAL also enhanced the interaction of complement component C3b with O1:K1 and O1:K2, but not O1:K⁻ strains. The relative concentration of cell-bound C3b in ELISA increased from <0.1 to 0.86 for O1:K1, from 0.62 to 1.58 for O1:K2, but remained 1.84 for O1:K⁻ cells treated with 5 μg/ml BisBAL.

269

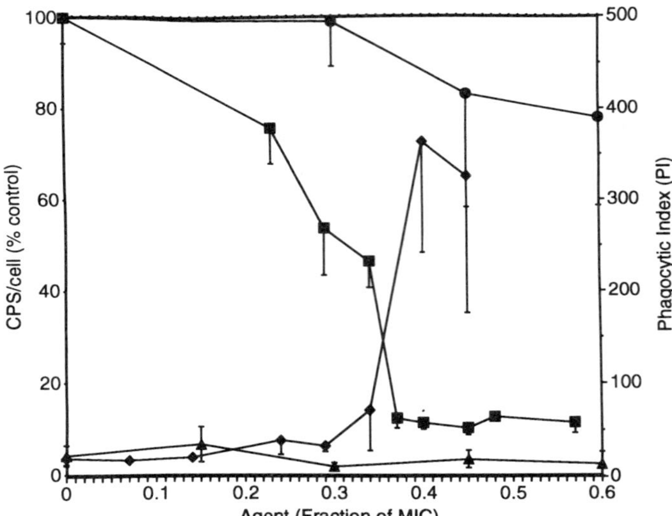

FIGURE 1. Effect of BisBAL or chlorhexidine on CPS expression and phagocytic uptake. *K. pneumoniae* O1:K2 was cultured for 18 hours in defined medium in the presence of subinhibitory concentrations of biocides. In phagocytic assays, bacteria were incubated at 37°C for 30 minutes with human polymorphonuclear (PMNL) leukocytes at a 10:1 ratio. The phagocytic index (PI; number of bacteria per 100 PMNL) was determined from stained preparations by light microscopy.[4] CPS was extracted with zwitterionic detergent and measured by its content of uronic acid.[4] Bacteria were enumerated by standard plating on agar medium. CPS/cell was expressed as a percentage of untreated control. Symbols: ■ = BisBal CPS; ● = CHX CPS; ◆ = BisBAL PI; ▲ = CHX PI.

Bactericidal activity of normal human serum was not neutralized by absorption with O1:K1 unless cells were first treated with 5 μg/ml BisBAL. At 3 hours' incubation, survival of O1:K⁻ cells was <0.1% using normal human serum absorbed with O1:K1, but increased to 107% using BisBAL-treated cells for absorption.

Capsules have the potential to interfere with complement or antibody-mediated host defenses.[1] At subMIC levels, BisBAL inhibited CPS expression, which promoted phagocytosis, enhanced monoclonal antibody reactivity specific for lipopolysaccharide O-Ag or core epitopes, and enhanced C3b binding to encapsulated cells. An unencapsulated mutant did not show these changes after BisBAL treatment. In conclusion, subMIC BisBAL renders encapsulated *K. pneumoniae* more susceptible to host defenses and may potentiate the immune response to these pathogens.

REFERENCES

1. MOXON, E. R. & J. S. KROLL. 1990. Curr. Topics Microbiol. Immunol. **150:** 65–82.
2. STRAUS, D. C. 1987. Infect. Immun. **55:** 44–48.
3. POLLACK, M. 1976. Infect. Immun. **13:** 1543–1548.
4. DOMENICO, P., R. J. SALO, A. S. CROSS & B. A. CUNHA. 1994. Infect. Immun. **62:** 4495–4499.

Use of Salt to Isolate *Legionella pneumophila* Mutants Unable to Replicate in Macrophages

JOSEPH P. VOGEL, CRAIG ROY, AND RALPH R. ISBERG

Howard Hughes Medical Institute
Department of Molecular Biology and Microbiology
Tufts Medical School
Boston, Massachusettes 02111

Legionella pneumophila is a respiratory pathogen that causes Legionnaires' disease, a sometimes fatal form of pneumonia.[1] This gram-negative bacterium replicates inside normally bactericidal, alveolar macrophages. *L. pneumophila* prevents macrophages from killing them by inhibiting fusion of the bacteria-containing phagosome with the bactericidal contents of the lysosome. Subsequently, it creates a novel organelle, called a replicative phagosome, where it multiplies and eventually lyses the cell.

One approach to understanding how *L. pneumophila* prevents phagosome-lysosome fusion and how it replicates inside macrophages is to isolate mutants defective in these processes. A commonly used method is to repeatedly passage wild-type cells on a suboptimal medium called supplemented Mueller-Hinton agar (SMH). Complementation of a mutant isolated by repeated passage on SMH agar identified the *icmWXYZ* operon which is required for intracellular growth.[2] Passage on SMH agar selects for avirulent cells by inhibiting the growth of wild-type cells. The inhibitory substance in SMH medium is a relatively moderate amount of sodium chloride (0.65% w/v final = 112 mM) introduced from the casein acid hydrolysate present in the SMH agar.[3] Inclusion of 0.65% sodium chloride in CYE plates is sufficient to inhibit the growth of virulent *L. pneumophila* in macrophages. A strong correlation appears to exist between salt sensitivity and ability to grow in macrophages, because most mutants isolated by insertion of Tn903*dIIlacZ* are both unable to replicate in macrophages and salt resistant.[4]

On the basis of these observations, we decided to exploit the sodium sensitivity of wild-type *L. pneumophila* to rapidly isolate a collection of mutants unable to replicate in macrophages. Wild-type cells were grown in media containing sodium chloride and subsequently were screened for inability to replicate in macrophages. From one liquid culture, 26 of 27 salt-resistant mutants were incapable of multiplying in macrophages. Of these, one mutant could be complemented for intracellular growth by a plasmid containing the *icm* locus, whereas eight mutants could be complemented by a plasmid containing *dotA,* a gene transcribed divergently from *icm* which is also required for intracellular growth.[5]

A mutant that was not complemented by either plasmid was chosen for further analysis. This mutant was examined for intracellular targeting and found to mistarget similar to *dotA* mutants.[5] Therefore, it was named *dotB* for *d*efective in *o*rganelle *t*rafficking. An *L. pneumophila* library was mated into the mutant, and a single clone was isolated which restored intracellular growth. By subcloning this plasmid, one open reading frame coding for a protein of 377 amino acids was identified which was responsible for the complementation. This locus was independently identified in

Howard Shuman's laboratory as a gene required for macrophage killing by *L. pneumophila* (unpublished communication).

The DotB protein is homologous to a family of nucleotide-binding proteins (e.g., PilT, PulE, and ComG) which are all components of related systems involved in transport of macromolecules into and out of the cell.[6] These systems include the secretion and assembly of type IV pili (e.g., pili in *Pseudomonas* and *Neisseriae*), the general secretion pathway (e.g., pullulanase secretion in *Klebsiella*), and even DNA uptake in *Bacillus*. Many of these systems are required for virulence. At present we do not know what this particular system is doing in *L. pneumophila* or why it is required for intracellular growth.

It remains unclear why the wild-type *L. pneumophila* is sensitive to moderate amounts of sodium chloride. One explanation is that *L. pneumophila* contains a large membrane complex required for intracellular growth which is leaky to sodium chloride. Because *L. pneumophila* is a fresh water organism and only replicates intracellularly, it probably exists primarily in low sodium environments. Therefore, it is possible that this organism is normally not challenged with the levels of sodium chloride used in the laboratory. Although we do not yet understand the mechanism of salt sensitivity of *L. pneumophila*, we are currently exploiting this apparent Achilles' heal to identify the additional factors required by this organism to cause disease.

REFERENCES

1. MARRA, A. & H. A. SHUMAN. 1992. Genetics of *Legionella pneumophila* virulence. Ann. Rev. Genet. **26:** 51–69.
2. MARRA, A., S. J. BLANDER, M. A. HORWITZ & H. A. SHUMAN. 1992. Identification of *Legionella pneumophila* locus required for intracellular multiplication in human macrophages. Proc. Natl. Acad. Sci. USA **89:** 9607–9611.
3. CATRENICH, C. E. & W. JOHNSON. 1989. Characterization of the selective inhibition of growth of virulent *Legionella pneumophila* by supplemented Mueller-Hinton medium. Infect. Immun. **57:** 1862–1864.
4. SADOSKY, A. B., L. A. WIATER & H. A. SHUMAN. 1993. Identification of *Legionella pneumophila* genes required for growth within and killing of human macrophages. Infect. Immun. **61:** 5361–5373.
5. BERGER, K. H., J. J. MERRIAM & R. R. ISBERG. 1994. Altered intracellular targeting properties associated with mutations in the *Legionella pneumophila dotA* gene. Mol. Microb. **14:** 809–822.
6. HOBBS, M. & J. S. MATTICK. 1993. Common components in the assembly of type 4 fimbriae, DNA transwfer systems, filamentous phage and protein-secretion apparatus: a general system for the formation of surface-associated protein complexes. Mol. Microbiol. **10:** 233–243.

Pathogenic Mechanisms of
Neisseria meningitidis

MUMTAZ VIRJI,[a] KATHERINE MAKEPEACE,[a]
IAN R. A. PEAK,[a] DAVID J. P. FERGUSON,[b]
AND E. RICHARD MOXON[a]

[a]*Departments of [a]Paediatrics and [b]Pathology*
University of Oxford
John Radcliffe Hospital
Oxford, OX3 9DU, UK

Neisseria meningitidis, a gram-negative bacterium, is highly adapted to its specific environment, the human nasopharynx, and may inhabit up to 30% of the normal population without causing adverse effects. However, in susceptible individuals it may invade deeper tissues and cause bacteremia and meningitis. The mechanisms that lead to pathogenesis are incompletely understood; however, certain features that are associated with disease isolates have been implicated in bacterial virulence.

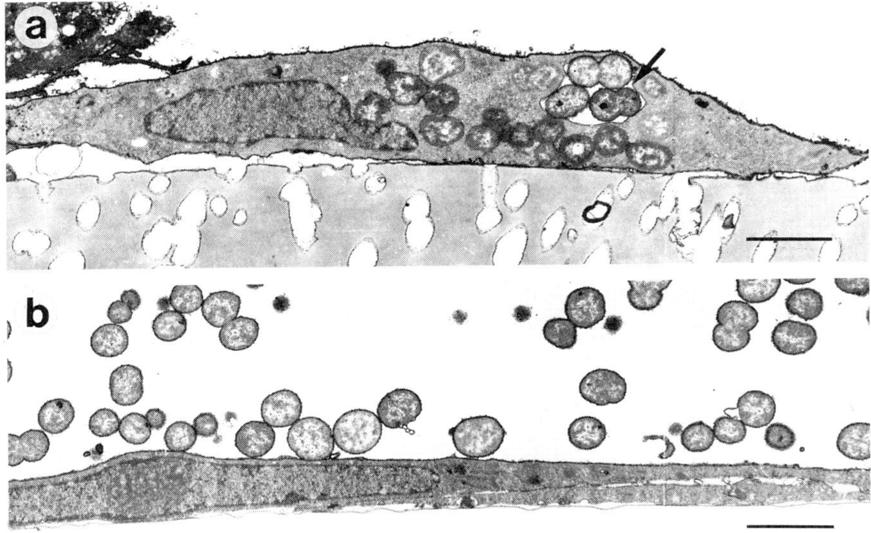

FIGURE 1. Transmission electron micrographs depicting the inhibitory effect of surface sialic acids on meningococcal invasion of human endothelial cells. (a) Acapsulate derivative $\not\subset 2$, P$^+$ OPC$^+$ L8 is highly invasive. (b) The expression L3 LPS immunotype (sialylated) in a P$^+$ Opc$^+$ derivative $\not\subset 3$ is sufficient to inhibit cellular invasion; pili remain effective in increasing bacterial adhesion. Ruthenium Red stain was used to show true intracellular location of bacteria. Several bacteria were stained within an incomplete vacuole (*arrow*). **Bar** represents 2 μm.

The organism elaborates capsular polysaccharide of which three different structures (A, B, and C) are often associated with disease. In addition, several phase and antigenically variable surface proteins (pili and opacity proteins) are expressed during carriage and disease. Pili, which are polymeric hair-like proteins that extend beyond the capsule, are effective as adhesins in numerous disease isolates. *In vitro* studies have shown a specific role for pili in adherence to human endothelial and some epithelial cells.[1] In addition, outer membrane opacity proteins (Opa, Opc) of a serogroup A strain C751[2,3] mediate adhesion and invasion. These studies indicated that surface sialic acids (capsule, sialylated lipopolysaccharide [LPS]) had a pronounced effect on interactions mediated by outer-membrane proteins.[2,3] In the current studies, we investigated the interplay between surface expressed virulence factors in modulating meningococcal interactions with host cells and the mechanisms of Opc-mediated invasion in defined phenotypic derivatives of a serogroup B strain (MC58) that was isolated from the blood of a patient during an outbreak of meningococcal disease in England.

To investigate the roles of surface-expressed virulence factors (capsule, LPS, pili,

TABLE 1. Derivation and Characterization of Phenotypic Variants of Meningococcal Serogroup B Strain MC58 (B:15, P.1, 7:16b)[a]

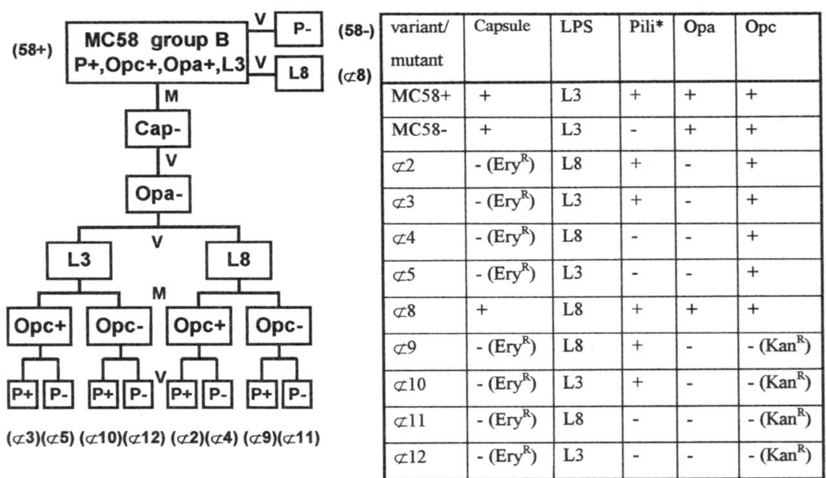

variant/ mutant	Capsule	LPS	Pili*	Opa	Opc
MC58+	+	L3	+	+	+
MC58-	+	L3	-	+	+
⊄2	- (Ery^R)	L8	+	-	+
⊄3	- (Ery^R)	L3	+	-	+
⊄4	- (Ery^R)	L8	-	-	+
⊄5	- (Ery^R)	L3	-	-	+
⊄8	+	L8	+	+	+
⊄9	- (Ery^R)	L8	+	-	- (Kan^R)
⊄10	- (Ery^R)	L3	+	-	- (Kan^R)
⊄11	- (Ery^R)	L8	-	-	- (Kan^R)
⊄12	- (Ery^R)	L3	-	-	- (Kan^R)

M= mutant derivation

V= variant selection

[a]An erythromycin cassette was inserted in the sialyl-transferase (ST) gene from MC58 and transformed into the capsulate parental phenotype 58[+]. Bacteria not expressing Opa proteins (not reacting with mAb B33 against Opa proteins) were used in further selection. The mAb SM82 was used to select L3 and L8 LPS immunotypes, because SM82 reacts with L3 but not L8 LPS. L3 but not L8 immunotype may be intrinsically sialylated in MC58. For mutation of Opc, a kanamycin resistance cassette was inserted into plasmid pBE501[4] containing the Opc gene which was then transformed into MC58. Colony immunoblotting with mAb SM1 was used to select nonpiliated variants. *Pilus expression was quantitated by electron microscopy.

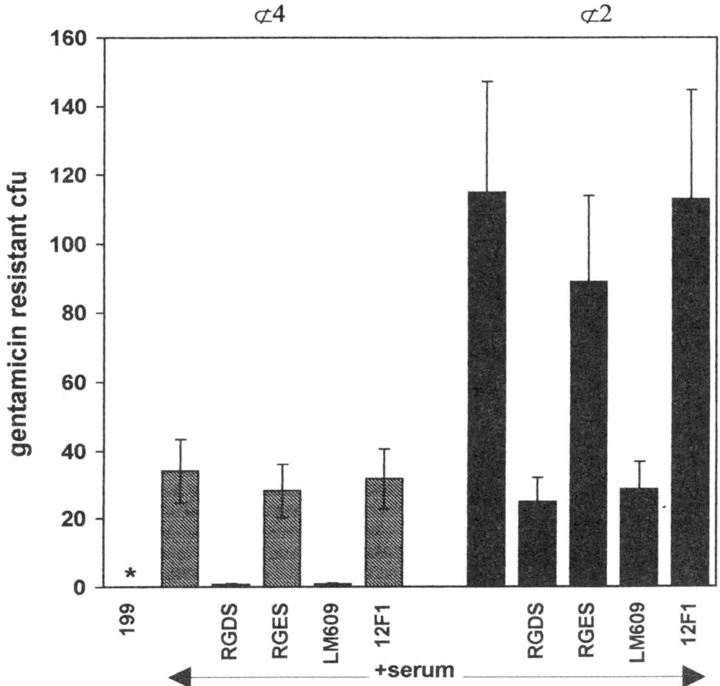

FIGURE 2. The role of serum factors and integrin αvβ3 in cellular invasion of P⁻ Opc⁺ variant ⊄4 (*hatched columns*) and of P⁺ OPC⁺ variant ⊄2 (*filled columns*). Relative numbers of gentamicin-resistant colonies ($\times 10^{-4}$) per monolayer in a typical experiment are shown. Data reflect relative internalization as confirmed by TEM. Other than column 1 (*: a mixture that contained variant ⊄4 and the medium 199 alone), all other mixtures contained 5% heat-inactivated human serum and further additions as shown. Antibodies against endothelial cell integrins were present at 5–30 μg/ml. LM609 is directed against vitronectin receptor and 12F1 against collagen receptor. RGDS and RGES were added at 50 μg/ml. The standard deviations of triplicate estimations in the experiment were less than 28% of mean values and are shown.

and Opc), a family of mutants and variants were isolated from MC58, as described in TABLE 1. To examine the role of Opc in piliated and pilus-deficient bacteria variants lacking the expression of Opa proteins were used. The effect of different LPS structures was examined in variants expressing either sialylated (L3 immunotype) or truncated nonsialylated (L8 immunotype) LPS. Studies showed that (a) pili were essential for meningococcal interactions with host cells in both capsulate and acapsulate bacteria with the sialylated L3 LPS immunotype; (b) the Opc-mediated invasion of host cells by piliated and nonpiliated bacteria was observed only in acapsulate organisms with L8 LPS immunotype; and (c) expression of pili in Opc-expressing bacteria resulted in increasing invasion (FIG. 1). Investigations on the mechanisms of cellular invasion indicated that Opc-mediated invasion was dependent on the presence of serum in the incubation medium and was mediated by serum proteins with the arginine-glycine-aspartic acid (RGD) sequence. Cellular invasion in piliated Opc⁺ phenotype also required bridging molecules containing the

RGD recognition sequence and appeared to involve the integrin $\alpha v\beta 3$ as a target receptor on endothelial cells (FIG. 2). These studies extend the previous observations on variants of C751 and show that Opc mediates host cell invasion in distinct meningococcal strains. They provide confirmation that Opc-mediated invasion involves subversion of host cell integrin function via mimicry achieved by coating of bacteria with integrin ligands.

REFERENCES

1. VIRJI, M., H. KAYHTY, D. J. P. FERGUSON, C. ALEXANDRESCU, J. E. HECKELS & E. R. MOXON. 1991. The role of pili in the interactions of pathogenic *Neisseria* with cultured human endothelial cells. Mol. Microbiol. **5:** 1831–1841.
2. VIRJI, M., K. MAKEPEACE, D. J. P. FERGUSON, M. ACHTMAN, J. SARKARI & E. R. MOXON. 1992. Expression of the Opc protein correlates with invasion of epithelial and endothelial cells by *Neisseria meningitidis*. Mol. Microbiol. **6:** 2785–2795.
3. VIRJI, M., K. MAKEPEACE, D. J. P. FERGUSON, M. ACHTMAN & E. R. MOXON. 1993. Meningococcal Opa and Opc proteins: Their role in colonisation and invasion of human epithelial and endothelial cells. Mol. Microbiol. **10:** 499–510.
4. OLYHOEK, A. J. M., J. SARKARI, M. BOPP, G. MORELLI & M. ACHTMAN. 1991. Cloning and expression in *Escherichia coli* of *opc*, the gene for an unusual Class 5 outer membrane protein from *Neisseria meningitidis*. Microb. Pathog. **11:** 249–257.

Identification of Genes Specifically Expressed by *Mycobacterium haemophilum* in Association with Human Epithelial Cells

LAURA J. FISCHER, FREDERICK D. QUINN,
LYNNE KIKUTA-OSHIMA, EFRAIN M. RIBOT,
AND C. HAROLD KING

Division of AIDS, STD, and TB Laboratory Research
National Center for Infectious Diseases
Centers for Disease Control and Prevention
Atlanta, Georgia 30333

Myocobacterium haemophilum is a facultative, intracellular pathogen that is emerging as a serious disease of immunocompromised populations (reviewed in ref. 1). Infections are characterized by painful cutaneous lesions and occasional tuberculosis-like granulomas in the lungs.[2] We developed an *in vitro* model to study the intracellular growth and temperature-regulated cytotoxicity of *M. haemophilum* in cultured Hec1B human epithelial cells.[3] *M. haemophilum* bacilli associated with and invaded Hec1B epithelial cells at both 33°C and 37°C, but multiplied intracellularly to a greater extent at 33°C in the presence of amikacin (FIG. 1). Disruption of the epithelial monolayers was observed only at 33°C, suggesting the presence of a temperature-regulated cytotoxin.

A cDNA substractive hybridization method (cDNA-SH) was used to identify genes that are expressed by *M. haemophilum* bacilli when associated with epithelial cells at 33°C. Total RNA was isolated from bacterial cultures grown in broth with the Hec1B epithelial cells at 33°C and 37°C using the FastPrep RNA isolation system (Bio101, Vista, California) and then converted to cDNA using the cDNA synthesis kit for RT-PCR (Boehringer Mannheim, Indianapolis, Indiana). The cDNA molecules reverse transcribed from the *M. haemophilum* RNA were tailed at the 3′ end with dATP (for cDNA from the 33°C cultures) or dGTP (for cDNA from the 37°C cultures) using terminal transferase (Boehringer Mannheim). The 5′ end of the cDNA was ligated with specific primer pairs using T4 RNA ligase (Boehringer Mannheim). Double-stranded cDNA was made by amplification of these cDNAs using the polymerase chain reaction (PCR).

Subtractive hybridization of the resultant cDNA products was then performed to remove identical transcripts. Briefly, double-stranded cDNAs from epithelial cell cultures grown at 37°C were biotinylated and hybridized at 70°C for 48 hours to the cDNAs from the epithelial cell cultures grown at 33°C at a 3:1 ratio. After incubation, hybrids were removed by repeated treatment with streptavidin-coated magnetic beads, and the cDNAs remaining in the supernatant were amplified with the same complementary primers used to make double-stranded cDNA from the 33°C cultures. This procedure removed most of the eukaryotic cDNA (data not shown). Southern blots of cDNA produced from RNA isolated from *M. haemophilum* in association with epithelial cells indicated that the cDNA-SH probe hybridized

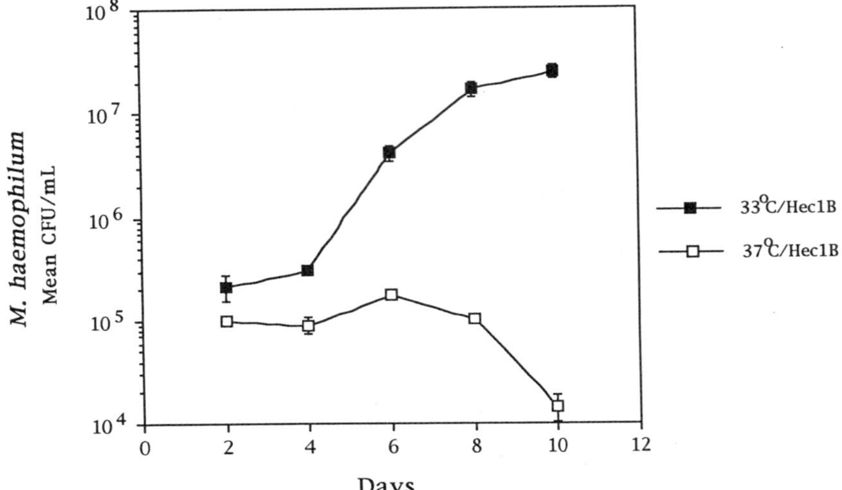

FIGURE 1. Mean colony forming units of *M. haemophilium* from Hec1B epithelial cells at 33°C and 37°C after the addition of amikacin. The multiplicity of infection was 10 bacilli/Hec1B cell. Bacterial inoculum was added for 3 hours, after which the supernatants were removed and tissue culture medium with 200 μg amikacin/ml (Sigma) was added to the wells to inhibit the growth of extracellular bacteria. The minimum inhibitory concentration of amikacin for *M. haemophilium* in tissue culture medium was 100 μg amikacin/ml; bacteria did not grow on Middlebrook 7H10 agar after exposure to 200 μg amikacin/ml for 24 hours. After 2, 4, 6, 8, and 10 days, tissue culture medium was removed, monolayers were washed three times with 0.1M phosphate-buffered saline solution, pH 7.2, and fresh medium containing amikacin was added. In one set of wells, medium was removed, 1 ml of water was added, and the monolayer was scraped, resuspended in water, diluted in Middlebrook 7H9 broth, and plated onto 7H10 agar plates. Plates were incubated at 33°C in 5% CO_2 for 10 days before bacterial colonies were counted. Error bars represent the standard errors of two independent experiments.

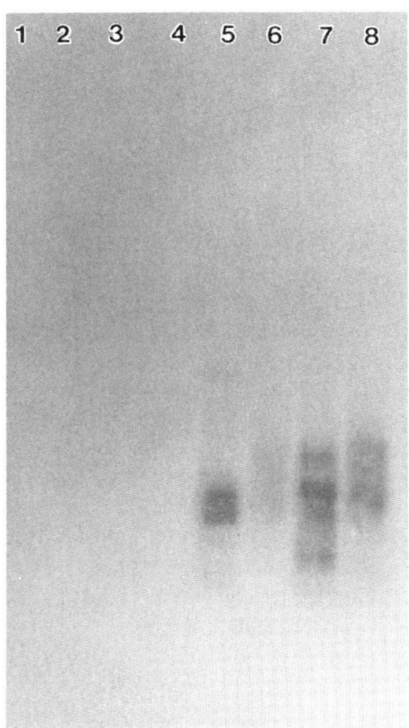

FIGURE 2. Southern blot of the subtractive hybridization product after hybridization to the cDNA produced from RNA isolated from *M. haemophilum* after broth culture and after association with Hec1B cells. *Lane 1*, eukaryotic cDNA digested with *Alu* 1 from Hec1B cells grown at 33°C; *lane 2*, eukaryotic cDNA digested with *Sau* 3A from Hec1B cells grown at 37°C; *lane 3*, cDNA digested with *Sal* I from broth-grown *M. haemophilum* bacilli incubated at 33°C; *lane 4*, cDNA digested with *Sau* 3A from broth-grown *M. haemophilum* bacilli incubated at 33°C; *lanes 5 and 7*, cDNA isolated from *M. haemophilum* bacilli in association with Hec1B cells grown at 33°C; *lanes 6 and 8*, cDNA isolated from *M. haemophilum* in association with Hec1B cells grown at 37°C.

preferentially to the cDNA isolated from *M. haemophilum* bacilli cultured with epithelial cells at 33°C, but it did hybridize to cDNA from the 37°C cultures to a lesser extent (FIG. 2). In addition, the cDNA-SH probe did not hybridize to cDNA from *M. haemophilum* grown in broth at 33°C. Because of this differential expression, genes identified by this method may be important for the growth of *M. haemophilum* in association with human epithelial cells. The genes encoding the RNAs identified by this method are now being isolated.

REFERENCES

1. KIEHN, T. E. & M. SMITH. 1994. *Mycobacterium haemophilum:* An emerging pathogen. Eur. J. Clin. Microbiol. Infect. Dis. **13:** 925–931.
2. KIEHN, T. E., M. WHITE, K. J. U. PURSELL, N. BOONE, M. TSIVITIS, A. E. BROWN, B. POLSKY & D. ARMSTRONG. 1993. A cluster of four cases of *Mycobacterium haemophilum* infection. Eur. J. Clin. Microbiol. Infect. Dis. **12:** 114–118.
3. FISCHER, L. J., F. D. QUINN, E. H. WHITE & C. H. KING. 1996. Intracellular growth and cytotoxicity of *Mycobacterium haemophilum* in a human epithelial cell line (Hec-1-B). Infect. Immun. In press.

Identification of Secreted Proteins of
Mycobacterium tuberculosis

IRMGARD BEHLAU AND ANDREW WRIGHT

Tufts University School of Medicine
Boston, Massachusetts 02111

Because of the resurgence of tuberculosis, which is the leading cause of death in the world due to an infectious disease, and the emergence of multidrug-resistant tuberculosis, we need to develop new strategies for its prevention and treatment. With recently developed methods that enable gene transfer in mycobacteria and allow expression of foreign genes, we can begin to study mycobacterial pathogenesis.

Secreted gene products play an important role in host-pathogen interactions; they have been identified as having a role in an organism's virulence, transport mechanisms, and antigenicity. Many virulence products either reside on the surface of the bacterium or are excreted into the extracellular milieu. We wish to take advantage of the observation that many virulence factors are secreted or membrane-associated proteins.

Alkaline phosphatase fusion systems have become a powerful tool in the analysis of protein secretion.[1] *Escherichia coli* periplasmic alkaline phosphatase (PhoA) is inactive while it resides in the bacterial cytoplasm, but it is active when it is secreted across the cytoplasmic membrane into the periplasm. This novel property of PhoA as a sensor for protein export signals makes it particularly useful in gene fusion reporter systems. Signals that will promote alkaline phosphatase export include cleavable signal sequences, such as those of lipoproteins, and appropriately oriented transmembrane segments of cytoplasmic membrane proteins.

We have used a PhoA fusion approach to identify membrane-associated and secreted proteins produced by *M. tuberculosis*. We constructed a *M. tuberculosis phoA* expression library by fusing 2–6 kb fragments of *M. tuberculosis* DNA upstream of the *Escherichia coli phoA* gene present in plasmids pAWLP-1, -2, and -3. These plasmids contain a *phoA* gene lacking the signal sequence coding region; therefore, it cannot give rise to active alkaline phosphatase unless it is fused to sequences that allow its secretion. The plasmids have a unique cloning site upstream of the *phoA* gene positioned in each of three possible reading frames relative to *phoA*. Plasmids containing *M. tuberculosis* inserts were transformed into a *phoA* deletion derivative of *E. coli*. Approximately 1.6% of the transformants were blue when plated on selective medium containing the chromogenic indicator XP (5-bromo-4-chloro-3-indolyl phosphate), indicating active alkaline phosphatase (AP) fusions. Further analysis of 16 of the most active AP fusions revealed that in 10, alkaline phosphatase was efficiently released by osmotic shock, indicating that they were in the periplasm. The other six showed less than 50% release of AP activity, suggesting that they may be membrane bound. Protein fusions of varied sizes were seen by Western immunoblot analysis using anti-PhoA antibody. Nine of the smaller protein fusions were chosen for further DNA sequence analysis. We found *M. tuberculosis* inserts with DNA and protein homology to a known secreted gene product and one with DNA sequence homology to an open reading frame in a *M. leprae* cosmid library. One of our fusions, D3-58:PhoA, specified a 48-kD protein, defined as a lipoprotein by ^{3}H-palmitate labeling. By sequence analysis, it appears to be a unique, newly identified mycobacterial lipoprotein. We retrieved the entire gene from a *M. tuberculosis* plasmid library. Further characterization of this potentially important lipoprotein is planned.

Results obtained in the preliminary screening of this *M. tuberculosis-phoA* expression library suggest that it may be a powerful tool to selectively identify *M. tuberculosis* secreted proteins that may be involved in the orgnaism's pathogenesis and confer antigencity.

REFERENCES

1. HOFFMAN, C. S. & A. WRIGHT. 1985. Proc. Natl. Acad. Sci. USA **82:** 5107.

Sequence Studies on the COOH-Terminal Region of the Merozoite Surface Protein-1 in Field Samples of *Plasmodium falciparum* from Diverse Geographic Areas

YANG KANG AND CAROLE A. LONG

Department of Microbiology and Immunology
Medical College of Pennsylvania and
Hahnemann University
Philadelphia, Pennsylvania 19102

Recent findings have focused attention on the COOH-terminal, cysteine-rich region of merozoite surface protein-1 (MSP-1) as one of the leading vaccine candidates against the erythrocytic stages of malaria.[1] However, sequence heterogeneity of this region may compromise its use as a vaccine candidate. Although the COOH-terminal region of MSP-1 from the two prototypic alleles of *Plasmodium falciparum* is relatively conserved in laboratory-maintained strains, little data exist on sequence heterogeneity of this region in field isolates from diverse geographic areas. To address this question, DNA encoding this region of *P. falciparum* MSP-1 from 15 field samples was analyzed by a polymerase chain reaction (PCR)-direct sequencing method. This strategy uses easily obtained finger-prick samples and does not require culturing of parasites, so that both culture-adapted and culture-nonadapted isolates can be sequenced. In addition, the PCR-direct sequencing method does not rely on cloning the PCR products into vectors and transforming bacteria, so that possible errors introduced in propagation of plasmodial DNA in *Escherichia coli* are minimized. Some difficulties have been reported in maintaining genomic clones of parasite DNA in bacterial hosts.

Parasite DNAs in field samples from different geographic regions (TABLE 1) were extracted with Chelex 100 and subjected to PCR amplification using allele specific 5′ primers, M5 and K5, and the conserved 3′ primer T3 independently on each sample (FIG. 1). Each of the PCR products was reamplified with two pairs of nested primers, M5 or K5 and S4, and S1 and T3. The products of reamplification were then purified by polyacrylamide gel electrophoresis and electroelution. The purified DNA fragments from each sample were sequenced directly. To minimize possible PCR errors and confirm the variations found, PCR amplifications on the same Chelex-treated samples were repeated using allelic specific primers M5 and K5 and primer T3. The same procedures were followed, but the complementary strand of the purified PCR products was sequenced.

Eventually, 20 double-stranded sequences were obtained from 15 field samples, indicating that at least 5 of 15 individuals tested were coinfected with more than one parasite clone. The deduced amino acid sequences were compared with the corresponding sequences of the two prototypic alleles, PfMAD20 and PfK1/Wellcome.[2] In 15 isolates, only a few nucleotide changes were found, leading to amino acid alterations at 4 positions out of 102 residues (TABLE 1 and ref. 3). The four changes

TABLE 1. Nucleotide and Putative Amino Acid Variations of the COOH-terminal Conserved Region of *Plasmodium falciparum* MSP-1 from Field Samples

Samples (Allele[a])	Geographic Area	At 1644[b]		At 1691		At 1700		At 1701	
		Nt	AA	Nt	AA	Nt	AA	Nt	AA
01 (M)	West Africa	GAA → CAA	E → Q,	—[c]		—		—	
03 (M), 04 (M), 06 (M)	Indonesia	—		—[c]		—		—	
07 (M)	Zimbabwe	GAA → CAA	E → Q,	—[c]		—		—	
08 (M)	Guatemala	—		—[c]		—		—	
09 (M)	Guatemala	GAA → CAA	E → Q,	—[c]		—		—	
10 (M)	Ghana	GAA → CAA	E → Q,	ACA → AAA	T → K,	AGC → AAC	S → N,	AGA → GGA	R → G
11 (M)	West Africa	—		—[c]		—		—	
12 (M), 13 (M), 14 (M), 15 (M)	China	—		—[c]		—		—	
02 (K), 05 (K)	Indonesia	GAA → CAA	E → Q,	—[c]		—		—	
03 (K), 04 (K), 06 (K)	Indonesia	GAA → CAA	E → Q,	ACA → AAA	T → K,	AGC → AAC	S → N,	AGA → GGA	R → G
09 (K)	Guatemala	GAA → CAA	E → Q,	ACA → AAA	T → K,	AGC → AAC	S → N,	AGA → GGA	R → G
11 (K)	West Africa	GAA → CAA	E → Q,	ACA → AAA	T → K,	AGC → AAC	S → N,	AGA → GGA	R → G

[a]Refers to the allele-specific oligonucleotide from block 16 used for initial amplification reactions—either M for PfMAD20 allele or K for PfK1/Wellcome allele.

[b]Number indicates the amino acid position at Png-MAD20 (ref. 2). Nt and AA refer to nucleotide and amino acid, respectively.

[c]Dash means that the residue is identical to that of the Png-MAD20 allele (ref. 2).

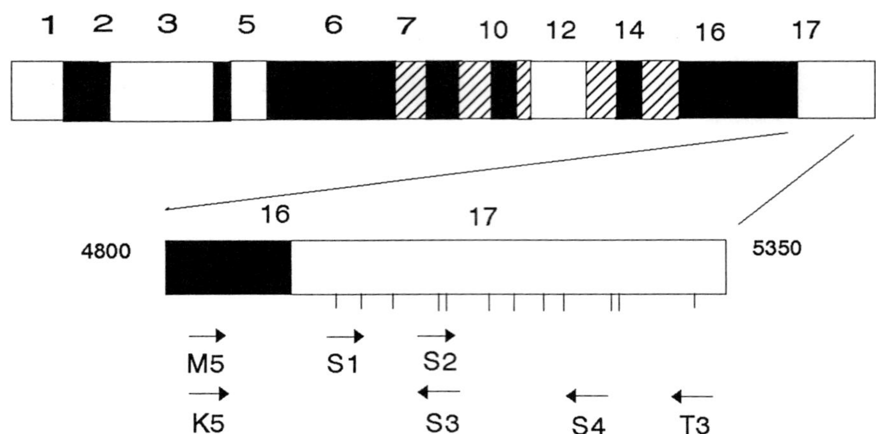

FIGURE 1. Schematic representation of the gene encoding the COOH-terminal region of *P. falciparum* MSP-1. The conserved, variable, and semivariable regions of the gene encoding PfMSP-1 are represented by *open, filled,* and *hatched* boxes, respectively. The COOH-terminal conserved region (block 17) and the variable region (block 16) which are amplified includes nucleotides 4800 to 5350 (ref. 2). The location of cysteine residues is indicated by *vertical lines.* The directions of primers used for PCR and sequencing are indicated by *arrows.* Primers M5, K5 and T3 were used in primary amplifications; M5, K5, T3, S4, and S1 were used for reamplifications; M5, K5, S2, T3, and S3 were used as sequencing primers. The sequences of primers are as follows: M5: 5′ GATACGAAAAAAGATATGCTTGGC 3′; K5: 5′ GCTGATT-TATCAACAGATTATAACC 3′; T3: 5′ TTAAGGTAACATATTTTAACTCCTAC 3′; S1: 5′ AATTCTGGATGTTTCAGACAT 3′; S2: 5′ CCAAATCCTACTTGTAACG 3′; S3: 5′ TTC-GTTACAAGTAGGATTTGG 3′; S4: 5′ AGAGGAACTGCAGAAAATACC 3′.

were E → Q at position 1644 and TSR → KNG, or KNG → TSR at positions 1691, 1700, and 1701. All the variations corresponded to the predicted amino acid sequence of the other prototype. Thus, only three patterns of the COOH-terminal, cysteine-rich region of MSP-1, E-TSR, Q-KNG, and Q-TSR, were detected. Of interest, this is the first evidence for the existence of the Q-TSR PfMSP-1$_{19}$ variant. The limited heterogeneity seen in these samples supports the potential utility of the COOH-terminal region of MSP-1 as a vaccine candidate.

REFERENCES

1. NUSSENZWEIG, R. S. & C. A. LONG. 1994. Malaria vaccines: Multiple targets. Science **265:** 1381–1383.
2. MILLER, L. H., T. ROBERTS, M. SHAHABUDDIN & T. F. McCUTCHAN. 1993. Analysis of sequence diversity in the *Plasmodium falciparum* merozoite surface protein-1 (MPS-1). Mol. Biochem. Parasitol. **59:** 1–14.
3. KANG, Y. & C. A. LONG. 1995. Sequence heterogeneity of the C-terminal, Cys-rich region of the merozoite surface protein-1 (MSP-1) in field samples of *Plasmodium falciparum*. Mol. Biochem. Parasitol. **73:** 103–110.

Prophylaxis with the Immunomodulator PGG Glucan Enhances Antibiotic Efficacy in Rats Infected with Antibiotic-Resistant Bacteria

ARTHUR O. TZIANABOS[a] AND RONALD L. CISNEROS

Channing Laboratory
Brigham and Women's Hospital
Harvard Medical School
180 Longwood Ave.
Boston, Massachusetts 02115

Previous studies have established the efficacy of soluble polymers of poly-(1-6)-β-glucotriosyl-(1-3)-β-glucopyranose (PGG) glucan, a biologic response modifier, in protecting against mortality associated with experimentally induced peritonitis in a rat model.[1] The antiinfective effect of PGG glucan (Betafectin, Alpha Beta Technology, Worcester, Massachusetts) has also been documented in phase II human clinical trials.[2] The experimental models of peritonitis employed in our studies have been used extensively to evaluate therapeutic regimens during an infectious process simulating intraabdominal sepsis in humans.[3,4] The peritonitis phase of the experimental disease process is characterized by a mortality rate of 50% or greater and septicemia. Studies of the antiinfective effect of PGG glucan demonstrated that mice challenged intraperitoneally with either *Escherichia coli* or *Staphylococcus aureus* were protected against mortality associated with experimental intraabdominal sepsis in rats. In addition, animals treated with PGG glucan showed enhanced clearance of bacteria from blood and increased total leukocyte counts. These studies suggested that the PGG glucan has no direct antibacterial activity per se and that protection is based on modulation of the host response to infectious challenge.[1]

The increase in the incidence of antibiotic-resistant strains of pathogenic bacteria has prompted reevaluation of the current treatment modalities for infectious diseases. The advent of methicillin-resistant *S. aureus* and vancomycin-resistant *Enterococcus faecalis* strains in the clinic has emphasized the need for new strategies in preventing infections due to these organisms. The current studies were designed to examine the ability of PGG glucan to act in combination with antibiotics to decrease mortality in a rat model of intraabdominal sepsis using antibiotic-resistant bacteria as infectious inocula.

RESULTS AND DISCUSSION

The effect of PGG glucan, a test antibiotic, or a combination of PGG glucan and antibiotic in decreasing mortality due to antibiotic-resistant strains of *E. coli* or *S. aureus* was assessed (TABLE 1). The antibiotics tested included cephalothin, gentamicin, and ciprofloxacin. Results of these experiments showed that prophylaxis with a

[a]Tel: 617/432-1610; fax: 617/731-1541.

TABLE 1. Prophylaxis with PGG Glucan and Selected Antimicrobial Agents

Treatment	Mortality n (%)	p Value vs Saline
Cephalothin		
Saline	15/17 (88)	—
Cephalothin	4/20 (20)	0.0001
PGG glucan	6/18 (33)	0.0012
PGG glucan + cephalothin	1/19 (5.2)	0.0001
Gentamicin		
Saline	14/20 (70)	—
Gentamicin	8/20 (40)	0.1111
PGG glucan	2/20 (10)	0.0002
PGG glucan + gentamicin	3/19 (16)	0.0011
Ciprofloxacin		
Saline	12/20 (60)	—
Ciprofloxacin	11/20 (55)	1.0
PGG glucan	9/22 (41)	0.35
PGG glucan + ciprofloxacin	3/21 (14)	0.0036

combination of PGG glucan and antibiotics provided enhanced protection against mortality induced by antibiotic-resistant strains of bacteria. Prophylaxis with a combination of PGG glucan and cephalothin or ciprofloxacin reduced mortality rates more than did PGG glucan or either antibiotic alone. In experiments with gentamicin, prophylaxis with PGG glucan alone yielded a reduction in mortality rates comparable to those of a combination of PGG glucan and gentamicin against a resistant strain of *E. coli.* Furthermore, treatment with PGG glucan alone was significantly better than that of gentamicin alone ($p < 0.03$). These data demonstrate that PGG glucan enhances the antiinfective properties of several antibiotics against antibiotic-resistant bacteria and supports the role of immunomodulators as potent new adjuncts to conventional antimicrobial therapies.

SUMMARY

The emergence of multiple antibiotic-resistant microorganisms has led to a search for alternatives to traditional therapeutic regimens. PGG glucan is a soluble β-glucan immunomodulator that selectively enhances the microbicidal activities of neutrophils and macrophages without stimulating proinflammatory cytokine production. In the present studies, we examined the ability of PGG glucan to act in concert with antibiotics to decrease mortality in a rat model of intraabdominal sepsis using antibiotic-resistant bacteria as infectious inocula. Results of these studies demonstrated that prophylaxis with PGG glucan in combination with antibiotics provided enhanced protection against lethal challenge with *Esherichia coli* or *Staphylococcus aureus* as compared with the use of antibiotics alone.

REFERENCES

1. ONDERDONK, A. B., R. L. CISNEROS, P. L. HINKSON & G. R. OSTROFF. 1992. Anti-infective effect of poly-β1-6 glucotriosyl β1-3 glucopyranose (PGG) glucan *in vivo.* Infect. Immun. **60:** 1642–1647.
2. BABINEAU, T. J., A. HACKFORD, A. KENLER, B. BISTRIAN, R. A. FORSE, P. G. FAIRCHILD, S.

HEARD, M. KEROACK, P. CAUSHAJ & P. BENOTTI. 1994. A phase II multicenter, double-blind, randomized, placebo-controlled study of three dosages of an immunomodulator (PGG-Glucan) in high-risk surgical patients. Arch. Surg. **129:** 1204–1210.
3. CISNEROS, R. L., R. BAWDON & A. B. ONDERDONK. 1990. Efficacy of ampicillin/sulbactam for the treatment of experimental intra-abdominal sepsis. Curr. Ther. Res. **48:** 1021–1209.
4. LOUIE, T. J., A. B. ONDERDONK, S. L. GORBACH & J. G. BARLETT. 1977. Therapy of experimental intraabdominal sepsis. A comparison of four cephalosporins with clindamycin and gentamicin. J. Infect. Dis. **135:** 518–522.

Cytoplasmic Proteins Involved in Thyroid Hormone Response Also Bind *Neisseria gonorrhoeae* Opa Outer Membrane Proteins

J. M. WILLIAMS AND R. F. REST

Department of Microbiology and Immunology
Allegheny University of the Health Sciences
Philadelphia, Pennsylvania 19102–1192

Gonococci bind to and invade human epithelial cells and appear to reside within the cytoplasm for at least part of their intracellular tenure.[1] Changes occurring to the host cell and to the gonococci upon and after invasion remain unknown. A family of phase and antigenically variable outer membrane proteins, called the opacity-associated or Opa proteins, are one of several surface components that mediate gonococcal adhesion to and invasion of human epithelial cells. In these studies, we looked for host epithelial cell proteins that interact with gonococcal Opa proteins to determine if gonococci, through Opa protein interactions, regulated host cell responses.

We used Clontech's MATCHMAKER yeast two-hybrid system to identify HeLa cell proteins that bind Opa proteins, probably by protein-protein (as opposed to protein-carbohydrate) interactions. In the MATCHMAKER system, yeast (*Saccharomyces cerevisiae*) is cotransformed with two plasmids, one containing the "bait" gene of interest and the other carrying the "fish" genes, generally comprising a cDNA library. The plasmid genes, which are fused to a transcriptional activator, are translated within the yeast and delivered to the nucleus. If a member of the cDNA "fish" library encodes a protein that interacts with the bait gene, the yeast grows and the plasmid containing a cDNA of interest can be isolated, sequenced, and analyzed.

We inserted a gonococcal *opa* gene (*opaP* from strain F62SF) into the bait plasmid and a HeLa cell cDNA library into the "fish" plasmids. We identified 56 cotransformed yeast, which yielded 15 different plasmid restriction maps containing HeLa cell cDNA encoding for potential *O*pa-*I*nteracting *P*roteins (OIPs). Sequences of HeLa cell genes in five of these restriction map families revealed three unknown OIP genes and two OIP genes that encode proteins known to modulate thyroid hormone (triiodothyronine [T3]) function. Both of these proteins are cytoplasmic, not membrane, proteins. T3, through transcriptional and metabolic control, regulates some key cellular functions including oxygen utilization and glucose metabolism. OIP1 possesses a region that is nearly 100% homologous to human TRIP6, a cytoplasmic *T*hyroid hormone *R*eceptor *I*nteracting *P*rotein, that interacts with nuclear thyroid hormone receptors.[2] OIP1 contains three LIM (specialized zinc finger) domains, which are thought to regulate gene transcription and protein-protein interactions. OIP3 is pyruvate kinase, subtype M2, a cytoplasmic thyroid hormone receptor.[3] These results suggest that Opa⁺ gonococci can actively modulate host cell physiology and metabolism upon or after internalization.

To confirm the yeast two-hybrid results, we investigated the ability of gonococci and *E. coli* expressing functionally active OpaP on their surface to bind rabbit muscle

PK subtype M1. Opa$^+$ gonococci and Opa$^+$ *E. coli* bound substantially more PK than did Opa$^-$ gonococci or Opa$^-$ *E. coli*. Observations were dose dependent for bacterial and PK concentrations. We are currently working to further define Opa binding of PK and of OIP1. These results suggest that (1) the yeast two-hybrid system can be used successfully to investigate host-parasite protein-protein interactions, and (2) gonococci have evolved mechanisms by which they interact with components of thyroid hormone utilization within human epithelial cells. Our observations suggest that gonococci regulate host cell physiology and metabolism to their own advantage, by parasitizing the thyroid hormone "pathway." To what end remains to be determined.

REFERENCES

1. MEYER, T. F., J. POHNER & J. P. M. VAN PUTTEN. 1994. Curr. Top. Microbiol. Immunol. **192:** 283–317.
2. LEE, J. W., H.-S. CHOI, J. GYURIS, R. BRENT & D. D. MOORE. 1995. Mol. Endocrinol. **9:** 243–254.
3. KATO, H., T. FUKUDA, C. PARKISON, P. MCPHIE & S.-Y. CHENG. 1989. Proc. Natl. Acad. Sci. USA **86:** 7861–7865.

Analysis of the Role of Invasin during *Yersinia pseudotuberculosis* Infection of Mice

ANDREA MARRA AND RALPH R. ISBERG

Department of Molecular Biology and Microbiology
Tufts University and Howard Hughes Medical Institute
136 Harrison Ave.
Boston, Massachusetts 02111

The goal of every pathogen is to gain access to its replicative niche. To do so, it must avoid the myriad host defenses put up to thwart that goal. Pathogens that can enter cells can potentially be protected from host defenses. Often cell invasion is the first step of a pathogen's infectious cycle. The enteric pathogen *Yersinia pseudotuberculosis* is a model pathogen for studying bacterial invasiveness. It usually causes self-limiting enteritis when contaminated food is ingested; the bacteria translocate across the intestinal epithelium of the Peyer's patches, probably via M cells, and migrate to the mesenteric lymph nodes and then to the liver and spleen where they replicate extracellularly. The translocation step can be viewed as essential to *Y. pseudotuberculosis's* infection process, as it is likely that bacteria that do not translocate will be swept away by intestinal contents and peristalsis and expelled from the host.

Y. pseudotuberculosis is easily manipulated genetically, and several genes involved in its pathogenesis have been identified. One chromosomal gene, *inv*, encodes a 986 amino acid surface protein, invasin, which is capable of conferring an invasive phenotype on noninvasive *Escherichia coli*. Invasin binds β_1-chain integrins on the surfaces of mammalian cells in culture with a much higher affinity than do the natural ligands for these receptors,[1] which are extracellular matrix proteins such as fibronectin and vitronectin.

The goal of this work is to examine events that take place soon after infection, especially to identify the cell types recognized by invasin in the small intestine and the receptors it binds. If invasin is involved in the translocation step of infection, then it is unclear what receptors it is recognizing. It was previously shown that the β_1-chain integrins that are presumably involved are not on the apical surface of intestinal epithelial cells, but instead are basolaterally localized and therefore inaccessible to bacteria invading from the intestinal lumen.[2,3] The most likely explanation for this apparent paradox points to a role for M cells, the specialized cells lining the Peyer's patches of the small and large intestines, as the target cells for *Y. pseudotuberculosis*. Localization of integrins on M cells has not been established.

Amino acid position 911 of invasin is important for invasin function. D911A and D911E mutations were separately introduced onto the *Y. pseudotuberculosis* chromosome, and the mutants have the following phenotypes: the D911E mutant shows a 10-fold decrease in binding to animal cells and the D911A mutant shows a complete loss of binding ability. Neither mutant is able to invade cells in culture.

Mouse infections were performed to analyze the behavior of these point mutants. In a Peyer's patch invasion assay, mice were fed bacteria intragastrically, sacrificed 90 minutes postinfection, and Peyer's patches from the small intestine were removed, homogenized, and titered for colony-forming units. Wild-type *Y. pseudotuberculosis* colonized the Peyer's patches efficiently, whereas both mutants were defective in their ability to invade this tissue (FIG. 1). This result suggests that both the binding and invasion functions of invasin are important for Peyer's patch penetration.

We then observed this event microscopically. The wild-type strain is very efficient at penetrating the Peyer's patch tissue, and using fluorescence microscopy, bacteria can be found deep within the tissue after only 30 minutes. At shorter time points, wild-type bacteria can be seen by electron microscopy to specifically bind to M cells on the Peyer's patch surface as well as inside these cells. By contrast, both microscopy methods indicate that neither mutant can penetrate this tissue; instead, both

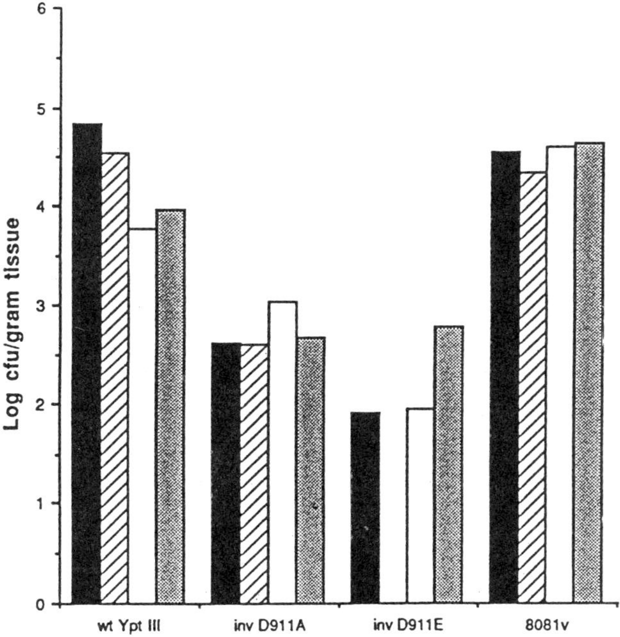

FIGURE 1. Peyer's patch invasion by different *Yersinia* strains. Four BALB/c mice per strain tested were fed intragastrically 5×10^8 bacteria and sacrificed after 2 hours. Peyer's patches were harvested and the number of bacteria per gram of Peyer's patch tissue was determined for each mouse. Wt Ypt III, *Y. pseudotuberculosis* wild-type strain; *inv* D911A and inv D911E, *Y. pseudotuberculosis* point mutants in *inv*; 8081v, *Y. enterocolitica* wild-type strain.

are found to be bound within mucus at the intestinal surface. No specific M cell-mutant interactions are seen on electron microscopy; instead, clusters of bacteria are seen along the brush borders of intestinal epithelial cells, not bound to cells but held there by a meshwork of mucus. This experiment indicates that invasin is the dominant ligand for efficient recognition and penetration of the Peyer's patch surface; however, when invasin's activity is diminished, other adhesins on the *Yersinia* surface may be unmasked as the primary adhesin.

One candidate for such an adhesin is YadA, a surface protein of *Y. pseudotuber-culosis* that binds collagen and mucus.[4] To determine if in the absence of mucus

TABLE 1. Colocalization of Invasin, Integrin, and M Cell Markers on Mouse Peyer's Patch Tissue Sections

Markers	% of Cells Staining with Both Markers
Invasin + α-VLA4	88
Invasin + α-VLA5	97
Invasin + α-β_1	88
Invasin + UEA-1	44
α-VLA4 + UEA-1	42
α-VLA5 + UEA-1	46

binding the *inv* mutants could efficiently translocate, a *yadA* deletion mutation was introduced into either of the *inv* mutants. The resulting double mutants were able to colonize the Peyer's patches slightly better than did the wild-type strain, indicating that another pathway must be available to the bacteria for translocation in the absence of *inv*. We are currently developing screens to identify bacterial factors required for the alternative pathway.

To identify the cells and receptors that invasin recognizes on the surface of the Peyer's patch, immunofluorescent staining of fixed, sectioned mouse Peyer's patch tissue was performed. Purified invasin or anti-mouse integrin antibodies were used to probe tissue sections for specific staining of cells at the Peyer's patch surface. In addition, a lectin, UEA-1, was shown to recognize M cells and mucus. In double- and triple-labeling experiments, purified invasin was observed to recognize specific cells at the Peyer's patch surface, and most of these cells are also labeled with antibodies to the α_4 and α_5 chains of integrins and with anti-β_1 chain antibodies. Approximately 50% of cells staining with these antibodies also label with UEA-1 (TABLE 1). These results indicate that (1) M cells can be recognized by invasin; (2) M cells have β_1-chain integrins; and (3) invasin is most likely binding to β_1-chain integrins of the M cell surface in order to mediate translocation. Whether the UEA^-, β_1^+ cells represent a new cell type or M cells that lack the lectin has yet to be determined.

REFERENCES

1. ISBERG, R. R. & J. M. LEONG. 1990. Cell **60:** 861–871.
2. DESTROOPER, B. *et al.* 1991. Eur. J. Biochem. **199:** 25–33.
3. DESTROOPER, B. *et al.* 1989. J. Histochem. Cytochem. **37:** 299–307.
4. PAERREGAARD, A. *et al.* 1991. Contrib. Microbiol. Immunol. **12:** 171–175.

In Vitro Models to Study Attachment and Invasion of *Helicobacter pylori*

K. A. BIRKNESS,[a] B. D. GOLD,[b] E. H. WHITE,[a]
J. H. BARTLETT,[a] AND F. D. QUINN[a]

[a]*Centers for Disease Control and Prevention and*
[b]*Emory University School of Medicine*
Atlanta, Georgia 30333

Helicobacter pylori, until recently an unknown organism, is now recognized as one of the most common human pathogens. In addition to causing chronic active gastritis in infected individuals, significant evidence also indicates that long-term infection may lead to peptic ulcer disease and perhaps to gastric cancer. The organism exhibits marked tissue specificity for the gastric mucosa. Following ingestion, *H. pylori* colonizes the mucous layer overlying the gastric epithelium and subsequently attaches to the epithelial cell surface, often in close proximity to the cellular tight junctions. Bacterial multiplication, invasion between cells, internalization, elaboration of toxins, and stimulation of potent inflammatory and immune responses follow. The chronic active gastritis seen in this disease is a consequence of the inflammatory responses mounted by the host gastric mucosa against *H. pylori* colonization. Although this inflammatory reaction, which is both acute and chronic, contributes to the disease process, it is not effective in eradicating the organism. *H. pylori* also elicits vigorous humoral and cellular immune responses, but there is little evidence to suggest that either is successful in spontaneous clearance of the organism.[1]

In histopathologic studies, tissue invasion by *H. pylori* is seldom reported; small numbers of bacteria have been seen within the lamina propria, but mucosal invasion is rare. The attraction and activation of inflammatory cells are more likely a response to cytokines produced by gastric epithelial cells. The bacterial invasion that does occur may allow presentation of bacterial antigens to the host immune system or may offer the organism protection from chemotherapeutic agents, leading to difficulty in eradication.[2] Although many questions remain unanswered, it is clear that the initial interaction between *H. pylori* and the gastric epithelium is of critical importance in understanding the pathogenesis of the disease spectrum caused by this organism. We have used AGS human gastric carcinoma tissue culture cell monolayers to study cell association and internalization of *H. pylori* using both viable cell count and electron microscopy. In addition, we have developed a novel tissue culture bilayer model[3]; it consists of human microvascular endothelial cells (HMEC-1) and AGS or mouse hepatic (NCTC) epithelial cells separated by a microporous membrane. The system allows observation of attachment and intra- or intercellular passage through the cell layers as well as enumeration of bacteria able to pass through both cell layers into the space below. The bilayer model resembles more closely than a monolayer the tissue that the bacterium may encounter in the human host. When *H. pylori* is added to these bilayers, light and electron microscopy shows the progression of infection from the first intimate attachment to the apical surface of the epithelial cells to passage through and between the epithelial cells, membrane, and endothelial cells and into the subendothelial space.

When AGS monolayers were infected with *H. pylori,* 9–17% of the inital inoculum associated with the tissue culture cells after a 3-hour incubation. With the addition of gentamicin to kill extracellular bacteria, only 0.6–2.0% of the inoculum was actually internalized by the host cells. Using the bilayer system we found that 0.1–2% of the inoculum was able to pass through both cell layers and into the lower chamber within 3 hours. Electron micrographs of both monolayer and bilayer infections showed evidence of intimate attachment of the organisms to the host cell surface. Bacteria were also seen within coated pits and appeared to be taken into the host cell by endocytosis. Once taken into the cell, *H. pylori* were seen within vacuoles in the epithelial cells (FIG. 1). Some of the organisms not internalized made their way into the tight junctions and were seen between cells. Electron micrographs of the bilayer showed both intracellular and intercellular organisms in the epithelial cell layer. Organisms were also found within the membrane and associated with both sides of the endothelial cell layer as they passed into the subendothelial space (FIG. 2). Preliminary eukaryotic cell inhibitor studies showed that in the presence of methylamine, which inhibits pinocytosis, internalization was only 0.04% of the inoculum, and in the presence of cytochalasin D, an inhibitor of actin polymerization and microfilament function, internalization was only 0.07%. When both inhibitors were present, internalization was reduced to 0.002%. This suggests that more than one mechanism may be involved in bringing *H. pylori* into these cells.

From these studies we hope not only to determine the path the organism takes from cell surface into or through the gastric epithelial cells during the initial phase of the infectious process but also to establish what role each step plays in stimulating cytokine production by the epithelial cells. Beyond this we must understand how the elicited immune and inflammatory responses contribute to the disease process and to

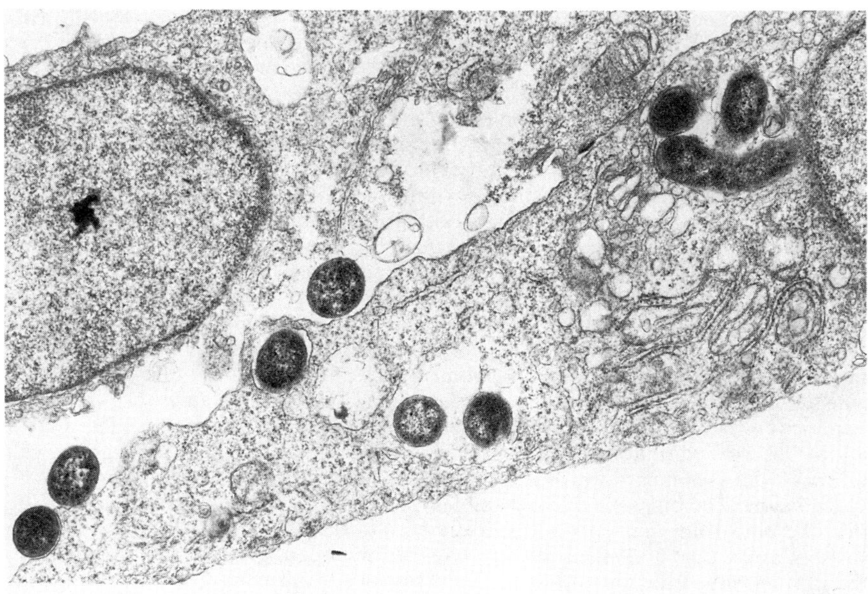

FIGURE 1. AGS gastric epithelial cell monolayer infected with *Helicobacter pylori*. Bacteria are attached to the cell surface, being drawn into the cell, and within an intracellular vacuole (magnification 23,000×).

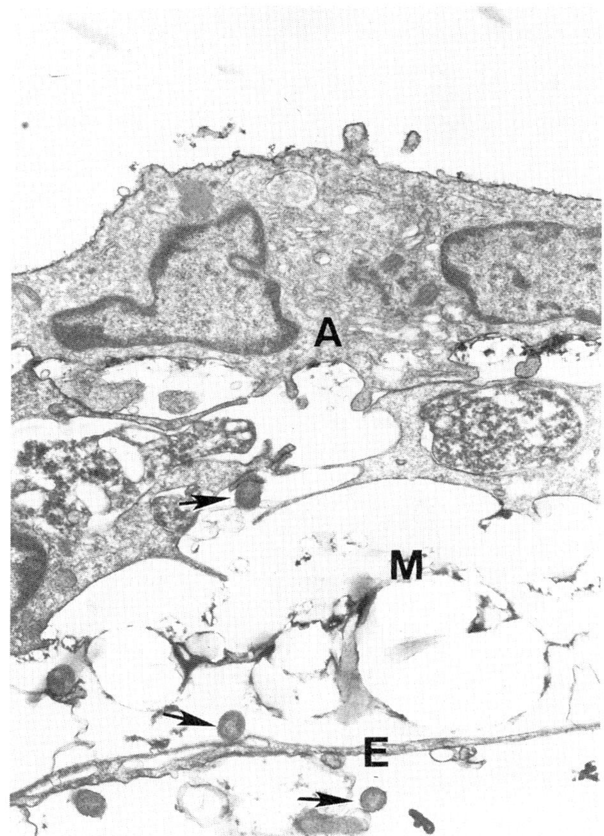

FIGURE 2. AGS and HMEC-1 bilayer infected with *Helicobacter pylori.* AGS epithelial cell layer (A), microporous membrane (M), and HMEC-1 endothelial cell layer (E) with bacteria (*arrows*) within the epithelial layer, within the membrane, attached to the endothelial cell surface, and emerging into the subendothelial space (magnification 13,500×).

the elimination or suppression of the infection. With this understanding we may be better able to develop more effective intervention and treatment strategies.

REFERENCES

1. SHERMAN, P. M. & B. D. GOLD. 1993. Can. J. Gastroenterol. **7:** 395–405.
2. DUNN, B. E. 1993. Gastroenterol. Clin. North Am. **22:** 43–57.
3. BIRKNESS, K. A., B. L. SWISHER, E. H. WHITE, E. G. LONG, E. P. EWING & F. D. QUINN. 1995. Infect. Immun. **63:** 402–409.

Impact of *in Vitro* Fatty Acid Uptake on Nitric Oxide Production and Antilisterial Activity of WEHI-3 Cells

U. S. BABU,[a,c] P. L. WIESENFELD,[a] V. K. BUNNING,[b]
AND R. B. RAYBOURNE[b]

[a]*Division of Science and Applied Technology*
Office of Special Nutritionals
and
[b]*Immunobiology Branch*
Division of Virulence Assessment
US Food and Drug Administration
Laurel, Maryland 20708

Several reports suggest that the type and concentration of individual fatty acids *in vivo* and *in vitro* modulate functions of cells of the immune system.[1–3] Among those cells, macrophages play a central role in ingesting and destroying microorganisms. This process, in turn, provides a source of processed bacterial antigens against which T-cell and antibody-mediated immune responses are directed.[4] This study compares the effect of uptake of commonly consumed fatty acids on immune functions of WEHI-3 cells. The use of WEHI-3 cells offers a convenient *in vitro* model to test the effects of fatty acids and other nutrients on the structure and functions of macrophages. These and other macrophage cell lines have also been used to develop methods for determining oxidative burst and nitric oxide (NO) production and, in turn, for examining antibacterial and antiinfective properties of these chemicals. Nitric oxide has also been shown to have immunoregulatory effects in some infections.[5]

WEHI-3 cells were incubated (24 hours) with 11 µM BSA-fatty acid complex prepared, as described previously.[6] Fatty acids included myristic (C14:0), plamitic (C16:0), linoleic (C18:2, n-6), alpha-linolenic (C18:3, n-3), and docosahexanoic (C22:6, n-3) acids. Total lipids from these cells were extracted, and methyl esters were prepared and analyzed by gas chromatography to determine the fatty acid profile.[7] Uptake of *Listeria monocytogenes* (LM), antilisterial activity, and NO production were assessed after fatty acid exposure. Phagocytic uptake and bacterial killing and/or survival by WEHI-3 cells were assessed by a FACS-based method, as described previously.[4] Phagocytic uptake of LM was determined after washing/ gentamicin addition (T = 0). Antilisterial activity of WEHI-3 cells was determined 24 hours after uptake by bacterial recovery from sorted and lysed replicates of infected macrophages. Production of NO by WEHI-3 cells was assessed using the Griess reagent protocol.[8]

The fatty acid profile of WEHI-3 cells indicated that C18:1 was the most abundant fatty acid followed by C16:0, C18:0, and C20:4 (TABLE 1). This fatty acid profile is similar to that reported for J774A.1 cells, except that a lower percentage of

[c]Address for correspondence: Dr. U. S. Babu, Division of Science and Applied Technology (HFS-465), Office of Special Nutritionals, U. S. Food and Drug Administration, Laurel, MD 20708 (tel: 301/594-5831; fax: 301/594-0517).

TABLE 1. Uptake of BSA-Fatty Acid Complexes by WEHI-3 Cells

Culture Condition	% of Total Fatty Acids								
	C14:0	C16:0	C16:1	C18:0	C18:1	C18:2	C18:3	C20:4	C22:6
RPMI-BSA	2.24[b]	19.1	5.49[a,b]	17.2	40.0[a]	4.18[b]	0.0[b]	12.5	0.0[b]
BSA-C14:0	4.66[a]	19.8	6.5[a]	15.7	39.2[a]	3.75[b]	0.0[b]	10.4	0.0[b]
BSA-C16:0	2.08[b]	21.4	5.48[a,b]	16.7	38.0[a]	3.85[b]	0.0[b]	10.7	0.0[b]
BSA-C18:2	2.71[b]	19.7	3.08[c]	16.0	28.1[c]	18.7[a]	0.0[b]	11.7	0.0[b]
BSA-C18:3	3.18[a,b]	21.4	4.51[b,c]	15.9	34.4[b]	4.17[b]	4.85[a]	11.6	0.0[b]
BSA-C22:6	3.07[a,b]	19.6	3.5[c]	15.7	29.5[c]	3.43[b]	0.0[b]	10.0	14.4[a]

Note: WEHI-3 cells were cultured in RPMI-1640 medium supplemented with 11 μM BSA-fatty acid complex. After 24 hours, cells were harvested, total lipids extracted, and methyl esters analyzed by gas chromatography. Values are means from three separate experiments. Standard errors were within 10% of the means. Different superscripts within the column indicate that the means are different at $p < 0.05$.

C18:1 was found in J774A.1 cells.[7] In WEHI-3 cells, uptake of saturated fatty acids, namely, C14:0 and C16:0, was lower than that of unsaturated fatty acids. Among unsaturated fatty acids, C18:2 and C22:6 uptake was identical and significantly higher than that of C18:3 (TABLE 1). Similarly, others have also reported differences in uptake of fatty acids by mouse peritoneal macrophages.[3] These variations in the incorporation of fatty acids may indicate not only differences in the rate of uptake but changes in metabolism or turnover.

Uptake of LM (T = 0) was significantly greater in the presence of C18:3 than in the presence of C16:0 or C22:6, but not when compared to the BSA control culture. However, the number of LM recovered at T = 24 was significantly lower in the presence of C18:3 than in the presence of BSA alone or C14:0, C16:0, and C18:2 (TABLE 2). A possible mechanism for increased antilisterial activity in the presence of C18:3 may involve enhanced production of tumor necrosis factor-alpha, interleukin-1 (IL-1), and IL-6, which are known to be involved in antilisterial activity.[9] Some of these factors are elevated by dietary n-3 fatty acids.[2,10] Concentration of NO was determined because, theoretically, it has shown immunoregulatory and direct antimicrobial effects in some infections.[5] Nitric oxide production by WEHI-3 cells, however, was not influenced by any of the fatty acids tested and did not correlate with antilisterial activity (TABLE 2).

TABLE 2. Impact of Fatty Acid-BSA Uptake on Nitric Oxide Production and Antilisterial Activity of WEHI-3 Cells

Culture Condition	LM (T = 0)	LM (T = 24)	NO Production (T = 24)
RPMI-BSA	148 ± 38[a,b]	196 ± 19[a,b]	1.30 ± 0.09
BSA-C14:0	135 ± 9[a,b]	325 ± 87[a]	1.14 ± 0.08
BSA-C16:0	100 ± 8[b]	285 ± 68[a]	1.24 ± 0.08
BSA-C18:2	130 ± 8[a,b]	237 ± 44[a,b]	1.10 ± 0.12
BSA-C18:3	199 ± 59[a]	20 ± 11[c]	1.39 ± 0.09
BSA-C22:6	82 ± 15[b]	117 ± 8[b,c]	0.66 ± 0.10

Note: WEHI-3 cells were cultured for 24 hours in the presence of 11 μM fatty acid-BSA complexes. Antilisterial activity was determined at T = 24 hours, and uptake was determined at the end of 60 minutes, (T = 0). Ratio of WEHI-3 to LM was 1:100. Production of NO was measured 24 hours after the uptake of LM by 2.5×10^4 WEHI-3. Values shown are the means ± standard errors from three experiments. Different superscripts within the column indicate that the means are different at $p < 0.05$.

We demonstrated that the uptake of alpha-linolenic acid (C18:3, n-3) by WEHI-3 cells resulted in significantly lower recovery of LM at T = 24 hours (i.e., increased antilisterial activity). Production of NO was not affected by the fatty acids used in this study. Overall, these results suggest that uptake of LM and antilisterial activity are, in part, influenced by the availability and metabolism of specific fatty acids. Antilisterial activity was independent of NO production.

REFERENCES

1. JOHNSTON, P. V. 1988. Nutrition and Immunology. R. K. Chandra, Ed.: 37–86. Alan R. Liss, Inc. New York.
2. TUREK, J. J., I. A. SCHOENLEIN & G. D. BOTTOMS. 1991. Prostaglandins Leukotrienes and Essential Fatty Acids **43:** 141–149.
3. CALDER, P. C., J. A. BOND, D. J. HARVEY, S. GORDON & E. A. NEWSHOLME. 1990. Boichem. J. **269:** 807–814.
4. RAYBOURNE, R. B. & V. K. BUNNING. 1994. Infect. Immun. **62:** 665–672.
5. YAMAMOTO, Y., H. FRIEDMAN & T. W. KLEIN. 1994. Ann. N. Y. Acad. Sci. **730:** 342–344.
6. MAHONEY, E. M., A. L. HAMILL, W. A. SCOTT & Z. A. COHN. 1977. Proc. Natl. Acad. Sci. USA **74:** 4895–4899.
7. SHICHIRI, G., M. KINOSHITA & Y. SAEKI. 1993. Arch. Biochem. Biophys. **303:** 231–237.
8. GOODRUM, K. J., L. L. MCCORMICK & B. SCHNEIDER. 1994. Infect. Immun. **62:** 3102–3107.
9. SZALAY, G., J. HESS & S. H. E. KAUFMANN. 1995. Infect. Immun. **63:** 3187–3195.
10. LOKESH, B. R., T. J. SAYERS & J. E. KINSELLA. 1990. Immunol. Lett. **23:** 281–286.

Pathogenesis and Immune Responses in Shigellosis

RUBHANA RAQIB,[a,b] BENGT WRETLIND,[a]
ALF A. LINDBERG,[a] ÅKE LJUNGDAHL,[c]
AND JAN ANDERSSON[d]

[a]Division of Clinical Bacteriology F82
Karolinska Institutet
Huddinge Hospital
S-14186 Huddinge, Sweden

[b]International Center for Diarrhoeal Disease Research
Bangladesh
GPO Box 128
Dhaka 1000, Bangladesh

[c]Division of Neurology R54
Karolinska Institutet
Huddinge Hospital
S-14186 Huddinge, Sweden

[d]Department of Immunology
The Arrhenius Laboratories for Natural Sciences
Stockholm University
S-10691 Stockholm, Sweden

Shigellosis, an invasive disease of the human colon, is a major cause of childhood morbidity in developing countries. It is estimated to affect about 250 million people world wide and is responsible for at least 650 thousand deaths annually. The pathogenesis of shigellosis leading to acute inflammation involves destruction of tissue caused by the bacteria itself as well as by host responses to the pathogen. Immunopathology and development of natural immunity were studied by assessing 14 different cytokines and associated receptors in adults with shigellosis. Comparative analyses were carried out using blood, stool, and rectal biopsy specimens from healthy controls from Bangladesh, a *Shigella* endemic area, as well as from Sweden, a *Shigella* nonendemic area.

During the acute stage of shigellosis, marked inflammation of the rectum was associated with increased infiltration of granulocytes, T lymphocytes, macrophages, and natural killer cells and upregulation of activation markers. The increased staining pattern of major histocompatibility HLA-DR antigens in colonic epithelial cells during the acute stage suggested the potential for increased antigen presentation.[1]

Extensive production of proinflammatory cytokines (interleukin 1α [IL-1α], IL-1β, tumor necrosis factor-α [TNF-α], IL-6, and IL-8) was observed at the local site during the acute stage, which persisted up to 1 month after the onset of the disease even after the disappearance of clinical symptoms. Analysis of cytokine production at the single cell level showed that increased frequencies of cytokine-producing cells closely correlated with the histologic grade of severity.[2] The concomitant production of Th1 (gamma interferon [IFN-γ], TNF-α, and TNF-β) and Th2 (IL-4 and IL-10) type of cytokines was seen during the study period. The secretion of cytokines was directed to stool (IL-1β, IL-1ra, TNF-α, IL-6, IL-8, IFN-γ, GM-CSF, and TGF-β$_{1-3}$), its cytokine concentrations being 100 times greater than those of plasma. Increased stool concentration of cytokines correlated with the severity of inflammation in the gut as well as with clinical markers of disease activity. By contrast, very low concentrations of IFN-γ were observed in stool during the acute stage with a progressive increase in levels during the convalescent stage.[3] Deposition of extracellular IFN-γ was gradually increased in the colon tissue during recovery from shigellosis. IFN-γ was entrapped in the colonic mucosa, particularly to its specific receptor located in the epithelial lining. Several-fold higher frequencies of cytokine mRNA-expressing cells were observed for most cytokines than for the corresponding

TABLE 1. Secretion and Expression of Cytokine Receptors in Patients with *Shigella* Infection Compared to Healthy Controls

Cytokine Receptors	Acute Stage (2–6 days after onset)		Convalescent Stage (30–40 days after onset)	
	Cell Surface Receptors	Soluble Receptors	Cell Surface Receptors	Soluble Receptors
IL-1 RI	⇓	ND	↓	ND
IL-1 RII	⇓	ND	↓	ND
IL-2 Rα	ND	Plasma ⇑ Stool ⇑	ND	Plasma ↑ Stool N
IL-2 Rβ	↓	ND	↓	ND
IL-3 Rα	⇓	ND	N	ND
IL-4 R	↓	ND	↑	ND
IL-6 Rα	N	Plasma N Stool ⇑	↑	Plasma N Stool UD
IFN-γ Rα	⇓	ND	↓	ND
TNF RI	⇓	Plasma N Stool ↑	↓	Plasma N Stool ↑
TNF RII	↓	Plasma ↑ Stool ↑	N	Plasma N Stool UD
GM-CSF Rα	↓	ND	↓	ND
TGF-β RI	⇓	ND	↓	ND
TGF-β RII	N	ND	N	ND

Abbreviations: N = normal compared to control levels; ND = not done; UD = undetectable; ↑ = higher than controls; ⇑ = significantly higher than controls; ↓ = lower than controls; ⇓ = significantly lower than controls.

protein-producing cells at the local site during the course of *Shigella* infection. Shiga toxin inhibits protein synthesis at the level of translation. *In vitro* stimulation of peripheral blood mononuclear cells with a superantigen in combination with Shiga toxin showed a dose-dependent decrease in IFN-γ protein production, whereas the combination of superantigen, SEA, with lipopolysaccharide from *Shigella dysenteriae* type 1 did not show any difference. These findings suggest that the abnormal accumulation of cytokine-specific mRNA was probably mediated by *Shigella*-derived toxins impairing translation.

Healthy controls constitutively expressed cell-surface cytokine receptors in the rectum. By contrast, during the acute stage of shigellosis, the loss of cytokine receptors (IL-1 type I, TNF type I, IL-3, IL-4, IFN-γ, and TGF-β type I) was observed[4] (TABLE 1). The findings suggest that the loss may be a consequence of internalization and shedding of receptors during signaling. In patients, soluble cytokine receptor levels in plasma were 100-fold higher than those of corresponding cytokines. By contrast, soluble receptors in stool were four to six fold lower in concentration than were cytokines at the acute stage. Counterregulatory actions of soluble receptors at the local site were overcome by excessive local production of cytokines, thereby promoting immune activation as well as tissue damage. These data suggest that the development of cell-mediated immunity was important for the eradication of *Shigella*. The expression and secretion of cytokines and cytokine receptors in the acute and convalescent stage were differentially regulated in order to modulate systemic immune activation.

REFERENCES

1. RAQIB, R., F. P. REINHOLT, P. K. BARDHAN, A. KÄRNELL & A. A. LINDBERG. 1994. Immunopathological patterns in the rectal mucosa of patients with shigellosis: Expression of HLA-DR antigens and T-lymphocyte subsets. APMIS **102:** 371–380.
2. RAQIB, R., A. A. LINDBERG, B. WRETLIND, P. K. BARDHAN, U. ANDERSSON & J. ANDERSSON. 1995. Persistence of local cytokine production in shigellosis in acute and convalescent stages. Infect. Immun. **63:** 289–296.
3. RAQIB, R., B. WRETLIND, J. ANDERSSON & A. A. LINDBERG. 1995. Cytokine secretion in acute shigellosis is correlated to disease activity and directed more to stool than to plasma. J. Infect. Dis. **171:** 376–384.
4. RAQIB, R., A. A. LINDBERG, L. BJÖRK, P. K. BARDHAN, B. WRETLIND, U. ANDERSSON & J. ANDERSSON. 1995. Down-regulation of gamma interferon, tumor necrosis factor type I, interleukin 1 (IL-1) type I, IL-3, IL-4, and transforming growth factor β type I receptors at the local site during the acute phase of *Shigella* infection. Infect. Immun. **63:** 3079–3087.

Index of Contributors